Advanced Laser Surgery in Dentistry

Advanced Laser Surgery in Dentistry

Georgios E. Romanos

D.D.S., Ph.D., PROF. DR. MED. DENT.
Stony Brook University
School of Dental Medicine
Stony Brook, NY, USA
and
Johann Wolfgang Goethe University
School of Dentistry - Carolinum
Frankfurt, Germany

WILEY Blackwell

Registered Office
John Wiley & Sons, Inc., 111 River Street, Hoboken, NJ 07030, USA

Editorial Office
111 River Street, Hoboken, NJ 07030, USA

For details of our global editorial offices, customer services, and more information about Wiley products visit us at www.wiley.com.

Wiley also publishes its books in a variety of electronic formats and by print-on-demand. Some content that appears in standard print versions of this book may not be available in other formats.

Library of Congress Cataloging-in-Publication Data

Names: Romanos, Georgios, author.
   Title: Advanced Laser Surgery in Dentistry / Georgios E. Romanos.
Description: First edition. | Hoboken, NJ : Wiley-Blackwell, 2021. |
   Includes bibliographical references and index.
Identifiers: LCCN 2020028457 (print) | LCCN 2020028458 (ebook) | ISBN
   9781119583301 (hardback) | ISBN 9781119583356 (adobe pdf) | ISBN
   9781119583349 (epub)
Subjects: MESH: Oral Surgical Procedures | Laser Therapy
Classification: LCC RK501 (print) | LCC RK501 (ebook) | NLM WU 600 | DDC
   617.6/05 dc23
LC record available at https://lccn.loc.gov/2020028457
LC ebook record available at https://lccn.loc.gov/2020028458

Cover Design: Wiley
Cover Images: Courtesy of Georgios E. Romanos, © MIKHAIL GRACHIKOV/Shutterstock

Set in 9.5/12.5pt STIXTwoText by SPi Global, Pondicherry, India
Printed in Singapore
M002457_260421

To my focused beam, little star, my daughter Stella

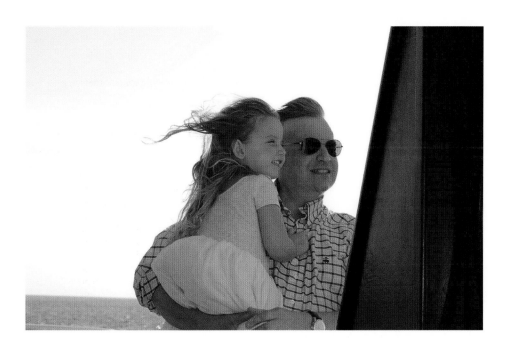

Contents

About the Author *xi*
List of Contributors *xiii*
Preface *xv*
Acknowledgement *xvii*

1 Laser Fundamental Principles *1*
Georgios E. Romanos
1.1 Historical Background *3*
1.2 Energy Levels and Stimulated Emission *3*
1.3 Properties of the Laser Light *3*
1.4 The Laser Cavity *4*
1.4.1 Active Medium *4*
1.4.2 Pumping Mechanism *5*
1.4.3 Lenses – Resonator *5*
1.5 Laser Application Modes *5*
1.5.1 Beam Profiles *7*
1.6 Delivery Systems *7*
1.6.1 Direct Coupling *7*
1.6.2 Articulated Arms *7*
1.6.3 Fiber Systems and Flexible Hollow Guides *8*
1.7 Applicators *9*
1.7.1 Handpieces *9*
1.7.2 Fiber Applicators *10*
1.8 Laser Types Based on the Active Medium *11*
1.8.1 Gas Lasers *11*
1.8.2 Crystal Lasers *14*
1.8.3 Liquid (Dye) Lasers *17*
1.8.4 Semiconductor (Diode) Lasers *17*
1.8.5 New Developments in Laser Technology *19*
1.8.6 Lasers for Research Applications *24*
1.9 Laser and Biological Tissue Interactions *24*
1.9.1 Photochemical Effects *27*
1.9.2 Photothermal Effects *29*
1.9.3 Ionizing or Nonlinear Effects *33*

2 Lasers and Wound Healing *41*
Georgios E. Romanos
2.1 Introduction *41*
2.2 Wound Healing and Low Power Lasers *42*
2.3 Wound Healing and High-Power Lasers *44*
2.3.1 Wound Healing and CO_2 Laser *44*
2.3.2 Wound Healing and the Nd:YAG Laser *47*

2.3.3   Wound Healing and Other Laser Wavelengths   *50*
2.4   Lasers and Bone Healing   *51*

3   **Lasers in Oral Surgery**   *57*
         Georgios E. Romanos
3.1   Introduction   *57*
3.2   Basic Principles   *57*
3.3   Excision Biopsies   *58*
3.4   Removal of Benign Soft Tissue Tumors   *59*
3.4.1   Surgical Protocol for Removal of Small Tumors   *59*
3.4.2   Surgical Protocol for Removal of Larger Soft Tissue Tumors   *62*
3.5   Removal of Drug-Induced Gingival Hyperplasias and Epulides   *80*
3.5.1   Removal of Drug-Induced Gingival Hyperplasias   *80*
3.5.2   Removal of Epulides   *81*
3.6   Removal of Soft Tissue Cysts   *83*
3.7   Frenectomies and Vestibuloplasties   *87*
3.7.1   Frenectomies   *87*
3.7.2   Vestibuloplasties   *92*
3.8   Removal of Precancerous Lesions (Leukoplakia)   *99*
3.9   Surgical Removal of Malignant Soft Tissue Tumors   *106*
3.10   Laser Coagulation   *106*
3.11   Lasers in Vascular and Pigmented Lesions   *107*
3.11.1   Laser Types   *107*
3.11.2   Removal of Vascular Alterations with the "Ice Cube" Method   *108*
3.12   Exposure of Impacted, Unerupted Teeth   *121*
3.12.1   Exposure of an Unerupted Teeth for Orthodontic Reasons   *122*
3.13   Removal of Sialoliths Using the Laser   *123*

4   **Lasers and Bone Surgery**   *129*
         Georgios E. Romanos
4.1   Introduction   *129*
4.2 CO_2 Laser   *129*
4.3   Excimer Laser   *130*
4.4   Er:YAG and Ho:YAG Lasers   *130*
4.5   Laser Systems for Clinical Dentistry   *131*

5   **Lasers in Periodontology**   *139*
         Georgios E. Romanos
5.1   Introduction   *139*
5.2   Laser-Assisted Bacteria Reduction in Periodontal Tissues   *140*
5.3   Removal of Subgingival Calculus   *142*
5.4   Removal of Pocket Epithelium   *144*
5.5   Retardation of the Epithelial Downgrowth   *149*
5.6   Laser Application in Gingivectomy and Gingivoplasty   *152*
5.7   Laser-Assisted Hemostasis in Periodontics   *154*
5.8   Photodynamic Therapy in Periodontology   *156*
5.9   Gingival Troughing for Prosthetic Restorations   *165*
5.10   Fractional Photothermolysis in Periodontology   *165*
5.11   Education and Future of Lasers in Periodontal Therapy   *178*

6   **Lasers and Implants**   *185*
         Georgios E. Romanos
6.1   Introduction   *185*
6.2   Laser-Assisted Surgery Before Implant Placement and Implant Exposure   *185*

6.3   Laser Application During Function *187*
6.4   Laser Applications in Peri-implantitis Treatment *188*
6.5   Recent Laser Research on Implants *199*
6.6   Implant Removal *204*
6.7   Laser-Assisted Implant Placement *204*
6.8   Future of Laser Dentistry in Oral Implantology *204*

7   Photodynamic Therapy in Periodontal and Peri-Implant Treatment *209*
         Anton Sculean and Georgios E. Romanos
7.1   Biological Rationale *209*
7.2   Use of PDT as an Alternative to Systemic or Local Antibiotics *211*
7.3   Conclusions *212*

8   Understanding Laser Safety in Dentistry *215*
         Vangie Dennis, Patti Owens and Georgios E. Romanos
8.1   Laser Safety *215*
8.2   International Laser Standards *215*
8.3   Regulatory Agencies and Nongovernmental Organizations *215*
8.3.1   Food and Drug Administration *215*
8.3.2   FDA Center for Devices and Radiological Health *216*
8.3.3   American National Standards Institute *216*
8.3.4   Occupational Safety and Health Administration *216*
8.4   State Regulations *218*
8.5   Nongovernmental Controls and Professional Organizations *218*
8.5.1   American Society for Lasers in Medicine and Surgery *218*
8.5.2   Association of periOperative Registered Nurses (AORN) *218*
8.6   The Joint Commission (TJC) *218*
8.7   Standards and Practice *218*
8.7.1   Laser Safety Officer *218*
8.8   Hazard Evaluation and Control Measures *219*
8.9   Administrative Controls *219*
8.10   Procedural and Equipment Controls *219*
8.11   Laser Treatment Controlled Area *220*
8.12   Maintenance and Service *221*
8.13   Beam Hazards *221*
8.13.1 Eye Protection *221*
8.13.2 Skin Protection *223*
8.14   Laser Safety and Training Programs *223*
8.15   Medical Surveillance *223*
8.16   Nonbeam Hazards *223*
8.17   Electrical Hazards *224*
8.18   Smoke Plume *224*
8.19   Fire and Explosion Hazards *224*
8.20   Shared Airway Procedures *225*
8.21   Conclusion *226*

         Appendix A: Suggested Reading *227*
         Appendix B: Physical Units, Laser Parameters, Physical Parameters, Important Formulas *229*

         Index *231*

About the Author

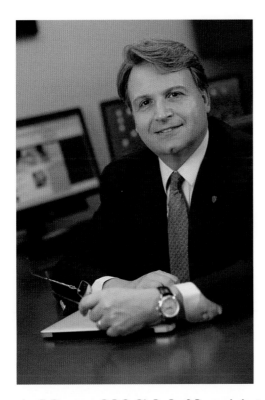

Georgios E. Romanos, D.D.S., Ph.D., Prof. Dr. med. dent.

- Professor of Periodontology and Director of Laser Education at Stony Brook University (SBU), School of Dental Medicine
- Professor (Prof. Dr. med. dent.) of Oral Surgery/Implant Dentistry in Frankfurt/Germany
- Fully trained in Periodontics, Prosthodontics and Oral Surgery in Germany and in USA

- Board Certified in Oral Surgery and Implant Dentistry in Germany
- Diplomate by the American Board of Periodontology
- Certified Medical Laser Safety officer (CMLSO) by the Board of Laser Safety (BLS)
- former Associate Dean for Clinical Affairs at SBU
- former Professor of Clinical Dentistry at the Univ. of Rochester/NY and Professor and Director of Laser Sciences at NYU
- Past President of the Academy of Osseointegration Foundation and the Implantology Research Group of the IADR
- Fellow of the American Association for Dental Research, the Academy of Osseointegration, Int. College of Dentists, ICOI, ITI Foundation, Pierre Fauchard Academy, American Society for Laser Medicine and Surgery, Great of NY Academy of Prosthodontics, Int. Academy for Dental Facial Esthetics, American College of Dentists
- Editorial Board Membership in various peer-reviewed journals
- More than 400 publications (h-Index: 66; over 14,000 citations, 6 books)
- Over 700 presentations worldwide; International scientific collaborations and teaching activities globally
- Lecturer in more than 50 countries

2016 Award Recipient for Excellence in Dental Laser Research (T.H. Maiman) by the Academy of Laser Dentistry

List of Contributors

Vangie Dennis, MSN, RN, CNOR, CMLSO
Executive Director Perioperative Services
Atlanta Medical Center
Downtown Campus
Atlanta
Georgia
USA

Patti Owens, BSN, MHA, RN, CNOR, CMLSO
President of Aesthetic Med Consulting International,
LLC
Laser Training
Rancho Mirage
California
USA

Anton Sculean, DDS, MS, PhD, Dr hc, Prof Dr med dent
Executive Director and Chairman
Department of Periodontology
School of Dentistry
Berne
Switzerland

Preface

Lasers are novel and innovative technologies with many benefits for clinicians, patients, and applications in surgical dentistry. It is a significant contribution to the modern medical field that laser light can be used effectively in clinical dentistry based on present scientific developments and technological advances.

Scientific evaluation of this technology presents a lack of strong evidence in specific areas of dentistry, but there is no doubt that lasers are beneficial as clinical tools in a variety of clinical scenarios based on the appropriate laser-tissue interactions and the challenges in daily practice.

The first part of the book will provide the fundamental and advanced uses of lasers as surgical tools for improvement of clinical outcomes and is focused on the intraoral applications of a variety of laser wavelengths and devices.

The book presents the clinical impact of the use of lasers on the different fields of surgical dentistry in a modern way with clinical photographs and step-by-step documentation. The strength of the book is the discussions of the use of different lasers and novel fiber-optics in the treatment of a variety of clinical problems and the contribution of top specialists in the field of antimicrobial, photodynamic therapy, and laser safety.

For instance, the use of laser light to excise or coagulate tumors, the impact of lasers on periodontal surgical procedures, as well as in implant dentistry, from the implant uncovering to the treatment of peri-implant diseases, are discussed. The highlights of the book for the new decade are the modification of traditional concepts of treatment and using a patient friendlier method leading to less postoperative complications and excellent wound healing.

The book explains systematically the protocols of treatment with clinical cases and illustrates the way of thinking and treatment methodology in the different surgical fields. It is an excellent resource for clinicians who want to improve their experience in surgical dentistry and advance their practice. In addition, the book is a strong foundation for the specialist who wants to learn more about this novel technology and how it can fit in their practice.

Enjoy reading but also practice, and you will recognize the pearls and jewels in *Advanced Laser Surgery in Dentistry*.

Georgios E. Romanos, DDS, PhD, Prof Dr med dent

Acknowledgement

Special thanks and appreciation to Mr. Hammaad R. Shah for the preparation of the schematical drawings presented in the Figures 3.1, 5.5, 5.6 and 5.8.

1

Laser Fundamental Principles

Georgios E. Romanos

Stony Brook University, School of Dental Medicine, Stony Brook, NY, USA

LASER is an acronym of "Light Amplification by Stimulated Emission of Radiation." Laser is light with specific properties and may interact with tissues and materials. Light is an electromagnetic wave, which is a coupling of electric and magnetic fields, traveling as waves at a speed equal to the known speed of light (velocity, c). Both fields oscillate at the same frequency, with a number of oscillations per second, which is well known as frequency (f). The speed of light is a universal constant, which is about 300 000 km/s.

Since medical professionals are interested in the applications of laser devices and not the internal physics, here we describe fundamental information, which is foundation knowledge, before the use of lasers in clinical settings.

A laser light is a *monochromatic, coherent* light in the visible and nonvisible (infrared or ultraviolet [UV]) parts on the electromagnetic spectrum. Laser light is optical radiation and is termed non-ionizing radiation to be differentiated from ionizing radiation, such as gamma- and X-rays, which may cause biological effects in the cells and tissues. The human eye associates a color to a group of specific wavelengths from violet, blue, green, yellow, orange, red based on the increase of the wavelengths. Invisible wavelengths for the human eye are wavelengths of radios and television (infrared) or in the UV parts of the spectrum, the gamma- and x-rays (Figure 1.1).

The spectrum is divided into two major zones: the short wavelength ionizing radiation (nonvisible to the human eye) and the non-ionizing radiation (visible light and non-visible infrared radiation) with longer wavelengths. The ionizing radiation can penetrate tissue and damage cells. In low doses it can be used for diagnostic purposes (i.e. X-rays). The non-ionizing range of radiation can be used for superficial heating of tissues, and for treatment of skin disorders and musculoskeletal injuries.

The power of lasers can range from milliwatts to almost 20 W for commercial lasers. In addition, higher levels of power in megawatts may be used for military purposes.

The sizes of lasers can have dimensions larger than 100 m. Lasers in this size can be used for nuclear experiments using laser beams to squeeze hydrogen atoms in order to release a high amount of energy (laser fusion). The biggest facilities in the world so far are the NIF (National Ignition Facility) in California and the Laser Megajoule (LMJ) in France, near Bordeaux.

In contrast to large lasers, the smallest lasers today are 5000 times smaller than the tip of a pen. Scientists have created the world's smallest laser after they squeezed light into a space smaller than a protein molecule. The so-called "spacer" generates stimulated emission of surface plasmons (oscillations of free electrons in metallic nanostructures) in resonating metallic nanostructures adjacent to an active medium. It is anticipated that, at least experimentally, the spacer (wavelength of 531 nm) will advance our fundamental understanding of nano-plasmonics and the development of new opportunities due to the photothermal properties in the therapy of malignant lesions (Chon et al. 2014).

In general, there is a broad diversity in laser applications, which can be used for industrial, commercial, research, and military interests.

Some areas where lasers can be used are:

- Material cutting and welding
- Measurements
- Communications
- Entertaining and performing arts
- Holography
- Spectroscopy and atomic physics
- Environment protection
- Plasma diagnostics
- Medical applications

Advanced Laser Surgery in Dentistry, First Edition. Georgios E. Romanos.
© 2021 John Wiley & Sons, Inc. Published 2021 by John Wiley & Sons, Inc.

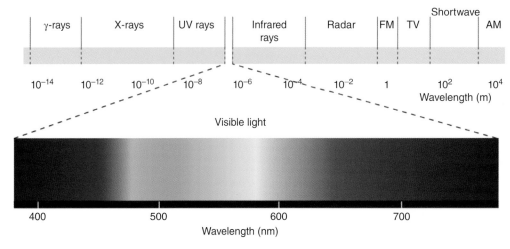

Figure 1.1 Electromagnetic spectrum and the different wavelengths.

There is no way to think about modern life without the internet, mobile phones, and technology. Therefore, lasers are everywhere in our lives since lasers are fundamental in all these technological advances.

Lasers can do a lot, for example measuring distances, such as the depth of oceans and in aerospace, based on the principle that laser light is sent to a target, which will then be reflected and sent backward. For instance, laser light can be sent to the moon, collecting a few photons reflected back by mirrors placed on the lunar surface (such as during the Apollo missions), and then we know the distance between the moon and the Earth.

The coherent properties of laser light will be used in ring laser gyroscopes allowing distance measurement in aircrafts, helicopters, missiles, ships, etc. Bar code readers and scanners exist only in conjunction with diode lasers. Also, optical storage capacity from compact discs (CDs) to digital video discs (DVDs) and today Blu-ray discs depends on the density of coding elements (pits) and the laser spot after focusing. The shorter the wavelength, the smaller the laser spot and the engraved surface of the disc. In addition, partial or complete absorption of the light can be at resonance with the material medium and create distinguished resonance frequencies (signals), characterizing the medium composition (spectroscopy).

In medicine, cornea surgery, removal of wrinkles, and coagulation of blood vessels in abdominal surgery accommodate lasers in daily practice. Also, other applications in laser medical imaging, like the phenomena of scattering and absorption of light by tissues, have been used extensively the last few years establishing excellent opportunities in the field of diagnostics. Specifically, optical coherence tomography (OCT) today allows a

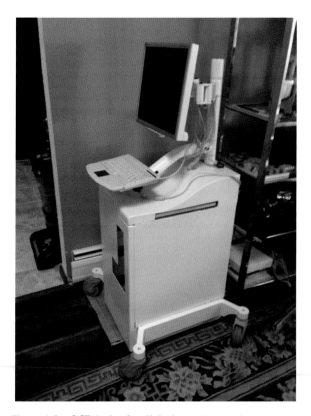

Figure 1.2 OCT device for clinical and diagnostic applications. *Source:* Dr. Georgios E Romanos.

high-resolution cross-sectional imaging compared to the conventional diagnostics due to the reflected light by a mirror and by measuring backscattered or back-reflected light.

OCT (Figure 1.2) can provide cross-sectional images of tissue structure on the micron scale in situ and in real time. This relatively new technology is very helpful today in biomedical and clinical sciences. Especially in ophthalmology, it provides treatment guidance for glaucoma and diseases of the retina, including age-related macular degeneration (AMD) and diabetic eye disease (Fujimoto et al. 2000).

1.1 Historical Background

The precursor of the laser, namely the "Maser," was developed in the United States by the physicist Theodore H. Maiman (1960). It consisted of an one-crystal-rod from artificial ruby and could emit red light with a wavelength of 694 nm in the microwave band. The Maser, an acronym for Microwave Amplification by Stimulated Emission of Radiation, is today generally known under the name *laser*. In its name is summarized the basic principle after which all laser systems work. Charles H. Townes (1964) received the Nobel Prize for the development of the laser; Townes was the first to achieve, due to stimulated emission, the fortification of the radiation in the microwave band.

Moreover, Albert Einstein (1917) had already argued in his thesis "Quantum Theory of Radiation," that parts of the electromagnetic field can be stimulated in such a way that through it fortified light originates. The first lasers were called optical masers.

1.2 Energy Levels and Stimulated Emission

Based on Niels Bohr and the Planck-quantum hypothesis, the following two postulates were formulated:

- Electrons move only on certain, firm orbits around the nuclear core

- Electrons can jump only from orbit to orbit and deliver energy in the form of radiation, as for example light (emission of radiation), or take up energy (absorption of radiation).

Therefore, in the interaction between light and matter three different optical concepts may occur: *absorption*, *spontaneous emission*, and *stimulated emission*.

Absorption is the process when electrons transfer from a low energy level (E1) (stable) to a higher energy level (E1) (unstable). Energy levels E1 are called the ground state and E2 called the excited state.

Spontaneous emission is the process, when electrons transit from a higher energy level (E2) to a lower energy level (E1). When E2 > E1, the energy difference satisfies the relation E2-E1 = h ν. The constant h ($= 6.63 \times 10^{-34}$ J/s) is known as Planck's constant, and ν is the radiation frequency. Spontaneous emission is responsible for the production of conventional visible sunlight.

Stimulated emission is the process when atoms initially from the excited stage fall down to the ground state emitting photons. An atom can be stimulated (excited stage) by an external source, so that its electrons of a low energy can jump to a higher energy orbit. This source can be of an electric kind, e.g. a flashbulb, and serves as "a pumping mechanism." Other pumping methods can be also chemical or optical, depending on the energy source (Figure 1.3).

1.3 Properties of the Laser Light

With the term *laser* is identified a physical principle leading to the production of electromagnetic radiation, which differs from the usual light in the following properties (Figure 1.4):

- *Coherence:* Wave streaks remain parallel and well-defined even in large distances. The light has spatially the same phase (the waves are "in tune").

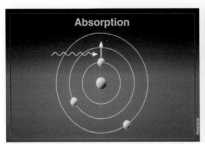 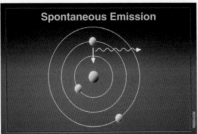 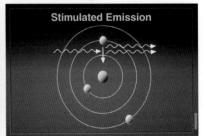

Figure 1.3 Spontaneous and stimulated emission principles.

- *Collimation:* The laser beam can give a localized spot when something is in its way. This has the practical advantage that the light can be well focused.
- *Monochromatism:* All wave streaks have the same wavelength, the same frequency, and thus the same energy. The wavelength of the light plays a critical role in medicine and determines today the exact clinical ranges of application.

A high energy density is produced when the generated electromagnetic radiation bundles in the narrowest space, due to the coherence and the collimation. The light can be focused precisely and have, because of its high energy density, different effects on the tissues. Therefore, vaporization, coagulation, and also carbonization of tissues are possible. Light with such qualities does not exist in nature. The photons of usual light exhibit different wavelengths, and they are emitted in all directions (Figure 1.4) of space (polychromatic, incoherent light).

The concurrent combination from the above-mentioned physical properties permits very high capacity density. In this way, for example, the sunlight striking our earth has power of on an average $0.1\,W/cm^2$; on the contrary, surgical laser systems easily reach a power of $100\,000\,W/cm^2$. Lighting a match produces energy of $200\,J$. With the energy of only $1\,J$ of coherent light generated by a ruby laser – focused by means of a plane optical lens – it is possible to cut a hole in a metal plate (Frank 1989).

The three basic criteria of light are: brightness (amplitude), color (frequency), and polarization (angle of vibration).

1.4 The Laser Cavity

From the practical standpoint, a laser device (Figure 1.5) contains the following components:

- The laser medium (active medium), which generates the laser light (this is the "brain" of the system).
- The optical resonator (reflecting system)
- The laser pumping mechanism

1.4.1 Active Medium

Atoms are stimulated to the production of the laser radiation. These atoms are components of the so-called **"active (gain) medium."** This can be a gas, a solid body (crystal), a liquid, or a semiconductor. Different lasers systems can be classified based on the active medium.

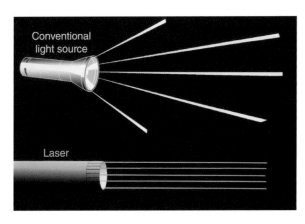

Figure 1.4 Collimated light of the laser versus non-collimated light of the conventional light source

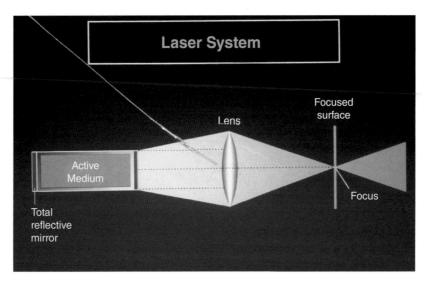

Figure 1.5 Schematic demonstration of a laser device.

1.4.2 Pumping Mechanism

The **laser pumping mechanism** is the act of energy transfer from an external source into the active medium of the laser. The pump energy is usually provided in the form of light (optic) energy, or electrical current, but also other sources have been used, such as chemical or nuclear reactions.

1.4.3 Lenses – Resonator

The **optical resonator** is the reflecting system of the laser device. With the use of two parallel, arranged mirrors (mostly concave shaped) at a specific distance, the light will be reflected. The exact radius of curvature characterizes the optical resonator. A certain curvature controls better the light reflections, modifying the distribution of light within the laser output beam.

The resonators with a stable reflecting distance are also called also stable resonators and differentiate themselves from the unstable ones, which obtain a variable reflecting distance. According to the distance and shape of the mirrors as well as their position, there are concentric, confocal, hemi-confocal, and hemispherical resonators. Energy loss can happen if mirrors (especially output mirrors) do not perfectly reflect light, and this should happen as much as possible. Concave mirrors are needed in order to focus light transversely.

The simplest laser cavity is formed by two parallel mirrors facing each other. This is called a *Fabry-Perot Cavity*.

The laser resonator has two different types of modes: transverse and longitudinal. Transverse modes can be explained by the cross section of the beam profile and represents the intensity pattern. This distribution of power is also referred to as transverse electromagnetic mode (TEM).

1.5 Laser Application Modes

The operation mode of a laser can be switched to *pulsed* or *continuous* (Figure 1.6). The pulsed mode is also known as normal mode. A continuous beam is referred to as continuous wave ("continuous-wave laser") or *CW laser*, when light will be constantly emitted over an uninterrupted period of time due to continuous pumping. These lasers have usually low peak energy and low power. They are usually gas lasers, i.e. CO_2 lasers.

The type of the operating mode, namely the length or width of a pulse is dependent on the pumping mechanism and the laser medium. The pulsed laser light (gated, chopped) can be achieved when a mechanical shutter opens and closes in front of the beam.

Pulses can be short or ultrashort dependent on the pulse duration. A superpulse mode is associated with good ablation and wide residual thermal damage (RTD) compared to the ultrapulse mode, where the ablation is precise and the RTD is shallow. The latter may be also called char-free mode.

Usually pulses have a pulse duration in the µs-ms range. *Free-running (FR) lasers* are pulsed lasers with shorter pulse durations than the conventional pulsed lasers. Such lasers can be used in areas when risk of overheating has to be avoided. For instance, a FR-Nd:YAG is used for the LANAP protocol in periodontal therapy (see also Chapter 5).

Shorter pulses with pulse duration from microseconds (10^{-6}) to nanoseconds (10^{-9}) define the *Q-switched* lasers (*Q-switching*). Compression or shortening of pulses can be done with this technique. This kind of laser can be used in industry for metal drilling, cutting, and marking with extremely high peak power.

The second compression technique of pulses is to create pulses with extremely short duration; sometimes referred to as *ultrashort pulses*. These are pulses with a width in picosecond (10^{-12} seconds), femtosecond (10^{-15} seconds), or attosecond (10^{-18} seconds) defining the *mode-locking*. This can be used for cutting or melting of metals due to the high penetration depth. Pulse repetition rate (frequency) also varies widely.

Pulse modes control the heat transfer to the tissues, providing vaporization without overheating and, as a consequence, melting. High peak power pulses can create defects with sharp edges in the matter (or tissues) without damage.

There is great interest in the *pulse duration,* also called pulse width, of the laser beam in order to avoid negative effects and damage in biological tissues.

Chopped (shuttered) pulses usually have a duration of 100–500 ms. Superpulses have a shorter width, usually of 60–200 µs and higher peak power. The width can be controlled electrically using mechanical shutters and other devices, like shutters and Q-switches. These devices are placed in the laser cavity.

The pulse width must be shorter or equal than the *thermal relaxation time (TRT)* of the target chromophore. This time is directly proportional to the square size of the chromophore. Therefore, small objects cool

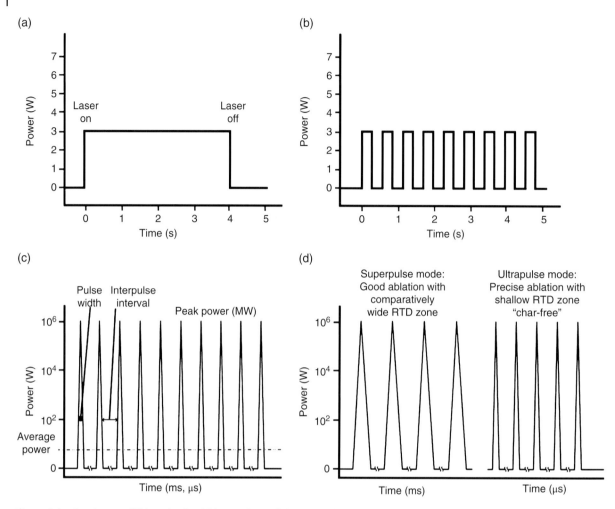

Figure 1.6 Continuous (CW) and pulsed (chopped, gated) laser application modes compared to pulsed, superpulse, and ultrapulse mode.

faster than large ones, while larger chromophores have a longer TRT than smaller chromophores.

The TRT is defined as the time needed for the target chromophore to dissipate 63% of its peak temperature. Bogdan Allemann and Kaufman (2011) showed different TRTs of importance based on the chromophore size in dermatology (see Table 1.1).

Contact and *non-contact laser* modes can be defined dependent on the position of the optic fiber or tip in relation to the tissue or material.

Important parameters, when continuous lasers are used, are the irradiation period, power, and spot size. In contrast, for pulsed lasers maximum energy per pulse, pulse duration, frequency, and spot size are fundamental. Power (in watts) is defined by the transmitted energy (in joules) per unit time.

Therefore,

$$P = E/t \, (\text{Frequency} = 1/t, \text{in Hz})$$

Also:

$$\text{meanP} = \text{Pmax} \times \text{tpulse} \times \text{frequency}$$
Pmax is the maximum power (watt)
tpulse is pulse duration (second)
frequency (Hz)

Table 1.1 Thermal relaxation times for different chromophores of various size.

	Size, µm	Thermal relaxation times (approx.)
Tattoo ink particle	0.5–4	10 ns
Melanosome	0.5–1	1 µs
Erythrocyte	7	2 µs
Blood vessel	50	1 ms
Blood vessel	100	5 ms
Blood vessel	200	20 ms
Hair follicle	200	10–100 ms

The energy per area is the power density (PD, or fluence) and expressed in joules/cm^2

PD = meanP/S
PD is Power Density (watt/cm^2); mean power (watt); S is the irradiated surface (cm^2)
r is the radius of the glass fiber; (S = $\pi \cdot$ r^2), π = 3.14

All parameters that must be included in different laser studies should be: power density, energy of the laser beam, pulse width and frequency, irradiation period, diameter of the glass fiber (or tip), beam profile, distance to the irradiation object, and tip angulation.

Peak Power is the energy flow in every pulse

Ppeak : E/Δt

Average Power is the energy flow over one full time period.

Pavg = E/T

Therefore:

Ppeak Δt = Pavg T

Also, *Duty Cycle* is the fractional amount of time the laser is "on" during a specific given period.
Therefore:

Duty Cycle = Δt/t = Pavg/Ppeak

1.5.1 Beam Profiles

The energy distribution across the beam (transverse electromagnetic mode) determines the nature of laser focus (focal spot size). This focus can have a circular, clean pattern (TEM$_{00}$), or an irregular pattern (multimode, TEM$_{xx}$). The circular spot is the fundamental mode, with Gaussian (normal distribution) in the beam profile, which has the highest concentration of power and can be focused into the smallest, most concentrated focal spot (Figure 1.7). The TEM$_{00}$ mode is the most desirable beam. The fundamental mode with the maximum intensity peak at the center of the beam is the TEM$_{00}$ and contains roughly 86% of the power in the spot.

Longitudinal modes correspond to different resonances along the length of the laser cavity which occur at different frequencies or wavelengths. The transverse modes are classified according to the number of nulls that appear across the beam cross-section. However, multimode beams can have high power but lower quality.

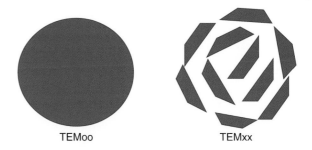

TEMoo   TEMxx

Figure 1.7 Transverse electromagnetic modes with regular, high concentrated beam (TEM$_{00}$) and irregular (TEM$_{xx}$) pattern with less concentration of the maximum energy in the beam.

1.6 Delivery Systems

The laser beam is used as a handpiece by means of different guide systems (the so-called beam guide systems), allowing the surgeon to perform a perfect, with minimal complications, and practical, laser application. A direct coupling, an articulated arm, a flexible hollow guide as an optical fiber, or a fiber system are currently available for this purpose.

1.6.1 Direct Coupling

A direct coupling is possible only in extremely compact systems (e.g. He:Ne target lasers, soft lasers, laser pointers). In such systems the laser unit corresponds to the handpiece of the system.

1.6.2 Articulated Arms

The laser beam can be used as a handpiece by means of articulated arms (Figure 1.8) at specific wavelengths (e.g. in the UV range and the wavelength of the CO$_2$ laser). In such systems, mirrors are used for beam deflection. For this reason, such articulated arms are also called transmission arms.

Articulated arm beam delivery dates back to the 1970s; it features a cumbersome four-elbow, seven-mirror articulation, which can rotate to different angles for the transmission of the laser beam, but it can have limitations in accessibility. A lens in the base of the handpiece focuses the laser beam 2–3 cm from the exit aperture of the handpiece. An articulated arm is unusable without an aiming beam – the only visible indicator of the focused CO$_2$ laser beam location on the target tissue.

Although, the beam quality can be described as a very good one, disadvantages are the large weight of the articulated arm and thus the entire laser unit, the

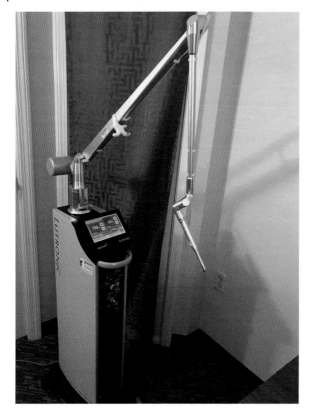

Figure 1.8 Articulated arm for a CO_2 laser application in the modern CO_2 laser (Denta 2, Lutronic, GPT dental, Fairfield, NE, USA).

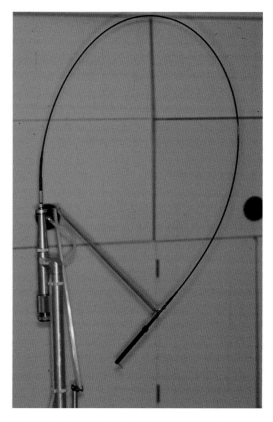

Figure 1.9 Hollow guide of a CO_2 laser presenting the flexible delivery system for oral applications. *Source:* Dr. Georgios E Romanos.

relatively inflexible operation, and the relatively expensive reconstruction. To reduce the heavy weight, a technical modification is needed. A weight balance with gas pressure springs or counterweights can also positively affect the clinical use of endoscopes, surgical microscopes, or handpieces.

1.6.3 Fiber Systems and Flexible Hollow Guides

These fiber systems are flexible light guides made of glass fibers (high-purity fused quartz glass) coated with transparent plastic or piping systems, the so-called waveguides (Figure 1.9).

Flexible hollow guides are also used in the construction of CO_2 lasers, instead of more expensive and relatively inflexible articulated arms. The flexible hollow fiber for CO_2 laser wavelength was developed in the 1990s; it features an unprecedented reach and accessibility unattainable with articulated arm lasers. A pen-size, scalpel-like handpiece is held very close to the target tissue. It focuses the CO_2 laser beam 1–3 mm away from handpiece's distal end; no aiming of the

beam is needed. The handpiece is autoclavable, and the latest designs use no disposable tips.

The optical fiber (Figure 1.10) works by a total internal reflection in which the index of reflection inside the core of the fiber is higher than the index of reflection of the cladding (Ghatak and Thyagarajan 1998). They are currently used in many laser systems, because they are reasonably priced. These light pipes can be quite long, so that the laser unit and the surgical area can be physically separated.

They have a broad clinical application possibility, among others in gastroenterology, vascular surgery, gynecology, and also in dentistry.

A disadvantage of these waveguides is the relative loss of power at high deflection of the fiber and the limitations in focusing. Of particular clinical importance is the intracorporeal application of the fiber, due to the high quartz fiber flexibility. Flexible fibers can nowadays be inserted, by means of endoscopy, in difficult to access areas, and there they can be therapeutically used.

For intracorporeal clinical use an optical fiber is essential. Waveguides are not currently used intracorporeally, as combustion products in the case of not-with-window-closed waveguides can contaminate the inner surfaces. Technological efforts for the optimization of beam control systems are intensively carried out in the various fields of clinical medicine.

1.7 Applicators

Applicators are technical devices of the laser unit, which allow direct transmission of the laser beam in the tissue. They have the shape of a handpiece or a tube (fiber applicator).

1.7.1 Handpieces

Handpieces are primarily used for mirror swivel arms and make possible the transmission and focusing of the beam on a tissue area without contact (noncontact). They can shrink the irradiated area considerably, depending on the manufacturer and by means of special tips made of ceramic or metal (Figures 1.11–1.14). Bent

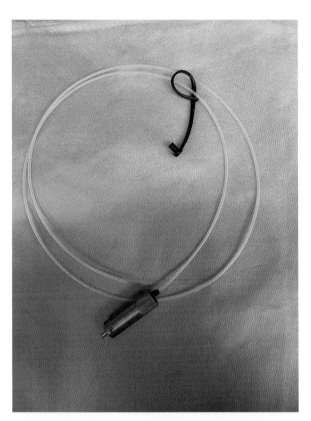

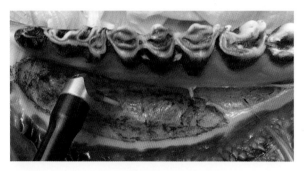

Figure 1.11 Irradiation of soft tissues in the lamb vestibule using a ceramic tip and CO_2 laser (left) and a glass flexible fiber of a diode laser (right). Observe the superficial carbonization of the CO_2 laser excision compared to the diode ablation. Different diameter applicators were used (ceramic cylindrical tip for the CO_2 and narrow glass fiber for the diode laser). *Source:* Dr. Georgios E Romanos.

Figure 1.10 Flexible optical fibers for medical and dental applications. *Source:* Dr. Georgios E Romanos.

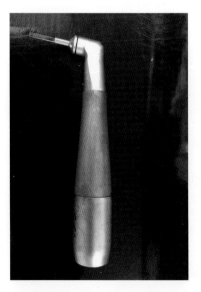
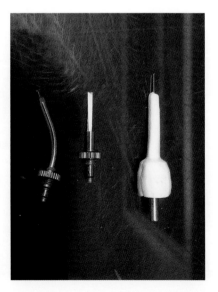
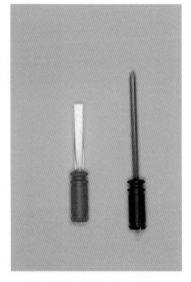

Figures 1.12–1.14 Special tips for direct connection with the hand piece (left) for Er:YAG laser made by sapphire or glass fiber for Er:YAG or diode lasers (middle) and for Er,Cr:YSGG laser (right). *Source:* Dr. Georgios E Romanos.

metal spikes can be also used for less accessible regions of the oral cavity. Likewise, there are handpieces with beam deflection.

1.7.2 Fiber Applicators

Fiber applicators are straight or curved tubes that allow contact of the flexible fibers with the tissues. The fiber can be fixed in the applicator by a simple screw. During a contact application, the fiber tip is worn out over time, which reduces the beam profile and decreases the available power density (Figures 1.15 and 1.16). Thus, an optimal ablation is prevented.

A fiber cable consists of the main core (8 μm), the cladding (125 μm) covered by the coating (approx. 250 μm), and the jacket (400 μm), which protects the entire fiber optic.

Laser manufacturers have special tools (Figure 1.17) for cutting the glass fibers after removal of the plastic coating (clearing).

With new laser developments, the industry grows, and laser devices become smaller and more powerful every day. An example is the growth of the Er,Cr:YSGG lasers (Biolase Inc.) over the last 20 years demonstrating a significant reduction of the size of the devices.

The spot size is very important since smaller spot sizes are associated with higher fluence. Thermal transfer in small spot sizes can be more effective without damage to the surrounding tissues. In contrast to this, a larger spot size requires higher energy levels or longer irradiation periods, which may have side effects to the surrounding tissues (i.e. carbonization or overheating). In this case, when clinicians try to avoid overheating

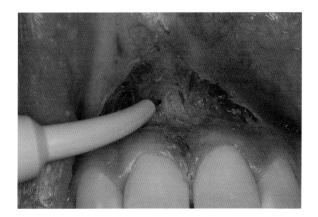
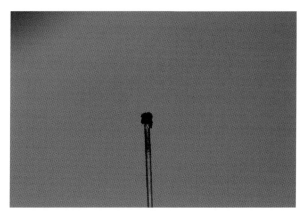

Figures 1.15 and 1.16 Diode laser irradiation during frenectomy and partial vestibuloplasty using a contact of the fiber tip with the tissues (left). This may allow damage of the tip, decrease of the power density, and, due to overheating, potential scar tissue formation. For this specific indication, initiated tips are strongly recommended (right). *Source:* Dr. Georgios E Romanos.

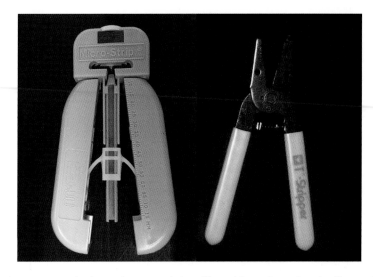

Figure 1.17 Special tools to remove plastic coating around glass fiber without damaging the fiberoptic. *Source:* Dr. Georgios E Romanos.

tissues, the therapeutic energy level cannot be achieved and, therefore, the final outcome is insufficient.

1.8 Laser Types Based on the Active Medium

The currently known laser systems are, according to their active medium, divided into the following types (Table 1.2):

- Gas lasers (He:Ne, CO_2, excimer [ArF or KrF] or argon laser)
- Solid state lasers (Nd:YAG, Ho:YAG, Er:YAG, Er,Cr:YSGG, rubin, alexandrite laser)
- Liquid (dye) lasers (containing liquid colorant as the medium, e.g. Rhodamine G6, Coumarin, etc.)
- Semiconductor (diode) lasers, so-called GaAs, GaAlAs lasers (containing semiconductor as the medium)
- "Free-electron" lasers (using an electron accelerator, not available for dentistry)

Physically seen, the change of energy levels of electrons in an atom produces the laser radiation. With the gas and solid-state lasers, the atoms are stimulated by electron collisions. On the contrary, in the excimer, or in the dye lasers, a transition of electrons to molecules takes place.

All lasers used in medicine, including their wavelengths, are in the Table 1.2.

Below are described those types of lasers, which are primarily used in surgical dentistry.

1.8.1 Gas Lasers

Such lasers use gas as the active medium. These lasers are relatively inexpensive and can achieve high power in continuous wave mode. Known systems are the CO_2, the argon, the He:Ne, and the excimer laser. In these types of lasers, the active medium is stimulated by an optical pumping mechanism or by electrical discharge. Flowing gas is required, and usually there is no need for gas refill for a long lifetime. Such lasers are the main

Table 1.2 Laser systems with applications in medicine.

Wavelength (nm)	Laser	Active Medium	Mode	Application
193	Argon fluoride Excimer	ArF	Pulsed	Ophthalmology
308	Xenon chloride Excimer	XeCl	Pulsed	Vascular surgery
488	Argon ion	Ar	CW	Various surgeries
511	Copper vapor	Cu ions	Pulsed	Dermatology
514	Argon	Ar	CW	Various surgeries
532	KTP (frequency doubled Nd:YAG)	Nd:YAG KTP crystal	Pulsed	Various surgeries
627.3	Gold vapor	Au ions	Pulsed	PDT
632.8	Helium-neon	Neon gas	CW	Biostimulation
647	Krypton	Ionized Kr gas	CW	Retinal coagulation
694.3	Ruby	$Cr^{3+}:Al_2O_3$	Pulsed	Dermatology
500–800	Dye	Dyes	CW/pulsed	PDT, Dermatology
670–1550	Diode	Ga-As	CW/pulsed	various surgeries
798	Alexandrite	Crystal	Pulsed	Research
1064	Neodymium:YAG	Crystal	Pulsed	Various surgeries
1070	Ytterbium:YAG	Crystal	Pulsed	Dermatology
2010	Thulium	Tm:YAG crystal	Pulsed	Urology
2140	Holmium	ThHoCr:YAG crystal	Pulsed	Cartilage surgery
2940	Er:YAG	Er:YAG crystal	Pulsed	Ophthalmology
10 600 (or 9300)	CO_2	CO_2	CW/pulsed	Various surgeries

lasers for general surgery especially the carbon dioxide laser. However, the bulky size of these devices and the fragile construction make these lasers not the first choice of application in private practices.

1.8.1.1 CO$_2$ Laser (10 600 nm)

This type of laser was developed in the US between the early 1960s and the early 1980s. The active medium consists of carbon dioxide (CO_2), nitrogen, and helium. The mixing ratio of the laser medium is 4.5% CO_2, 13.5% N_2, and 82% He and represents a nontoxic gas mixture. Nitrogen molecules are pumped by an external energy source, which by its energy activates the molecules of the active medium (CO_2). For this reason, this type of laser is also called a molecular laser.

Depending on the type of discharge, they are currently operated as continuous (CW) or pulsed systems. During the production of the laser light, an excessive overheating of the optical resonator is prevented by the cooling effect of helium. Optical materials for the CO_2 laser are, among others used, germanium, zinc selenide, and gallium arsenide. Even the slightest dirt on the lenses can cause destruction.

In terms of CO_2 laser construction characteristics, there are different types of CO_2 lasers including glass tubes dating back to the 1960s; this technology features a relatively short lifetime and high maintenance costs; it requires up to 20 000 volts and flowing liquid coolant, both of which are expensive in service. Innovative technology with all-metal tubes was developed in 1990s; it features rugged an all-metal air-cooled resonator design, long lifetime (up to 45 000 hours), low cost, low voltage RF transistor-operated power supplies, and excellent laser pulsing capabilities (Figure 1.18).

With a wavelength of 10 600 nm (invisible infrared range), the beam can be well absorbed by the enamel, so that at first it was considered to use this type of laser in the cavity preparation, the conditioning of dental enamel, and treatment of caries (Lobene and Fine 1966; Lobene et al. 1968; Stern et al. 1972). Significant increases in temperature on the tooth surface strongly limited the use of conventional CO_2 lasers (CW or pulsed) at the processing of hard tissues (Stewart et al. 1985). On the contrary, Melcer et al. (1984) demonstrated in a clinical trial with 1000 patients positive observations in the removal of caries. In an animal study Melcer et al. (1987) histologically confirmed the formation of secondary dentin and the sterilization of dentin and pulp during the application of CO_2 laser.

The absorption of the laser beam increases by water. Since its penetration depth is low (ca. 0.1–0.3 mm) and the surrounding tissue is hardly heated, modern CO_2 lasers can be primarily used in the superficial manipulating of soft tissues (Figure 1.19). The coagulating effect on small blood vessels allows a blood-free and clear surgical field.

1.8.1.2 CO$_2$ Laser (9300 nm)

This is a relatively new development of the CO_2 (9300 nm) laser with applications in hard and soft tissues in dentistry. Due to the relatively high absorption by hydroxyapatite, this wavelength can be used for removal of enamel and dentin.

The first laser with FDA clearance for soft and hard tissue applications in dentistry is the SOLEA (Convergent Dental). Compared to the conventional CO_2 lasers and the Er:YAG lasers, which vaporize water and enamel, this new laser uses an oxygen-18 isotope

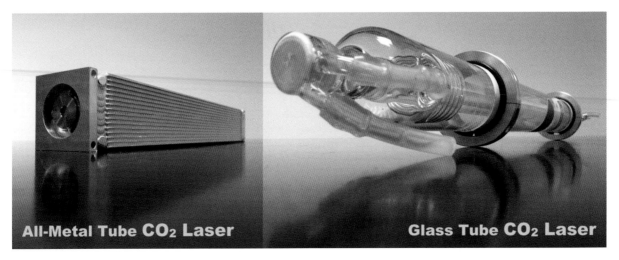

Figure 1.18 Innovative all metal-tube compared to the classic old glass tube of CO_2 laser systems (courtesy: LightScalpel, Inc.).

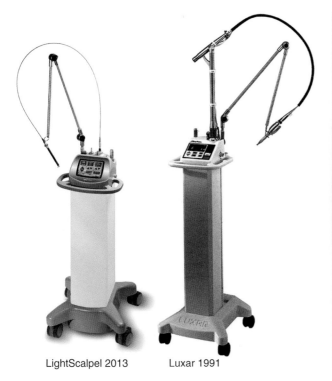

LightScalpel 2013   Luxar 1991

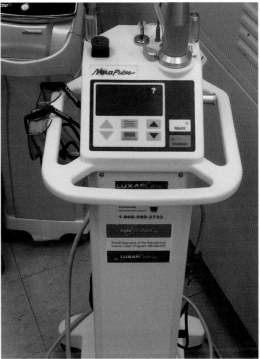

Luxar (MegaPulse, Lightscalpel)

Figure 1.19 Development of CO$_2$ lasers over time by LightScalpel, Inc. demonstrates the modern and robust design for surgical applications using hollow guide technology. Luxar (MegaPulse, Lightscalpel)

and other modifications to emit 9.3 µm, matching the peak absorption of hydroxyapatite. Therefore, it can be used for removal of decay and also soft tissue excisions with controlled bleeding. Since this wavelength is relatively new in dentistry, more case series and clinical applications are needed to demonstrate the long-term effects of this wavelength on the tissues.

1.8.1.3 Argon-Laser

The argon laser is an ion laser and is currently not popular in dentistry. Its wavelength is in the visible range of light (488 nm blue or 514.5 nm green light) and its capacity is up to 30 W. Almost all its power is converted into heat, which is why adequate water cooling is necessary.

Initially in the 1960s the argon laser was introduced in gynecology, dermatology, ENT, and ophthalmology. In dentistry, it is useful for caries diagnosis; it reduces the polymerizing time in the therapy with hybrid or micro-filled composite fillings (Kelsey et al. 1989; Powell et al. 1989; Severin and Maquin 1989; Blankenau et al. 1991a, 1991b; Powell et al. 1995) and can also be used in surgery for the removal of vascular lesions (White et al. 1993) (Figure 1.20).

The high absorption of the argon laser light from hemoglobin, hemosiderin, and melanin allows both

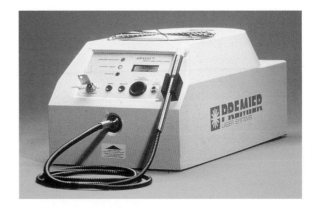

Figure 1.20 Argon laser device (Premier, Irvine, CA).

intra- and extraoral, a complication-free hemostasis of strongly vascular tissues, and the removal of pigmented lesions (Dixon et al. 1986; Hohenleutner and Landthaler 1990; Kutsch and Blankenau 1995; Poetke et al. 1996). Vessels up to a diameter of 1 mm can be coagulated. The optical penetration depth of the argon laser is limited to about 1 mm. The superficial water cooling allows a doubling of the thermal impact depth by about 2 mm. Thermal damage to the skin can be minimized by the use of saline solution and pressing with a glass spatula (Poetke et al. 1996).

1.8.1.4 He:Ne Laser

This laser is a neutral atom laser. It contains neon as the active medium and helium as pumping gas at a ratio of 1 : 10. The light is emitted at a wavelength of 633 nm. He:Ne lasers operate in continuous wave mode. The output power is at 0.5 to 50 mW relatively low. Reliability, manageability, and a relatively low price compensate for the low working efficiency of this laser. The He:Ne laser is currently used as a target (the so-called pilot laser), as well as a laser light pointer in holography. In medicine, it belongs to the group of soft lasers that are used to support wound healing and pain reduction. Further possible applications are found in the counting of cells and measuring of the eye in ophthalmology.

1.8.2 Crystal Lasers

Crystal lasers (usually named as "solid-state" lasers) are lasers with a crystal as an active medium. Usually, the YAG (yttrium-aluminum-garnet) crystal is used in these lasers. Approximately 1% of the yttrium atoms is replaced ("doped") with neodymium, to have the Nd:YAG (Neodymium: yttrium, aluminum, garnet) laser, which is the most known laser type of this group. The invisible 1064 nm wavelength penetrates deeply into biological tissues, compared to the 532 nm (half of 1064 nm) which penetrates far less and is visible. Such crystals are KTP (potassium triphosphate), producing the frequency-doubled Nd:YAG (KTP) lasers (green output) with many applications in the treatment of vascularized tissues due to the high absorption by hemoglobin.

Similarly, there are Er:YAG (erbium: yttrium, aluminum, garnet), Er,Cr:YSGG (erbium, chromium: yttrium, scandium, gallium, garnet) and the alexandrite lasers. Less popular crystal dental lasers and some no longer commercially available are the Ho:YAG (holmium: yttrium, aluminum, garnet; 2120 nm), the ruby (694.3 nm), the Nd:CGSGG (neodymium: chromium, gadolinium, scandium, gallium, garnet; 1061 nm) and the Nd:YAP (neodymium: yttrium, aluminum, perovskite; 1340 nm) laser.

These lasers or any glass lasers cannot operate in a CW mode in order to avoid risks of overheating and damage of the laser crystal.

1.8.2.1 Nd:YAG Laser

The Nd:YAG laser was used in dentistry for the first time in 1977 in animal studies in order to test its effect on the pulp (Adrian 1977). Nowadays, it is the most important known solid-state laser with a wavelength of 1064 nm. In the normal pulse mode, it provides energies up to 50 J, and has as a continuous beam (CW laser) and an output power up to 150 W. It is also used as an industrial laser for material processing (Abdurrochman et al. 2014). However, in dentistry the Nd:YAG laser can be used only in pulsed mode due to the high risk of tissue overheating and deep tissue penetration. The laser beam is absorbed from only a small amount of water and works in contact with the tissue. The heat effect occurs deep in the tissue of the irradiated area and has a strong coagulation effect. This leads to the shrinkage of the tissue, and vessels up to a diameter of 2– 3 mm can be closed. This hemostatic effect of the Nd:YAG laser is used in many ways in clinical surgery. Its biological effects are coagulation, carbonization, and vaporization (Frank 1989).

The application of Nd:YAG laser in medicine was tested by extensive clinical studies and is scientifically validated. One can currently use it in hepatectomy and in the removal of hemorrhoids and highly vascularized tissues, as hemangiomas, without major complications in contact with the tissue used in a fiber optic system (Kiefhaber et al. 1977; Iwasaki et al. 1985; Joffe 1986; Joffe et al. 1986; Poetke et al. 1996).

The first studies in dentistry were carried out by Myers and Myers (1985), and their purpose was the removal of dental caries, concluding that superficial carious enamel lesions can be removed with the Nd:YAG laser. The fine fiber of the Nd:YAG laser system can be used both in the excision of soft tissue, as well as for coagulation (Figures 1.21 and 1.22). In endodontics the positive effect of the laser was shown by means of bacterial reduction in the root canal (Dederich et al. 1984, 1985; Melcer et al. 1987; Hardee et al. 1994; Gutknecht et al. 1996). In various clinical articles it was shown that the application of the Nd:YAG laser is also possible in the surgical excision of the labial frenulum (frenectomy) in periodontology and in the excision of benign tumors in the oral cavity (Romanos 1994; Goldstein et al. 1995).

1.8.2.2 Er:YAG Laser

The Er:YAG laser with a wavelength of 2940 nm plays an important role in medicine and dentistry. Its active medium is as for the Nd:YAG laser, a crystal, although the Er:YAG laser with 30–40 wt% is relatively high doped, and yttrium atoms are replaced by erbium atoms. In total the Er:YAG system, including the pumping mechanism (using a pulsed linear xenon flash lamp), is similar to the Nd:YAG laser system (Figures 1.23 and 1.24).

The penetration depth of the radiation in the tissue is only approx. 1 μm (10^{-3} mm), so that a selective photoablation occurs, and the tissue is removed layer by layer.

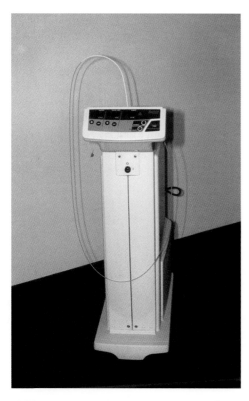

Figure 1.21 Classic Nd:YAG laser (Pulsemaster 1000; American Dental Technologies, Southfield, MI, USA). *Source:* Dr. Georgios E. Romanos.

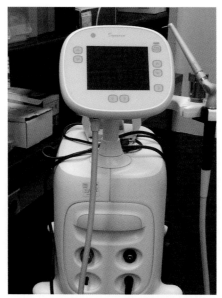

Er:YAG (Syneron, Israel)

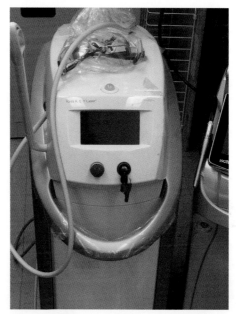

Er:YAG (KaVo Key III, Germany)

Figures 1.23 and 1.24 Representative Er:YAG laser devices for dental clinical applications. *Source:* Dr. Georgios E. Romanos.

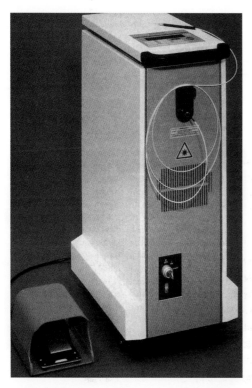

Figure 1.22 Nd:YAG laser device (American Dental Technologies, Southfield, MI, USA). *Source:* Dr. Georgios E. Romanos

This wavelength is used primarily in the field of microsurgery and hard tissue surgery. Soft tissue incisions and removal can be achieved due to the low penetration depth. Due to the high absorption rate of the laser beam in water, this wavelength can be used for the ablation of enamel, dentin, or bone. Discoloration and carbonized zones appear in the tissue only at the margins of the irradiated area. This can be prevented through an integrated water-cooling (Keller and Hibst 1995).

Although different experimental animal and clinical studies have been conducted (Keller and Hibst 1990; Keller et al. 1990, 1991), the scientific substantiation through a broad clinical application of this system is lacking, in contrast to other dental lasers.

In osteotomies with the Er:YAG laser, Keller et al. (1991) observed a minimal zone of necrosis, which compared to the osteotomies made with the CO_2 laser, and led to no wound healing delay. In contrast to these studies, Nelson et al. (1989) found a delay of wound healing (similar to the CO_2 laser) after the application of the Er:YAG laser, when no water cooling was utilized.

Regarding the treatment of the soft tissue, the wavelength of this laser is recommended for the ablation of oral mucosa (e.g. surgical removal of leukoplakia or lichen planus) (Keller et al. 1990). A clinical application in areas where there is no major bleeding tendency (Keller et al. 1990) (e.g. in the removal of benign soft tissue tumors, gingivoplasty, and extraorally on the skin) is possible without the need of additional suturing (Kautzky et al. 1992). The Er:YAG laser can be also applied, as shown in in vitro studies in periodontology, for the removal of calculus from the root surface (Aoki et al. 1994).

Experimental tests with this wavelength were also performed successfully in temporomandibular-joint (TMJ) arthroscopy, as conventional arthroscopy is highly time consuming and complex and is associated with significant trauma (Mordon et al. 1995).

1.8.2.3 Er,Cr:YSGG Laser

Great efforts have been made with the development of the Er,Cr:YSGG laser (2780 nm) for bone cutting. This wavelength has been used in oral surgery for osteotomies, osteoplasties, and removal of supernumerary teeth utilizing water and air spray in different ratios. Further applications in implant dentistry, like the preparation of the lateral maxillary sinus window, the implant uncovering, and implant site preparation have also been reported (see also Chapter 6). In addition, in pediatric dentistry and orthodontics, for removal of the frenum, gingivectomies, and operculectomies, is an opportunity for soft tissue excisions with low complication rates. The Er,Cr:YSGG laser has a lower water absorption coefficient compared to the Er:YAG laser and therefore a better penetration depth in the soft tissues. Therefore, the cutting efficiency is better. Furthermore, this wavelength can be used in operative dentistry for enamel conditioning before etching and cavity preparation. Due to the increased interest for use, the company Biolase, Inc. has developed numerous devices for different clinical applications (Figures 1.25–1.27).

1.8.2.4 Ho:YAG Laser

The Ho:YAG laser has a wavelength of 2.1 μm or 2.01 μm and in the water a penetration depth of 0.3 mm. It is used for hard and soft tissue excisions. Currently there is only the Ho:YAG laser for dental applications in some countries. This unit contains two laser sources, making

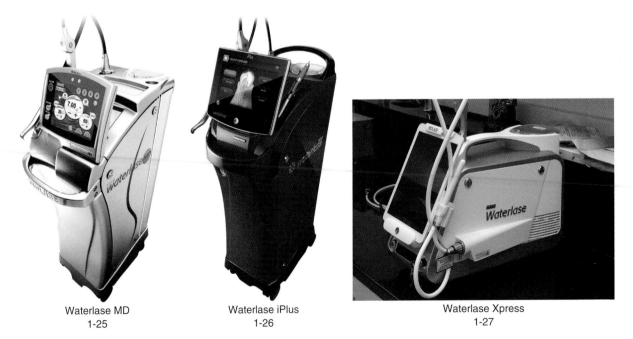

Waterlase MD
1-25

Waterlase iPlus
1-26

Waterlase Xpress
1-27

Figures 1.25–1.27 Different Er,Cr:YSGG laser devices developed in the last 20 years by Biolase, Inc. The size of the device has been decreased, providing innovative opportunities for clinical settings. *Source:* Biolase, Inc.

the application of two different wavelengths possible. A Ho:YAG (2090 nm) and a Nd:YAG (1064 nm) laser can be adjusted for use, depending on the therapeutic requirements, at the touch of a button. The Ho:YAG laser (formerly DuoPulse®) system can achieve up to 4 W output power, and it also allows easier handling through a flexible silica fiber. This type of laser is in used in the fields of vascular surgery (Mehmet et al. 1989; Hardee et al. 1994), ophthalmology (Iwasaki and Inomata 1986), urology (Johnson et al. 1992), ENT (Shapshay et al. 1990; April et al. 1991; Oswald and Bingham 1992), gastroenterology (Nishioka et al. 1989; Bass et al. 1991; Rubio 1991), gynecology (Rosenberg et al. 1990), and orthopedics, especially for arthroscopy (Trauner et al. 1990; Shi et al. 1993).

In the arthroscopic surgery of the TMJ, the use of this laser type was tested and clinically studied by Hendler et al. (1992) and Koslin and Martin (1993). It has been proven that the Ho:YAG laser is currently a low-invasive treatment alternative in arthroscopic surgical procedures. Examinations of the irradiated tissue and the adjacent areas showed only a slight thermal effect.

In dentistry, the Ho:YAG laser is used for the conditioning of dentine, the removal of the dentin surface (White et al. 1993), the effective ablation of dentine from the root canal (Stevens et al. 1994), and for in vitro root apex resections (Komori et al. 1997). Under certain circumstances it can remove enamel, dentin, and calculus (Mani 1992).

Physically seen, the Ho:YAG laser beam is very well absorbed by water, although its absorption coefficient is about 19 times lower in comparison to the CO_2 laser. Due to the high amount of water in enamel and dentin, the removal of hard tissue is minimally possible. One can achieve with it an efficient management of soft tissue without complications, either highly pigmented or white (with or without contact with the tissue). In regard to the coagulation of vessels, the coagulation zone is in comparison to CO_2 laser bigger, but smaller than the one of Nd:YAG laser.

1.8.2.5 Alexandrite Laser

The design principle of the frequency-doubled alexandrite laser (comprised of a $Cr:BeAl_2O_4$ crystal) corresponds to the Nd:YAG laser. The alexandrite laser has a fundamental wavelength between 720 and 800 nm (typically 755 nm). The frequency-doubled Alexandrite laser corresponds to ca. 578 nm. Its application, which was previously only experimental, takes place in the salivary duct stone lithotripsy. Its advantages are the high stone fragmentation rate and the low trauma, as it is a minimally invasive procedure (Gundlach et al. 1995).

1.8.3 Liquid (Dye) Lasers

Liquid (dye) laser systems have a dye as the active medium. They need other lasers or intense light for optical pumping. The laser light has a wavelength ranging from UV, through the visible, to infrared spectral range. A medium is used, usually rhodamine 6G, which flows at high velocity through the pump beam. In this way heating during the operation is avoided. The concentration of the dye is 10^{-4} mol/I. Another laser (e.g. an excimer laser) or a flash lamp is used as the pumping mechanism. This allows a pulse mode, and the corresponding output power ranges from a few mW to 10^6 W. When an argon or krypton laser is used as a pump laser, a continuous laser beam (CW) with a capacity of up to 1 W is possible. The wavelength of the laser beam is then in the range of 570–620 nm.

In medicine, such laser systems are used in the field of ophthalmology (for surgeries of the retina, for instance, coagulation of the retina) and in dermatology (e.g. in pigmentation and tattoo removal).

1.8.4 Semiconductor (Diode) Lasers

Laser dentistry has specific, sometimes unique, other times rather standard requirements for laser parameters and design of laser systems. Common desired features of laser systems for such widespread procedures as hard and soft tissue microsurgery, bacteria reduction, tissue regeneration, and tooth whitening are small size and low cost of ownership. These demands stimulated the growth in popularity of semiconductor (diode) lasers due to their high efficiency, small package size, convenient ergonomics, high reliability, and reasonable costs. Such lasers fulfill the needs of the vast majority of dental practices very well.

A semiconductor (diode) is a crystal in which the individual atoms are arranged periodically and has an electrical conductivity, which stands between insulators and metals. Semiconductor lasers are relatively small, compact, and practice-friendly devices (Figure 1.28) and have as the active medium semiconductors (diodes). This diode can be a GaAlAs (gallium aluminum arsenide) or GaAs (gallium arsenide) diode. Such lasers are relatively small, but relatively high-energy densities can be achieved. Therefore, they can also be used for medical purposes. Diode lasers have been used widely outside the United States as therapeutic devices for pain control with controversial efficacy.

The GaAs diode lasers generate pulses with an average power of 10–20 mW and are used for biostimulation. The GaAlAs diodes can be modulated and pulsed as

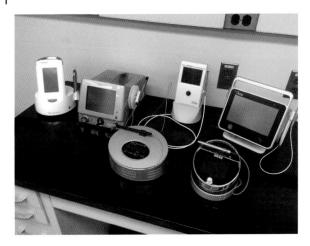

Figure 1.28 Various diode lasers for oral applications (from left to right): Sirona blue light; KaVo 980 nm; Spectralaser (980 nm); Ivoclar 810 nm; Epic (940 nm, Biolase); and the Alta Diode (975 nm) laser with automatic power control (APC) (Biolase). *Source:* Dr. Georgios E. Romanos.

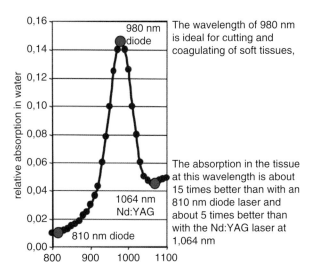

Figure 1.29 Water absorption spectrum in the wavelengths of 980, 810, and 1064 nm.

desired. In the continuous mode, the performance is lower than in the pulsed mode. The lifetime of the diode in continuous operation is approximately 500 hours.

Diode lasers can be used not only as biostimulation devices (soft lasers), but also as surgical (hard) lasers (Cetinkaya et al. 2015; Hermann et al. 2015; Arroyo-Ramos et al. 2019; Serra and Silveira 2019).

The laser light is generated in semiconductors at a suitable geometry of a semiconductor (parallel end surfaces as a resonator) under the application of electric energy. By applying an operating voltage, the electrons are injected into the different transition zone between two mirrors, and for this reason, such laser systems are referred to by some authors as "injection laser diodes." The wavelength of this laser light is typically in the range of 810–980 nm, but it can be, however, substantially lower (635 nm) when used as a low power (soft) laser. The working mode is both "continuous" and "pulsed." An external cooling of the laser system is not necessary because usually the performance is low.

In microsurgery (e.g. vascular surgery) they are used for an effective vascular anastomosis with minimal complication (Tang et al. 1994; Mordon et al. 1995), in ophthalmology for surgery of the retina, and very early in dentistry (Bach and Krekeler 1996). The diode laser is currently unsuitable for the manipulation of the hard tissue, due to the thermal load on the pulp and the periodontal tissues. Pilot studies showed potential benefits in the treatment of peri-implantitis (Bach et al. 2000).

New diode lasers have been developed recently in order to control the potential risk of thermal collateral tissue damage (overheating), allowing at the same time an efficient cutting of soft tissues. The tissue will be excised faster with sufficient hemostasis in a contact surgery mode compared to the other surgical lasers working in noncontact mode. The new advances in diode laser technology will definitely provide more opportunities in the future for the dental profession.

Currently available mainstream diode lasers are not free of limitations. Specifically, their peak power is usually low, whereas selection of available wavelengths is narrow and limited to spectral regions with low absorption of light by soft and hard tissues. Until very recently, these factors seriously limited competitiveness of the diode lasers vs. other more expensive technological approaches. The absorption of water in the 980 nm is 15 times better than with an 810 nm diode laser and approximately five times better than in the Nd:YAG (1064 nm) laser (Figure 1.29).

Recent developments in laser technology have resulted in the advent of several new laser platforms with the same unique combination of small size and low cost as traditional diode lasers, but with power characteristics and wavelength versatility making them capable of replacing conventional flash-lamp-pumped solid-state Nd:YAG, Ho:YAG, and Er:YAG lasers as well as the CO_2 lasers.

1.8.4.1 Blue Light (445 nm)

The development of a diode laser in the blue wavelength range (445 nm) promises good energy coupling to pigmented cells and tissue, combined with low absorption in water, improves cutting quality for surgical procedures, and provides deep decontamination for periodontal and endodontic lesions (Braun et al. 2015).

Shuji Nakamura was the first person to present the gallium nitride laser diode in the blue light range with a wavelength of 405 nm. He and his colleagues, Isamu Aksaki and Hiroshi Amano, were awarded the Nobel Prize for Physics in 2014. In such procedures, one of the most important advantages of blue laser light (Figure 1.30) is that, due to its shorter wavelength, it penetrates less deeply into the tissues with minimal scattering (Wilson 2014). Due to this low penetration depth, the risk of accidental injuries in deeper layers is drastically reduced, and the beam can be guided more precisely. At the same time, the thermal input to surrounding tissue from the scattering of the laser light is reduced. The absorption maximum for blood cells is in the range of approximately 430 nm (Beard 2011; Niemz 2019), which leads to a high energy input and can thus cause rapid hemostasis.

The wavelength of 445 nm displays a high level of direct coupling to tissue during incision or excision that is achieved by the favorable biophysical properties of this radiation. Comparison of the cutting effectiveness

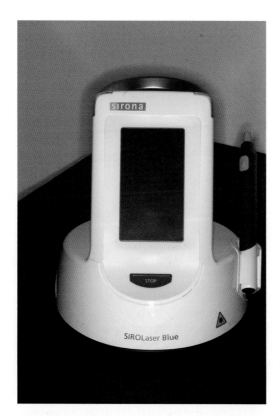

Figure 1.30 Blue-light laser (SIROLaser Blue, Dentsply Sirona, Charlotte, NC), the main market representative for blue laser diode laser in dentistry. *Source:* Dr. Georgios E. Romanos

shows advantages with 445 nm in comparison to 980 nm (Frentzen et al. 2016). The consistent results from the histological investigations and the cell culture tests showed that with both lasers tested, damage in the sense of an unspecific thermal interaction occurs. The width of the coagulation zone is, at the same cutting speed, larger at 980 nm compared to the 445 nm. With 445 nm, the width of the coagulation zone increases with rising power, in particular at a low cutting speed. At a high cutting speed, the cutting depth is the same for 445 nm at 2 W and 980 nm at 3 W (output power). The width of the coagulation zone is smaller with all 445 nm parameters than with 980 nm. Evaluation of the blue light incision quality in our lab showed minimal carbonization and good depth of the surgical incision, providing promising results in surgical applications (Figures 1.31 and 1.32).

The blue diode laser seems to be a promising technology for clinical application due to high absorption of blue light without major side effects in adjacent tissues even by reduced power settings. No increase of devitalized cells was documented with higher distances between laser tip and cell layer. Temperature development during laser irradiation was measured with a thermographic infrared camera and showed no negative thermal interactions (Reichelt et al. 2017).

1.8.5 New Developments in Laser Technology

1.8.5.1 Fiber Laser

A fiber laser is a laser in which the active gain medium is an optical fiber doped with active centers rare-earth elements such as ytterbium (Yt), neodymium (Nd), erbium (Er), thulium (Tm), and others. Unlike most other types of lasers, the laser cavity in fiber lasers (Figure 1.33) is constructed monolithically by fusion splicing rear and output reflectors (Bragg gratings), which replace conventional dielectric mirrors to provide optical feedback. Fiber lasers are pumped by pigtailed CW or QCW diodes with pumping wavelength λ_P typically in the range 960–975 nm or by other fiber lasers. Pumping light from the diode laser is propagated through a silica end cap of the fiber laser and is coupled into transparent cladding of the fiber laser with a typical diameter 100–300 μm. The core of the fiber laser has diameter of just 10–20 μm and is doped by active centers which absorb diode laser radiation. Diode laser radiation is propagated through the full fiber laser length (10–30 m) and is gradually absorbed in the core to create inversion and gain of active centers. Lasing-effect at the new laser wavelength λ_L is achieved by multipass circulation of the laser photons between rear and output

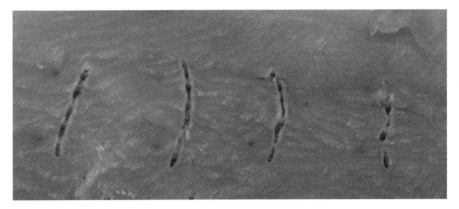

Figure 1.31 Incisions using blue laser light (445 nm) and average power of 2 W (continuous wave) in chicken breast showing minimal carbonization zone. *Source:* Dr. Georgios E. Romanos.

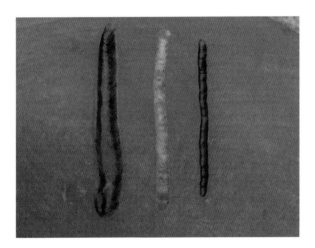

Figure 1.32 Comparative incisions using blue laser light (left), pulsed CO_2 laser with microsecond pulses (middle, char-free), and CO_2 laser (continuous wave and average power of 2 W (continuous wave) in chicken breast showing minimal carbonization zone but sufficient incision depth. *Source:* Dr. Georgios E. Romanos.

reflectors into core of the fiber laser. The fiber laser has several unique characteristics. Firstly, the fiber laser is the brightest (in terms of output radiance) laser due to the very small diameter of the output beam. It means than fiber laser beam can be focused at the smallest spot size and coupled into smallest-diameter silica fiber for delivery to the treatment zone. Secondly, fiber laser has a very high conversion efficiency and converts almost every pumping photon into laser photons. Thirdly, the fiber laser is the most stable and reliable laser design because it does not need mirror alignment; is not sensitive to variations in environmental conditions; and does not have mechanics for alignment, water flow, lamp, gas, electrodes, and other components that usually cause instability or failure regimes typical for solid-state

or gas lasers. Fourthly, the fiber laser, much like the diode laser, can be manufactured in a mass production environment with very high yield, stringent quality control, and low cost typical for the electronics industry. In short, fiber lasers offer a compact, electrically efficient, low-cost alternative to solid-state and gas laser technologies.

Fiber lasers can generate a variety of wavelengths, which can be used for standard and new medical applications. For medical applications, one of the most important considerations is that the fiber laser produces wavelengths which can be delivered through silica fibers transparent in wavelength range 300–2600 nm with high throughput. The Figure 1.34 shows the spectrum of absorption of water, which is a major tissue chromophore in NIR and MIR spectral ranges. Also shown are bands of emission of Yt (1020–1180 nm), Er (1530–1565 nm), and Tm (1900–2040 nm) fiber lasers. The ytterbium fiber laser (1070 nm) has been used in dentistry for debonding of ceramic orthodontic brackets without thermal increase and enamel damage (Sarp and Gülsoy 2011) or to treat zirconia surfaces before cementation (Unal et al. 2015). As one can see from this figure, these three lasers invoke three different mechanisms of light-tissue interaction with low (Yt), medium (Er), and high (Tm) tissue absorption. Tm line has the highest coefficient of tissue absorption in the band of transparency of silica fiber. This coefficient is about $160\,cm^{-1}$ at 1908 nm, which is almost five times higher than that for the Ho:YAG laser at 2140 nm. Fiber lasers can be used for laser pumping of external laser crystals to extend the output spectrum into the longer-wavelength IR range for even higher absorption in soft and hard tissues. Such hybrid systems can be packaged into a medical handpiece with pumping power delivered from a fiber laser through silica fiber. It has been demonstrated that such hybrid systems are feasible with standard laser crystals doped by Er, Ho, and other rare earth ions. IPG Photonics Corp. (Oxford, MA) has developed a new Cr^{+2}: Zn Ce laser crystal, which can be pumped by an Er or Tm fiber laser. These systems can generate wavelengths in the range 1800–3000 nm, which includes strong absorption bands of water (2700–2940 nm). This laser can be used for hard tissue cutting to achieve efficiency similar to classic Er:YAG or Er,Cr:YSSG and for soft tissue cutting with efficiency similar to that of the CO_2 laser.

Ytterbium high-power fiber lasers (YDF) in a power range from 1 to 10 kW, can be used in industry in continuous or pulsed mode in advanced materials-processing applications requiring extremely high power and brightness, such as fine cutting and surface structuring, cutting high-reflectivity metals, microwelding, sintering, and engraving, as well as remote processing and directed-energy applications (Figure 1.35).

1.8.5.2 Thulium (Tm:YAP) Laser

Relatively new laser systems have been developed recently and used in soft tissue dissections in ENT. The thermal damage is greater than that from the CO_2 laser, but the thulium laser (1940 nm wavelength) has the

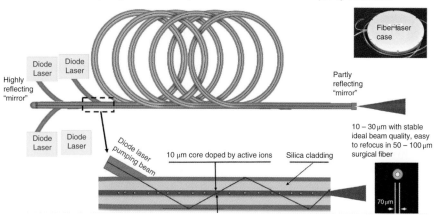

Figure 1.33 Basic concept of a fiber laser. *Source:* IPG Photonics (Oxford, MA).

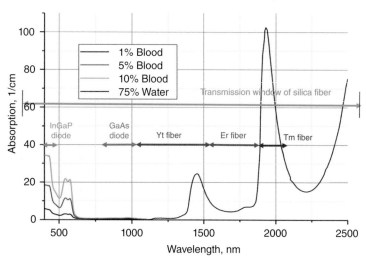

Figure 1.34 Absorption spectrum of water and blood. *Source:* IPG Photonics (Oxford, MA).

primary advantage of a silica fiber optic delivering thulium laser energy. The fiber-based delivery system offers the advantages of tangential cutting and office-based applications, because the laser energy is not delivered in a "line-of-sight" mode (Burns et al. 2007). Therefore, air-cooling has been used to reduce the extent of thermal trauma associated with thulium laser surgery of the vocal folds, and the high-temperature plume generated during laser cutting is effectively cleared.

In addition, the thulium laser has been used extensively in urology, especially in prostate surgery, providing benefits in comparison to the conventional methods. This new wavelength has been determined as a safe and effective method for the treatment of symptomatic benign prostate hyperplasia (Sun et al. 2015). Recent studies demonstrate much better outcomes in lithotripsy compared to the Ho:YAG laser applications (Traxer and Keller 2019).

In dentistry, two studies present applications of the thulium fiber laser in oral surgical procedures (Guney et al. 2014) and also for the debonding of ceramic brackets (Dostalova et al. 2011). The Tm:YAP fiber laser seems to be a promising tool for intraoral surgery, due to the excellent absorption by tissue, good coagulative qualities, easy to manipulate fiber output, and its use as an incisional tool with very little to no carbonization. Also promising solutions in hermetic connections

between metals with polymers seem to be new innovative industrial applications.

1.8.5.3 Superpulse Diode Laser

The superpulse (SP) diode or quasi continuous wave (QCW) diode laser can generate very high peak powers comparable to that of an Nd:YAG laser (on order of 100–400 W in the range of pulse widths 5 μs to 10 ms and duty cycle about 10%). It is a fundamental departure from a standard diode laser which normally operates either in a continuous wave (CW) mode with power up to 10 W or in a pulsed (modulated) mode with peak power not much different from that in CW mode (i.e. 10–15 W). The SP laser is characterized by a unique design featuring a special quantum structure of semiconductor emitters, high number of emitters coupled into single fiber (up to 12 vs. one or two of a typical mainstream dental diode laser), special packaging for efficient cooling, and a high threshold of optical damage of all light train materials.

Figure 1.36 shows a picture of a standard CW diode laser rated at 10 W of optical power and a new superpulse QCW diode laser with peak optical power up to 200 W, both emitting at wavelength of 975 nm. They are both produced by IPG Photonics Corporation (Oxford, MA), the largest manufacturer of high-power diodes and fiber lasers in the world. The 10 W laser, PLD-10, has a single CW diode laser emitter inside the package, its output coupled into a 110 μm core diameter fiber. The superpulse diode laser, PLD-120QCW, has six QCW diode laser emitters inside.

The superpulse diode laser can be expected to be similar in terms of optical output to a standard dental Nd:YAG laser, which has average power of about 6 W

Yt fiber laser with
output power 10 kW

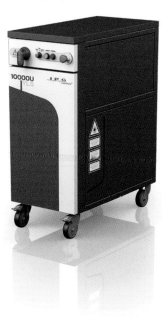

Figure 1.35 Ytterbium high-power laser developed by IPG Photonics Co. *Source:* IPG Photonics Co.

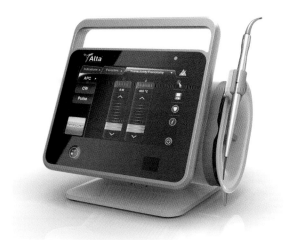

Figure 1.36 Superpulse diode laser (Alta-ST, Surgical Laser System, IPG Photonics Co.).

and peak power of about 400 W. These parameters (average and peak power) have been shown to be effective in terms of tissue heating and antibacterial effect. Table 1.2 compared optical output characteristics and heat generation efficiency on the major soft-tissue chromophores (water and blood) of CW diode, SP diode, and Nd:YAG laser with typical parameters for dental systems.

In Table 1.3, we used blood and water optical characteristics (Das et al. 1985; Edge and Carruth 1988; Feyh et al. 1989) and calculated temperature rise for 1 ms pulse width and spot size or fiber diameter 200 μm for the peak power of the respective laser. As one can see from Table 1.3, a CW laser in modulated pulse mode can produce negligible temperature rise in water and temperature rise in blood just on the threshold of blood coagulation. In contrast the SP diode laser can elevate temperature in water up to 45 °C, whereas the Nd:YAG laser achieves a water temperature rise of ~32 °C, which has been shown sufficient for bacteria deactivation. Both the superpulse diode and Nd:YAG laser with 1 ms pulse can be used for ablation of blood vessels as well.

Superpulse lasers can produce faster tissue cutting with lower collateral damage than standard CW or modulated diode lasers (Dahlman et al. 1983; Aronoff 1986; Anneroth et al. 1988; Castro et al. 1988; Basford 1990; Beer et al. 2012) because tissue ablation efficiency increases with peak power and a similar cutting effect can be achieved in pulse mode with lower average power, which in turn reduces collateral tissue heating and residual damage.

Superpulsed lasers with high-power pulses of short duration minimize the protein coagulation effects of the laser. The vaporization will be controlled without significant peripheral heating. In the surgical field, superpulsed mode permits the surgeon to advance the handpiece as slowly and as accurately as desired, while experiencing a fraction of the necrosis which occurs using conventional continuous-wave lasers. The superpulse feature may significantly change the way in which the carbon dioxide laser is used in cutaneous surgery. The superpulse diode laser has a stronger antibacterial effect than the CW diode laser because temperature elevation during biofilm illumination is higher.

However, superpulse mode was compared with ultrapulse mode of a fractional carbon dioxide laser on normal back skin of seven healthy Chinese women (split design). Clinical outcomes and side effects were evaluated. Biopsies were taken for histologic evaluation. There was no significant difference between the two sides with regard to pain, edema, crust formation, erythema, or pigmentation. The histopathological findings showed similar penetration depth for superpulse and ultrapulse mode (Xu et al. 2013).

In summary, advent of the superpulse diode lasers and fiber lasers opens up new opportunities for medical (and dental, in particular) applications. At the same time, these novel laser systems have a significant potential of competing with and eventually replacing existing solid-state and gas laser sources for many standard applications.

Table 1.3 Optical output characteristics and heat generation efficiency on the major soft-tissue chromophores (water and blood) of CW diode, SP diode, and Nd:YAG laser.

Laser type	CW Diode laser		Super Pulse Diode laser (PLD 120)	Nd:YAG laser
Wavelength, nm	800	975	975	1064
Maximum average power	10	10	60	6
Minimal pulse width, μs	5	5	5	100
Maximal pulse width, ms	100	100	100	1
Maximum average power	10	10	60	6
Maximal peak power for short pulse, W	15	15	220	1000
Maximal energy of 1 ms pulse, mJ	12	12	120	300
Water absorption coefficient, cm^{-1}	0.02	0.49	0.49	0.14
Maximal temperature increase, in water per 1 ms pulse	0.2	4.5	45	32
Arterial blood absorption coefficient, cm^{-1}	4.8	6.3	6.3	3.4
Maximal temperature increase, in blood per 1 ms pulse	44	58	575	776

1.8.6 Lasers for Research Applications

1.8.6.1 Free-Electron Laser

The free-electron laser (FEL) is a very large device, which extracts light energy from a beam of free very-high-speed electrons passing through a spatially periodic magnetic field. The electron beam must be maintained in a vacuum, which requires the use of numerous vacuum pumps along the beam path. While this equipment is bulky and expensive, FELs can achieve very high peak powers, and the tunability of FELs makes them highly desirable in many disciplines, including chemistry, structure determination of molecules in biology, and in medical diagnosis.

This laser type is not used in dentistry due to its size, high costs, and lack of practicality (more specialists are required for its application).

1.8.6.2 Nuclear-Pumped Gas Lasers

These are gas lasers in which the excitation energy is transferred from products of a nuclear reaction.

1.8.6.3 X-Ray Laser

An X-ray laser is a device that uses stimulated emission to generate or amplify electromagnetic radiation in the near X-ray or extreme UV region of the spectrum. Applications of coherent X-ray radiation include coherent diffraction imaging, research into dense plasmas (not transparent to visible radiation), X-ray microscopy, phase-resolved medical imaging, and material surface research.

1.9 Laser and Biological Tissue Interactions

The contact of the laser beam with tissue leads to different effects. These effects are distinguished in:

- photochemical
- photothermal
- ionizing or nonlinear (photoablation and photodisruption).

At the contact of light with a surface of body tissue, various optical phenomena occur (reflection, transmission, scattering, and absorption).

Depending on the surface of the irradiated object, a more or less pronounced *reflection* of the radiation takes place. This small part of radiation, which will be reflected remains without therapeutic effect. Smooth surfaces reflect the light very intensively; rough surfaces scatter it diffusely back (Figure 1.37).

The orientation of the reflection may be direct or diffuse depending on various factors, such as the surface structure, the tissue reflective index, and the angle of incidence. As an example, the reflection of the laser beam in the oral cavity on dental mirrors and metal restorations, such as amalgam fillings, crowns, and/or implant surfaces may lead to undesirable effects in not directly irradiated tissues.

The *absorption* of the ray is defined as an impairment of the radiation intensity during the transit through the substance. It is based on the transition of the radiation energy in another form of energy. The potency of the absorption is dependent on the absorption coefficient of the irradiated object. The wavelength of the laser light is an important factor in this correlation. For example, the absorption of hemoglobin under the wavelength of the argon laser light is high, and therefore this laser is clinically widely used for the coagulation of blood vessels and vascular lesions (Figure 1.37).

By definition, *scattering* of light means the deflection (dispersion) of a part of a bundled radiation from its original direction within the tissue in different directions. It takes place mainly within the irradiated body and can be deflected in every direction due to lack of homogeneity in the tissue or body structure (Figure 1.37).

The change of the path of the light (*refraction*) and the spreading of waves around an obstacle (*diffraction*) are additional phenomena in the interaction of light with matter or tissues.

At the irradiation of an object, apart from the reflection, *transmission* also occurs, which is the transfer of the light through the tissue (medium) without being absorbed or scattered. This is prominent for transparent objects, compared to opaque objects, because the high absorption of the beam is significantly reduced (Figure 1.37).

The interaction of laser light with biological tissues is always associated with the presence of chromophores within the tissues, which influence the absorption, transmission, scattering, and reflection from the tissues. We can talk about a phenomenon of "selective photothermolysis" between the wavelength and the chromophore. The absorption spectrum of water, (oxy) hemoglobin, and melanin (pigmented tissues) in relationship to the light wavelengths is presented in Figure 1.38. The absorption by (oxy)hemoglobin in the connective tissue is 1000 times weaker than the absorption by water at the CO_2 (10,600 nm) laser. A primary goal of laser therapy is to allow the maximum transmission to the target tissue (or chromophore) without conduction to the healthy surrounding tissues. For instance,

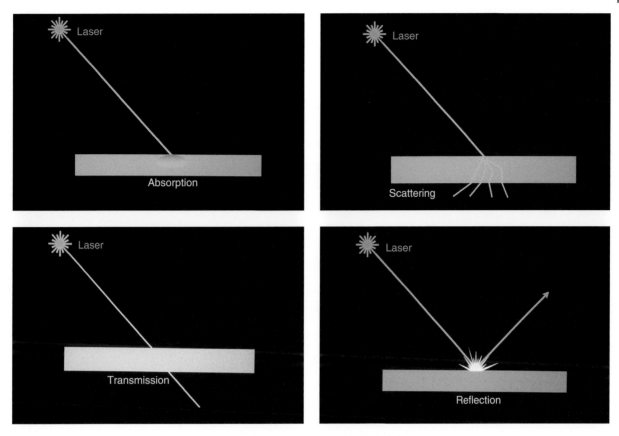

Figure 1.37 Physical properties of the light in contact with matter or biological tissues.

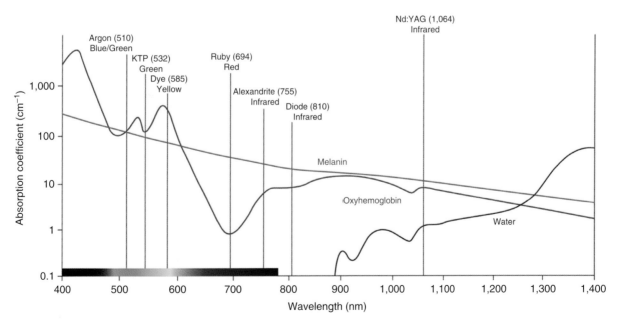

Figure 1.38 The absorption spectrum of water, (oxy)hemoglobin, and melanin depends on the different wavelengths, characterizing the specific laser-tissue interactions.

in clinical scenarios with vascular lesions, a selective irradiation of blood vessels to achieve effective coagulation without damage or structural alteration of the surrounding tissues is the primary goal of treatment. Similarly, hair removal is associated with the absorption of the laser by the melanin located in the hair follicle (and not the hair) as the main chromophore to have a therapeutic value.

The lasers and the interactions with the tissues have high importance especially in the interaction of the laser light with the eye. There are differences in the reflective and absorptive properties of the different laser wavelengths from the retina and the cornea. Since the cornea is highly concentrated in water, laser wavelengths in the mid-infrared and far infrared (1400 nm–1 mm) and middle UV (180–315 nm) and near UV (315–390 nm) wavelengths are highly absorbed. In contrast to these wavelengths, in the range of visible light and near infrared (400–1400 nm) light spectrum, there is absorption by the macula lutea of the retina (oval-shaped pigmented area near the center of the retina of the human eye and some other animal eyes) (Figure 1.39).

In order to avoid hazardous effects in the eye, special safety measures are followed. Use of goggles specific for

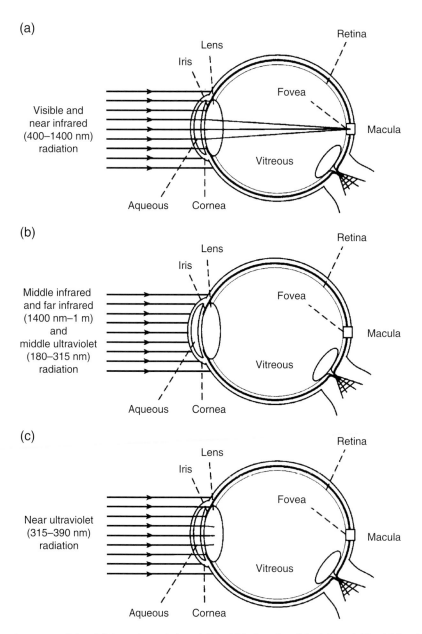

Figure 1.39 Absorption areas of the visible and near infrared (a), mid-infrared and far infrared (b), middle ultraviolet and near ultraviolet (c) wavelengths.

the individual wavelengths (see also Chapter 8), as well as curved mirror systems (reflectors) within the laser device, control direct reflections and irreversible eye damage (Figure 1.40).

1.9.1 Photochemical Effects

The laser beam can chemically change a tissue's molecules or warm a tissue, when higher power densities are applied. As a result, different effects may occur:

- formation of ions (photo-ionization)
- isomerization of the macromolecules (photo-isomerization)
- decomposition of the molecules (photo-dissociation).

These effects of the laser energy can be applied during biostimulation, photodynamic therapy, or also acupuncture.

The chemical changes of the tissue molecules due to the photochemical effect of the laser light can be shown schematically as follows:

- photo-ionization: $AB \rightarrow AB+$
- photo-isomerization: $AB \rightarrow BA$
- photo-dissociation: $AB \rightarrow A + B$

1.9.1.1 Biostimulation

The absorption of the laser light in the tissue is for biostimulation an essential condition. Within the cells, the light is absorbed in the area of the mitochondria, and thereby the tissue is stimulated. In contrast to the surgical use of the laser, there are no fabric-damaging side effects known during biostimulation.

For the phenomenon of the biostimulation (or "photobiomodulation"), only lasers with a low power are used (1–5 mW), the so-called "soft" lasers. Examples for this, are the He:Ne laser or the GaAs and the GaAlAs laser diodes. For this reason, these lasers are also called "low-level-therapy lasers" (LLTL) or "low power," "low-energy," "over-the-counter" lasers, or "low-intensity-laser therapy" (LILT) lasers, and the technology is noninvasive. The biomodulation has been used for pain reduction, acceleration of wound healing and blood flow, and treating a variety of inflammatory-related conditions (Chung et al. 2012). In this case, because the temperature in the tissue is slightly increased (less than 0.1–0.5 °C), the effect is only of a chemical (not thermal) nature.

The currently available trials of these laser types indicate no significant clinical effect. Anneroth et al. (1988) did not ascertain any difference in the wound healing of the rat skin between the test (with GaAs laser) and the control group.

On the other hand, other studies ascertained a stimulating effect of the laser light on wound healing or collagen synthesis with the He: Ne laser on pigs. Because of the stimulation of wound healing, this phenomenon is referred to as biostimulation. Moreover, in addition to the differentiation of the connective tissue, it has been proven that the migration of the epithelium cells is, under the effect of the He: Ne laser, more intensive, and the tissue's wound healing is thereby faster. Hargate (2006) showed in studies that using this technology, acute wounds (cold sores on the lips) as a result of herpes labialis can treated with complete closure. Nather et al. (2007) tried to treat chronic wounds in the legs of diabetic patients who did not respond to previous treatments

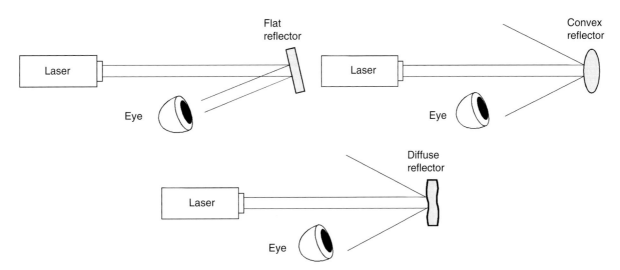

Figure 1.40 Use of flat reflectors can produce direct reflections having hazardous effects in the eye. Therefore, convex or diffuse reflectors are recommended.

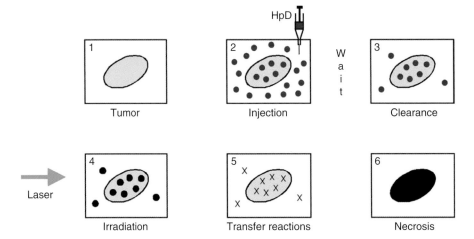

Figure 1.41 Concept of the photodynamic therapy of tumors (from Niemz 2019).

and showed favorable results after biostimulation. Usually the treatment period depends on the medical condition and ranges from a few days to several weeks.

The exact mechanism of biostimulation is still unknown. Some authors have implicated a "placebo," and furthermore there is a lot of speculative discussion about the biostimulatory effects of the light. More trials are necessary to better clarify the effect of biostimulation on tissues. Governments are encouraging programs that support self-management from home, reducing the load in the healthcare system (Renner et al. 2015).

Japanese researchers, focused on the phototherapeutic effects of the light, described the stimulation of specific light sensory receptors at the cell surface, which promote intracellular changes in the cell nucleus (Aleksic et al. 2010). Specifically, low level Er:YAG lasers may enhance the osteoblastic proliferation via MAPK/ERK pathway in the nucleus.

1.9.1.2 Photodynamic Therapy (PDT)

Photodynamic therapy represents a special technology of modern laser use, which finds its use particularly in the noninvasive treatment of superficial malignant tumors. The principle of photodynamic therapy is the resorption of a photosensitive substance (the so-called "photosensitizer") from the tumor's cells and later the selective destruction of the tumor with the help of a laser. First a photosensitizer is injected in the vein of the patient. The photosensitizer is distributed within a few hours in the entire soft tissue. After about 48–72 hours, the injected substance (photosensitizer) is eliminated by the healthy, normal cells; however, in the tumor cells, it remains for approximately seven to 10 days. With the help of a dye label of the tumor cells, they can be destroyed selectively by means of laser beams (Figure 1.41). The

pathological tissue will be rejected after successful PDT within 5–15 days. The resulting defect will be then – without leaving a scar – epithelialized (Herzog et al. 1992).

This therapy does not have the disadvantages of a chemotherapy or radiotherapy and provokes no damage to the normal tissue areas, but it has the disadvantage that patients have to stay in darkness for days.

Red coloring or diodes lasers are used for photodynamic therapy. The photosensitive substances can be derivatives of hematoporphyrin (HPD), merocyanine 540 (MC-540) or rhodamin-I23 (Rh-123). Lipson and Blades (1961) were the first to describe the photodynamic properties of hematoporphyrin and its derivatives, as well as its ability to provoke a rapid necrosis of the tumor tissue after exposition to light.

Although the effects of the PDT are already long known, the exact mechanism of action is not yet completely clear. Early on, Tappenier and Jesionek (1903) observed a positive therapeutic effect of skin carcinomas after use of eosin and fluorescein under simultaneous light radiotherapy.

Today the bonding of the sensitizer with different cellular components is controversial. The cell membrane, the nucleus, the mitochondria, the lysosome or microsome are decisive for the selective resorption of the photosensitizer.

In the maxillofacial surgery, the clinical value of photodynamic therapy has been often investigated. It could be used for the improvement of the surgical therapy result, particularly for hardly recoverable structures, like the carotid artery and the facial nerve, as well as other important anatomical structures.

A comprehensive review of the literature of the antimicrobial effects of photodynamic therapy in periodontal and peri-implant diseases with the entire spectrum of existing photosensitizers has been published by Takasaki et al. (2009). The review presents the existing preclinical and clinical evidence on the effects of photodynamic therapy in the treatment as a promising novel therapeutic approach for eradicating pathogenic bacteria in periodontal and peri-implant diseases.

A systematic review of the literature demonstrates also that photodynamic therapy in periodontology as an adjunctive treatment to the standard therapy enhances the antibacterial effects in dentistry (Javed and Romanos 2013).

1.9.2 Photothermal Effects

The photothermal effects of the laser beam on tissue are dependent on several factors (Niemz 2019). The power of the beam, its energy, and the respective exposure time can accordingly raise the temperature of the tissue and cause thereby coagulation, carbonization, or melting in the hard tissue and vaporization (Figure 1.42).

The irradiation of tissue by laser light results in the absorption of energy. This energy is expressed entirely as a heat transfer absorbed by the tissue. Laser light will be transferred to the tissues ablating inflamed soft tissues and supporting wound healing via photomodulation. Due to heat transfer, the liquid will boil into vapor, causing changes in the tissue. Since the main liquid in the tissues is water and, in case of inflammation, blood, the impact of heat transfer to the tissues is vaporization of water and later on denaturation of proteins. The tissue will become firm. Common example of this denaturation phenomenon is that boiled eggs become hard and cooked meat becomes firm (see Tables 1.4 and 1.5).

Thermal *conductivity* and thermal *diffusivity* are two tissue properties that are temperature dependent. The conductivity of the living tissues is higher compared to dead tissues, indicating the dominant role played by blood transfusion enhancing the heat transfer in living tissues (Bhattacharaya and Mahajan 2003). Water has the highest thermal conductivity of any liquid.

Considering the rules of physics, the *thermal conductivity coefficient K* is larger in muscles than in the liver and smaller in water and blood (Ponder 1962).

Also, the thermal *diffusivity* is the ability of an object to conduct heat during change of temperature. Thermal conductivity and diffusivity increase when temperature increases (Valvano 2011). Collagen has lower thermal properties and acts as a thermal insulator (Valvano 2011). Therefore, in clinical medicine it is more difficult to cut hypertrophic tissues and tissues containing more collagen using the laser beam.

However, thermal damage due to high temperature or longer heating time leads to collapse of the tissue. First, cellular death occurs and later on the extracellular matrix will be replaced by a scar.

In the laser-mediated tissue ablation high energy will be transferred with short pulses. Water vaporization appears as the temperature approaches 100 °C. When the water vaporization is faster than the diffusion of the heat out of the tissue, the vapor (steam) stays in the tissue forming steam vacuoles (Thomsen and Pearce 2011). This creates histologically a "popcorn" effect. When the temperature exceeds 200 °C, a carbonization (carbon formation) will be formed with a layer of a thin black membrane (5–20 μm) covering the defect.

The ablative effects of the laser radiation on the tissue are variously used in medicine. Thus, strong bleeding can be controlled and a blood-free operation area can be

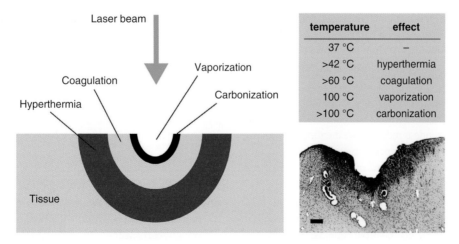

Figure 1.42 Effects of temperature distribution in the tissues (from Niemz 2019).

Table 1.4 Biological effects in soft tissues based on temperature increase (according to Niemz 2019).

Temperature (°C)	Effect
37	Normal
45	Hyperthermia
50	Reduction in enzyme activity, cell immobility
60	Protein (collagen) denaturation, coagulation
80	Permeability of membranes
100–140	Tissue vaporization, Thermal decomposition (ablation)
>150	Carbonization
>300	Melting

Table 1.5 Biological effects in hard tissues based on temperature increase (according to Bachmann et al. 2004).

Temperature (°C)	Effect
140	Elimination of water
200	Collagen denaturation
300–400	Organic material loss
400–1000	Carbonate loss
200–800	Cyanate formation
800–1000	Cyanate loss
200–1000	Changes in hydroxyapatite structure
1100	$Ca_4(PO_4)_2O$ formation
1300	Elimination of structural water, Hydroxyapatite melting

achieved. With the use of lasers it is also possible to remove superficial tissue alterations by means of carbonizing and vaporizing. Using different modes (i.e. continuous or pulsed mode and various pulse characteristics), we can have effects in the tissue of clinical significance (Figure 1.43). If during the laser use, the tissue reaches the temperature of approximately 150 °C, the tissue is carbonized (charred). From the clinical point of view, first a coagulation of the respective layers of the tissue is provoked, and afterwards a necrosis and carbonization. Higher temperatures alter the surface to a large extent and lead to pronounced irreversible changes, like melting of the hard tissue and vaporization.

Similar effects can be found in soft tissues. The use of water and air supply in different ratios can change the thermal effects and provide a reduced overheating, improving the cut efficiency. Some lasers can be used in conjunction with an air/water supply. The use of water and air provides new opportunities in clinical dentistry (Figure 1.44).

Recent studies on dental tissues showed that heat application changes the physicochemical properties of enamel contributing to positive effects due to the reduced adhesion of some bacterial species (Hu

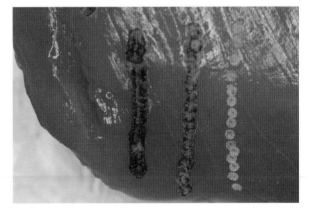

Figure 1.43 Photothermal effects of a 3 W-CO_2 laser on soft tissues (chicken breast) using a continuous wave (left), pulsed mode (middle), and superpulsed mode (right). The thermal effects demonstrate changes in the tissue. *Source:* Dr. Georgios E Romanos

et al. 2011). Specifically, heating reduced the adhesion force of both *Streptococcus mitis* and *Streptococcus oralis* to enamel (with or without saliva coating), but heating did not affect the adhesion of *Streptococcus sanguis* with or without saliva coating.

Bacterial photo-elimination has been described as a novel modality in the eradication of *Streptococcus mutans* colonies in the near future; significant reduction of *Streptococcus mutans* was observed in planktonic cultures after photodynamic and photothermal therapy (Fekrazad et al. 2013).

The penetration depth of laser light within the oral soft tissues depends on the laser wavelength and can schematically be demonstrated in Figure 1.45.

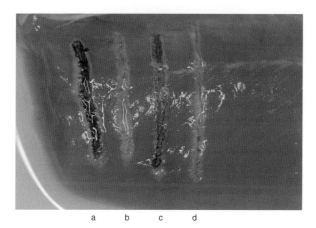

Figure 1.44 Photothermal effects of lasers on soft tissues (chicken breast) using a 6 W Er,Cr:YSGG laser (15 Hz, no air/no water, [a], pulsed mode, 70% air/30% water [b]). With higher frequency in pulsed mode (50 Hz) and no air or water, there is a carbonization effect due to overheating (c). This can be reduced significantly using a sufficient air/water (70%/30%) supply (d). *Source:* Dr. Georgios E Romanos.

Dependent on the contact or noncontact mode, but also the used wavelength, different thermal effects may occur within the tissues. Figure 1.46 demonstrates these effects as an example for clinical use. The glass fiber of the pulsed Nd:YAG or diode laser is associated with irradiation with deep penetration, creating a carbonized, coagulation, and stimulation zone. However, a carbonized fiber tip (on the 810, 940, 975 980, and the 1064 nm lasers) transforms the laser-tissue effect of a laser with high water absorption, i.e. the light is absorbed in the carbon layer, resulting in a "hot" fiber tip. This property should be carefully considered when using the 810–1064 nm lasers. When superficial ablation is needed, a carbonized tip is absolutely necessary. Therefore, initiated tips are recommended to avoid scattering and improve light absorption (see also Chapter 3).

1.9.2.1 Fractional (Photo)-Thermolysis

Fractional (photo)-thermolysis (FT) is a relatively new technique with applications in dermatology and plastic reconstructive surgery. This novel, nonablative method was introduced in the market by Dieter Manstein and Rox Anderson and published by Huzaira et al. (2003). Compared to conventional skin resurfacing methods, FT allows treatment of a fraction of the skin leaving up to 95% of the skin uninvolved.

Basically, FT is the production of an "injury pattern" to the soft tissue (i.e. skin) with skip areas repeated over and over again, which, as they heal, promote an

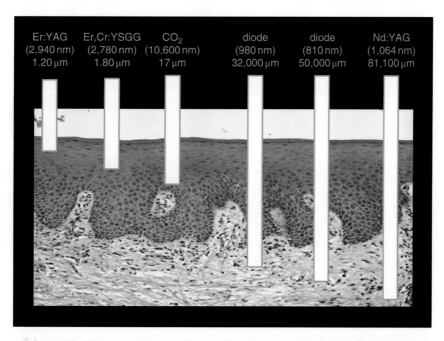

Figure 1.45 Schematic drawing of the penetration depth of different laser wavelengths in the oral mucosa based on the laser wavelength. *Source:* Dr. Georgios E Romanos.

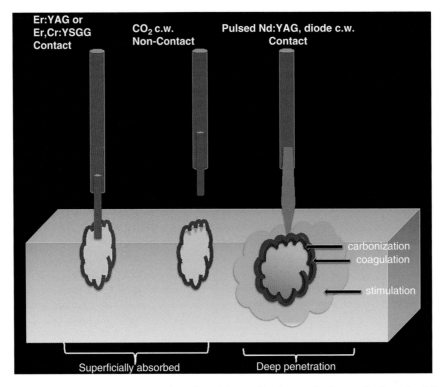

Figure 1.46 Laser-tissue effects based on the wavelength and the application mode. *Source:* Dr. Georgios E Romanos.

improvement in the tone and texture of the tissue. This technology triggers the body's natural healing process, accelerating the production of collagen and new, healthy skin cells.

In more technical terms, all of these devices produce small columns of thermal injury to the skin, which are known as microthermal zones (MTZs). These MTZs vary from device to device. Some are nonablative dermal injuries only; whereas, others are associated with ablative changes in the skin, causing both epidermal and dermal injury patterns. MTZs also vary greatly in their diameter of effect and in the degree of depth they achieve to create the injury. Once injured, the skin begins a very rapid process of repair (Figure 1.47).

In dermatology, lines and wrinkles, as well as pigmentary concerns including melasma, and in scars, especially acne and traumatic scars, can be removed and generally improve skin's appearance. This concept of therapy was applied using a prototype device (1.5 μm laser, Reliant MTZ SR prototype, Palo Alto, CA) for skin restoration of photoaged skin in the periorbital area of 30 subjects and 15 subjects with injuries in the forearm. These first clinical results showed 18% improvement of the wrinkle score after three months of therapy (Manstein et al. 2004).

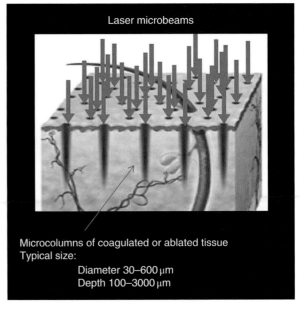

Figure 1.47 Principle of the fractional photothermolysis in the soft tissue. *Source:* IPG Photonics Inc.

Laser skin resurfacing began with the application of the carbon dioxide (CO_2) laser to facial rejuvenation, initiating a new era in the field of photorejuvenation (Alexiades-Armenakas et al. 2008). However, the major long-lasting side effect of nonfractionated CO_2 lasers is permanent skin hypopigmentation, although permanent hyperpigmentation can rarely occur (Ward and Baker 2008). In general, the CO_2 laser can vaporize the superficial epidermis without having an impact on the superficial dermal layer. Serious thermal damages can occur, especially if such procedures are performed by nonskilled clinicians. In contrast, Er:YAG or Er,Cr:YSGG lasers can ablate the epidermis superficially using short pulses and accomplish a "pure" ablation of the epidermis.

Recently, studies have looked at the use of FT in the treatment of hypertrophic scars, keloids, and burn hypertrophic scars. Ablative CO_2 fractional laser (Lumenis UltraPulse Encore, Fraxel re:pair) and ablative Er:YAG fractional lasers have been used with similar postoperative effects and comparable cosmetic improvements (Karsai et al. 2010; Preissig et al. 2012).

Erbium fiber lasers with wavelength 1550 nm (Fraxel, Reliant Technologies Inc., San Diego, CA) have been used in photomedicine for FT treatment of tissue. FT was developed as a way for laser surgeons to get closer to ablative laser resurfacing clinical outcomes with less patient downtime and fewer overall adverse events. Currently available devices vary in the way in which they produce their injury patterns, their wavelength, and their intensity. Recent studies showed that atrophic scars can be effectively and safely reduced with 1550 nm erbium-doped fiber laser treatment (Alster et al. 2007).

Of interest is the use of a similar concept in dentistry, as a minimally invasive microsurgical approach to initiate gingival and oral mucosal tissue regeneration. A *laser patterned microcoagulation (LPM)* was used in the rabbit oral mucosa using a diode laser at a wavelength 980 nm and a power of up to 20 W. The laser irradiation applied to the gingival and oral mucosa at multiple time points.

A single LPM treatment induces a wound healing response in the oral mucosa, showing the potential of LPM for the initiation of oral mucosa and gingival regeneration. This technology stimulates significantly the fibroblast activity and may lead to periodontal reattachment in periodontal tissues. Complete healing was observed in 3 months after treatment with no change in keratinization or scar tissue formation (Romanos et al. 2013).

Using this concept in clinical practice, ablation of soft tissues may be avoided and only coagulation zones underneath the epithelium surface may stimulate the matrix for new connective tissue formation. With the correct selection of laser wavelength, microbeam column diameter, and power and pulse width, there is a potential innovative mechanism to improve dense collagen fibers formation (Figure 1.48).

This concept has been initially used to improve the quality of periodontal tissues and increase the width of keratinized, attached gingiva (Figure 1.49). Clinical trials are encouraging to test this technology in specific patient populations.

1.9.3 Ionizing or Nonlinear Effects

1.9.3.1 Photoablation

The phenomenon of *photoablation* (nonlinear process) was until recently not clearly defined and was described for the first time by Srinivasan and Leigh (1982) (photodecomposition). A tissue ablation takes place as soon as

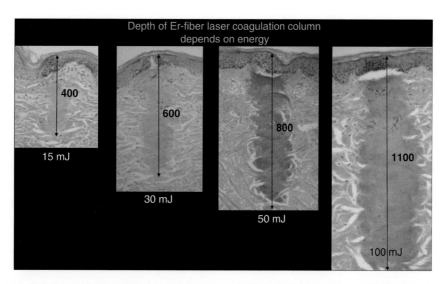

Figure 1.48 Histological demonstration of the coagulation zones in the soft tissues without ablation based on the concept of fractional photothermolysis. *Source:* Dr. Georgios E Romanos.

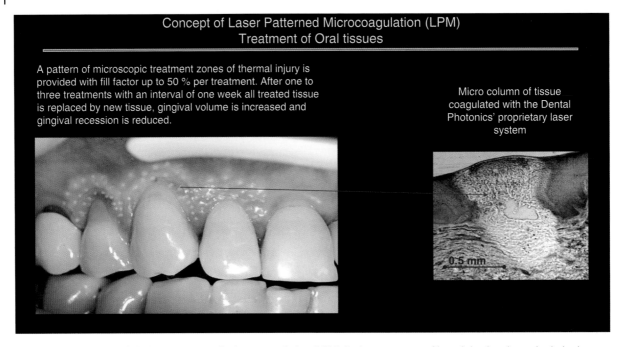

Figure 1.49 Concept of the Laser patterned micro-coagulation (LPM) for improvement of keratinized and attached gingiva. *Source:* Dr. Georgios E Romanos.

photons fall on the tissue. As a result, molecular connections are broken. The broken molecular structure suffers a volume enlargement and expands rapidly. An optimum photoablation can occur only with a wavelength of 193 nm (ArF, excimer laser). The extent of the photoablation increases with smaller wavelengths. This happens on the condition that the photon energy is greater than the molecular binding energy ($E = h \times r$). Free electrons are accelerated in the field of the laser beam and form a rise of free electrons as well as ions (formation of plasma and tissue overheating). At all other wavelengths a concurrent thermal change occurs in the tissue. It has been discussed that the ablative effect of the laser beam can lead to mutagen changes of the molecules. Studies showed that the 193 nm excimer laser beam does not transform corneal keratocytes and that the energies emitted by this beam will not cause cell transformation when the excimer laser is used as a surgical tool in human eyes (Gebhardt et al. 1990).

The conditions for photoablation are a short-pulse duration (in the area of nano- to microseconds) and a low penetration depth in the tissue, which is in the UV (<400 nm) and middle infrared (>2.5 pm) range of the spectrum. An ablative effect on the surface of the matter (e.g. dental surface) thereby takes place, and thermal damages of nonirradiated areas are avoided. This phenomenon is today clinically applied during caries removal with a laser using different (short, medium-short,

and supershort) pulses. According to recent studies the effect of supershort laser pulses was the most efficient in ablation of caries in dentin, providing a smear layer-free surface with open dentinal tubules (Baraba et al. 2012).

Other biomedical applications of the photoablative photodecomposition are the irradiation of a KrF excimer laser pulses (wavelength: 248 nm; fluence: 1J/cm^2 pulse) onto several polymer films resulting in the formation of an etched pit on the irradiated surface (Nakayama and Matsuda 1995).

1.9.3.2 Photodisruption

Plasma, in physics, is an electrically conducting medium in which there are roughly equal numbers of positively and negatively charged particles, produced when the atoms in a gas become ionized. It is sometimes referred to as the fourth state of matter, distinct from the solid, liquid, and gaseous states. Modifications to the process can be made by introducing different gases to the chamber. Commonly used gases include O_2, N_2, Ar, H_2, and CF_4. These five gases are used singularly or in combination in the majority of the labs around the world for plasma processing.

After the formation of plasma, a wave spreads out explosively and is able to destroy by means of mechanical forces the surrounding tissues. This phenomenon is known as *photodisruption* and is, as a nonlinear pro-

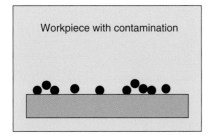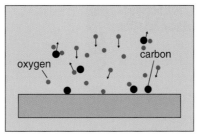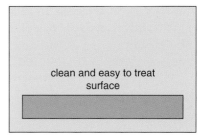

Figure 1.50 Principle of plasma cleaning process of a metal. *Source:* Thierry Plasma Science and Technology, Royal Oak, MI.

cess, closely related to the photoablative effect of the laser beam. No energy absorption has to take place for photodisruption in the tissue, because the laser energy is absorbed in the plasma of the tissue surface. Such phenomena can thereby also appear in transparent materials. Today, this interaction with the tissue is clinically applied in the ophthalmology (i.e. corneal surgery and cataract therapy) and in lithotripsy (e.g. the removal of salivary stones). The femtosecond laser especially (Sacks et al. 2003; Nuzzo et al. 2010; Rossi et al. 2015) but also the picosecond (ps) and nanosecond laser were used earlier (Vogel et al. 1994). Specifically, the use of ps pulses improved the precision of intraocular Nd:YAG laser surgery and diminished unwanted disruptive side effects.

Gas plasma technology has played a variety of roles in this scope of innovative work. These roles vary widely depending on the product market application. However, they do fall into the four categories of plasma cleaning, plasma activation, plasma etching, and plasma coating. Many plasma applications have been used in medicine for cleaning of metals using the so-called plasma cleaners (plasma treatment), but also using the plasma surface technology, there is the ability to change the surface of materials on the microscopic level, giving them different characteristics. One method that plasma *surface*

technology can employ to change a surface's traits is called micro-sandblasting. **Plasma cleaning** is the process of removing all organic matter from the surface of an object through the use of an ionized gas (so-called **plasma**). This is generally performed in a vacuum chamber utilizing oxygen and/or argon gas.

In plasma cleaning (Figure 1.50) the surface is cleaned by ion bombardment and chemical reactions. After plasma activation, the nonpolar surfaces are changed into adhesive surfaces, and the surface energy increases. To plasma etch or to remove material, the surface is etched with an etchant gas.

This innovative technology seems to have many applications in surgical dentistry in industrial but also clinical settings.

Low pressure plasma cleaners are an economical way to uniformly, safely, and completely plasma clean, removing contaminants from the surface of treated substrates without affecting the bulk material properties. This process of decontamination is used in industry before packaging and works for a large range of materials (metals, plastics, glass, ceramics, etc.). Plasma cleaning is an environmentally friendly procedure since there is no need for hazardous chemical solvents. The processing eliminates mold-releasing agents, antioxidants, carbon residues, oils, and all varieties of organic compounds.

References

Abdurrochman, A., Lecler, S., Mermet, F. et al. (2014). Photonic jet breakthrough for direct laser microetching using nanosecond near-infrared laser. *Appl. Opt. 53* (31): 7202–7207.

Adrian, J.C. (1977). Pulp effect of neodymium laser, a preliminary report. *Oral Surg. Oral Med. Oral Pathol. 44*: 301–305.

Aleksic, V., Aoki, A., Iwasaki, K. et al. (2010). Low level Er:YAG laser irradiation enhances osteoblast proliferation through activation of MAPK/ERK. *Lasers Med. Sci. 5*: 559–569.

Alexiades-Armenakas, M.R., Dover, J.S., and Arndt, K.A. (2008). The spectrum of laser skin resurfacing: nonablative, fractional, and ablative laser resurfacing. *J. Am. Acad. Dermatol. 585*: 719–737.

Alster, T.S., Tanzi, E.L., and Lazarus, M. (2007). The use of fractional laser photothermolysis for the treatment of atrophic scars. *Dermatol. Surg. 33* (3): 295–299.

Anneroth, G., Hall, G., Ryden, H., and Zetterqvist, L. (1988). The effect of low-red laser radiation on wound healing in rats. *Br. J. Oral Maxillofac. Surg. 26*: 12–17.

Aoki, A., Ando, Y., Watanabe, H., and Ishikawa, I. (1994). In vitro studies on laser scaling of subgingival calculus with an Er:YAG laser. *J. Periodontol. 65*: 1097–1106.

April, M.M., Rebeiz, E.E., Aretz, H.T., and Shapshay, S.M. (1991). Endoscopic holmium laser laryngotracheoplasty in animal models. *Ann. Otol. Rhinol. Laryngol. 100*: 503–507.

Aronoff, B.L. (1986). The state of the art in general surgery and surgical oncology. *Lasers Surg. Med. 6*: 376–382.

Arroyo-Ramos, H.H., Neri, L., Mancini, M.W. et al. (2019). Effects of diode laser setting for laryngeal surgery in a rabbit model. *Eur. Arch. Otorhinolaryngol. 276* (5): 1431–1438.

Bach, G. and Krekeler, G. (1996). Einsatz eines Dioden-Halbleiterlasers in der Zahnheilkunde. *Zahnärztl. Welt. Reform. 105*: 314–319. (German).

Bach, G., Neckel, C., Mall, C., and Krekeler, G. (2000). Conventional versus laser-assisted therapy of periimplantitis: a five-year comparative study. *Implant. Dent. 9* (3): 247–251.

Bachmann, L., Gomes, A.S.L., and Zezell, D.M. (2004). Bound energy of water in hard dental tissues. *Spectrosc. Lett. 37*: 565–579.

Baraba, A., Perhavec, T., Chieffi, N. et al. (2012). Ablative potential of four different pulses of Er:YAG lasers and low-speed hand piece. *Photomed. Laser Surg. 30* (6): 301–307.

Basford, J.R. (1990). The clinical status of low energy laser therapy in 1989. *J. Laser Appl. 2*: 27–63.

Bass, L.S., Oz, M.C., Trokel, S.L., and Treat, M.R. (1991). Alternative lasers for endoscopic surgery: comparison of pulsed thulium-holmium-chromium:YAG with continuous-wave neodymium:YAG laser for ablation of colonic mucosa. *Lasers Surg. Med. 11*: 545–549.

Beard, P. (2011). Biomedical photoacoustic imaging. *Interface Focus 1*: 602–631.

Beer, F., Körpert, W., Passow, H. et al. (2012). Reduction of collateral thermal impact of diode laser irradiation on soft tissue due to modified application parameters. *Lasers Med. Sci. 27* (5): 917–921.

Bhattacharaya, A. and Mahajan, R.L. (2003). Temperature dependence of thermal conductivity of biological tissues. *Physiol. Meas. 24*: 769–783.

Blankenau, R.J., Kelsey, W.P., Powell, G.L. et al. (1991a). Degree of composite resin polymerization with visible light and argon laser. *Am. J. Dent. 4*: 40–42.

Blankenau, R.J., Powell, G.L., Kelsey, W.P., and Barkmeier, W.W. (1991b). Postpolymerization strength values of an argon laser cured resin. *Lasers Surg. Med. 11*: 471–474.

Bogdan Allemann, I. and Kaufman, J. (2011). Laser principles. In: *Basics in Dermatological Laser Applications*. Curr Probl Dermatol, vol. *42* (eds. I. Bogdan Allemann and D.J. Goldberg), 7–23. Basel: Karger.

Braun, A., Berthold, M., and Frankenberger, R. (2015). The 445-nm semiconductor laser in dentistry – introduction of a new wavelength. *Quintessenz 66* (2): 205–211.

Burns, J.A., Kobler, J.B., Heaton, J.T. et al. (2007). Thermal damage during thulium laser dissection of laryngeal soft tissue is reduced with air cooling: ex vivo calf model study. *Ann. Otol. Rhinol. Laryngol. 116*: 853–857.

Castro, D.J., Saxton, R.E., Fetterman, J.R. et al. (1988). Phototherapy with argon lasers and Rhodamine-123 for tumor eradication. *Otolaryngol. Head Neck Surg. 98*: 581–588.

Cetinkaya, M., Onem, K., Rifaioglu, M.M., and Yalcin, V. (2015). 980-nm diode laser vaporization versus transurethral resection of the prostate for benign prostatic hyperplasia: randomized controlled study. *Urol. J. 12* (5): 2355–2361.

Chon, J.W.M., Taylor, A.B., and Zijlistra, P. (2014). Plasmonic nanorod-based optical recording and data storage. In: *Nanoplasmonics. Advanced Device Applications* (eds. J.W.M. Chon and K. Iniewski). Boca Raton, FL: CRC Press.

Chung, H., Dai, T., Sharma, S.K. et al. (2012). The nuts and bolts of low-level laser (light) therapy. *Ann. Biomed. Eng. 40*: 516–533.

Dahlman, A., Wile, A.G., Burns, R.G. et al. (1983). Laser photoradiation therapy of cancer. *Cancer Res. 43*: 430–434.

Das, M., Dixit, R., Mukhtar, H., and Bickers, D.R. (1985). Role of active oxygen species in the photodestruction of microsomal P-450 and associated monooxygenases by hematoporphyrin derivates in rats. *Cancer Res. 45*: 608–615.

Dederich, D.N., Zakariasen, K.L., and Tulip, J. (1984). Scanning electron microscopic analysis of canal wall dentin following neodymium-yttrium-aluminium-garnet laser irradiation. *J Endod. 10*: 428–431.

Dederich, D.N., Zakariasen, K.L., and Tulip, J. (1985). SEM analysis of dyed canal dentin following Nd:YAG laser irradiation (abstract). *J. Dent. Res. 64*: 239.

Dixon, J.A., Davis, R.K., and Gilbertson, J.J. (1986). Laser photocoagulation of vascular malformations of the tongue. *Laryngoscope 96*: 537–541.

Dostalova, T., Jelinkova, H., Sulc, J. et al. (2011). Ceramic brackets debonding using Tm:YAP laser irradiation. *Photomed. Laser Surg. 29*: 477–484.

Edge, C.J. and Carruth, J.A.S. (1988). Photodynamic therapy and the treatment of head and neck cancer. *Br. J. Oral Maxillofac. Surg. 26*: 1–11.

Einstein, A. (1917). Zur Quantentheorie der Strahlung. *Phys. Z. 18*: 121–128.

Fekrazad, R., Khoei, F., Hakimiha, N., and Bahador, A. (2013). Photoelimination of Streptococcus mutans with two methods of photodynamic and photothermal therapy. *Photodiagnosis Photodyn Ther. 10* (4): 626–631.

Feyh, J., Muller, W., and Luther, W. (1989). Photodynamic therapy of early stage cancer in head and neck surgery. *Photochem. Photobiol. 49* (Suppl): 1095.

Frank, F. (1989). Fundamental principles. In: *Lasers in Gastroenterology. International Experiences and Trends* (eds. J.F. Riemann and C. Ell), 3–11. Stuttgart: Thieme Publ.

Frentzen, M., Kraus, D., Reichelt, J. et al. (2016). A novel blue light diode laser (445 nm) for dental application. Biomedical testing and clinical aspects. *Laser 3*: 6–13.

Fujimoto, J.G., Pitris, C., Boppart, S.A., and Brezinski, M.E. (2000). Optical coherence tomography: an emerging Technology for Biomedical Imaging and Optical Biopsy. *Neoplasia 2* (1–2): 9–25.

Gebhardt, B.M., Salmeron, B., and McDonald, M.B. (1990). Effect of excimer laser energy on the growth potential of corneal keratocytes. *Cornea 9* (3): 205–210.

Ghatak, A. and Thyagarajan, K. (1998). *An Introduction to Fiber Optics*. Cambridge University Press.

Goldstein, A., White, J.M., and Pick, R.M. (1995). Clinical applications of the Nd:YAG laser. In: *Lasers in Dentistry* (eds. L.J. Miserendino and R.M. Pick), 199–216. Chicago: Quintessence.

Gundlach P, Leege N, Tschepe J, Hopf J, Linnarz M, Scherer H. Speichelsteinlithotripsie. In: *Angewandte Laserzahnheilkunde. Lehr- und Handbuch für Praxis und Klinik.* Müller G, Ertl Th (Hrsg.), III-2.3, 1-5, Ecomed, Landsberg/Lech, 1995. (German).

Guney, M., Tunc, B., and Gulsoy, M. (2014). Investigating the ablation efficiency of a 1,940nm thulium fiber laser for intraoral surgery. *Int. J. Oral Maxillofac. Surg. 43*: 1015–1021.

Gutknecht, N., Moritz, A., Conrads, G. et al. (1996). Bactericidal effect of the Nd:YAG laser in in vitro root canals. *J. Clin. Laser Surg. Med. Surg. 14*: 77–80.

Hardee, M., Miserendino, L., and Kos, W. (1994). Evaluation of the antibacterial effects of intracanal Nd:YAG laser irradiation. *J. Endod. 20*: 377–380.

Hargate, G. (2006). A randomized double-blind study comparing the effect of 1072nm light against placebo for the treatment of herpes labialis. *Clin. Exp. Dermatol. 31*: 638–641.

Hendler, B.H.H., Cateno, J., Mooar, P., and Sherk, H.H. (1992). Holmium:YAG laser arthroscopy of the temporomandibular joint. *J. Oral Maxillofac. Surg. 50*: 931–934.

Hermann, G.G., Mogensen, K., Lindvold, L.R. et al. (2015). Office-based transurethral devascularization of low grade non-invasive urothelial cancer using diode laser. A feasibility study. *Lasers Surg. Med. 47* (8): 620–625.

Herzog, M., Fellbaum, C., and Horch, H.H. (1992). Erste klinische Erfahrungen mit der photodynamischen Therapie (PDT) des Mundhöhlenkarzinoms. *Dtsch. Zahn-Mund-Kieferheilkd. Zentralbl. 80: 141–143.* (German).

Hohenleutner, U. and Landthaler, M. (1990). Traditional tattooing of the gingiva: successful treatment with the argon laser. *Arch. Dermatol. 126*: 547.

Hu, X.L., Ho, B., Lim, C.T., and Hsu, C.S. (2011). Thermal treatments modulate bacterial adhesion to dental enamel. *J. Dent. Res. 90* (12): 1451–1456.

Huzaira, M., Anderson, R.R., Sink, K., and Manstein, D. (2003). Intradermal focusing of near- infrared optical pulses: a new approach for non-ablative laser therapy. *Lasers Surg. Med. 32* (suppl. 15): 17–38.

Iwasaki, M., Sasaka, M., Konishi, T. et al. (1985). Nd:YAG laser for general surgery. *Lasers Surg. Med. 5*: 429–438.

Iwasaki, M. and Inomata, H. (1986 Dec). Relation between superficial capillaries and foveal structures in the human retina. *Invest Ophthalmol Vis Sci. 27* (12): 1698–1705.

Javed, F. and Romanos, G.E. (2013). Does photodynamic therapy enhance standard antibacterial therapy in dentistry? *Photomed. Laser Surg. 31*: 512–518.

Joffe, S.N. (1986). Contact neodymium:YAG laser surgery in gastroenterology: a preliminary report. *Lasers Surg. Med. 6*: 470–472.

Joffe, S.N., Bracket, K.A., Sankar, M.Y., and Daikuzono, N. (1986). Resection of the liver with the Nd:YAG laser. *Surg Gynecol Obstet 163*: 437–442.

Johnson, D.E., Cromeens, M., and Price, R.E. (1992). Use of the Ho:YAG laser in urology. *Lasers Surg. Med. 12*: 353–363.

Karsai, S., Czarnecka, A., Jünger, M., and Raulin, C. (2010). Ablative fractional lasers (CO_2 and Er:YAG): a randomized controlled double-blind split-face trial of the treatment of peri-orbital rhytides. *Lasers Surg. Med. 42* (2): 160–167.

Kautzky, M., Bigenzahn, W., Steurer, M. et al. (1992). Holmium:YAG Laserchirurgie. Anwendungsmöglichkeiten bei entzündlichen Nasenneben-höhlenerkrankungen. *HNO 40*: 468–471. (German).

Keller, U. and Hibst, R. (1990). Ultrastructural changes of enamel and dentin following Er:YAG laser irradiation on teeth. Laser surgery: advanced characterization, therapeutics and systems. *Proc SPIE 1200*: 408–415.

Keller, U. and Hibst, R. (1995). Er:YAG laser effects on oral hard and soft tissues. In: *Lasers in Dentistry* (eds. L.J. Miserendino and R.M. Pick), 161–172. Chicago: Quintessence.

Keller, U., Hibst, R., and Mohr, W. (1990). Tierexperimentelle Untersuchungen zur Laserablation von Mundschleimhauterkrankungen mit dem Er:YAG-Laser. *Österr. Z. Stomatol. 87*: 475–480. (German).

Keller, U., Hibst, R., and Mohr, W. (1991). Tierexperimentelle Untersuchungen zur Laserosteotomie mit dem Er:YAG-Laser. *Dtsch. Zahn-Mund-Kieferheilkd. Zentralbl. 15*: 197–199. (German).

Kelsey, W.P., Blankenau, R.J., Powell, L.G. et al. (1989). Enhancement of physical properties of resin restorative materials by laser polymerization. *Lasers Surg. Med. 9*: 623–627.

Kiefhaber, P., Nath, G., and Moritz, K. (1977). Endoscopical control of massive gastrointestinal hemorrhage by irradiation with high-power neodymium-YAG laser. *Prog. Surg. 15*: 140.

Komori, T., Yokoyama, K., Matsumoto, Y., and Matsumoto, K. (1997). Erbium:YAG and holmium:YAG laser root resection of extracted human teeth. *J. Clin. Laser Med. Surg. 15*: 9–13.

Koslin, M.G. and Martin, J.C. (1993). The use of holmium laser for temporomandibular joint arthroscopic surgery. *J. Oral Maxillofac. Surg. 51*: 122–124.

Kutsch, V.K. and Blankenau, R.J. (1995). Surgical applications of the argon laser. In: *Lasers in Dentistry* (eds. L.J. Miserendino and R.M. Pick), 129–143. Chicago: Quintessence.

Lipson, R.L. and Blades, E.J. (1961). Hematoporphyrin derivative: a new aid for endoscopic detection of malignant disease. *J. Thorac. Cardiovasc. Surg. 42*: 623–629.

Lobene, R.R. and Fine, S. (1966). Interaction of CO_2 laser radiation with oral hard tissues. *J. Prosth. Dent. 16*: 589.

Lobene, R.R., Bhussry, R., and Fine, S. (1968). Interaction of CO_2 laser with enamel and dentin. *J. Dent. Res. 47*: 311–317.

Maiman, T. (1960). Stimulated optical radiation in ruby. *Nature 187*: 493–494.

Mani, G.L. (1992). Holmium laser in dental applications of advanced lasers. *GJM Associates Inc.*: 11–13.

Manstein, D., Scott Herron, G., Kehl Sink, R. et al. (2004). Fractional photothermolysis: a new concept for cutaneous remodeling using microscopic patterns of thermal injury. *Lasers Surg. Med. 34*: 426–438.

Mehmet, C., Oz, M.D., Treat, M.R. et al. (1989). A fiberoptic compatable midinfrared laser with CO_2 laser-like effekt: application to atherosclerosis. *J. Surg. Res. 47*: 493–501.

Melcer, J., Chaumette, F., Melcer, F., and Dejardin, J. (1984). Treatment of dental decay by CO_2 laser beam: preliminary results. *Laser Surg. Med. 4*: 311–321.

Melcer, J., Chaumette, F., and Melcer, F. (1987). Dental pulp exposed to the laser beam. *Laser Surg. Med. 7*: 347–352.

Mordon, S., Martinot, V., and Mitchell, V. (1995). End-to-end microvascular anastomoses with a 1.9-μm diode laser. *J. Clin. Laser Med. Surg. 13*: 357–361.

Myers, T.D. and Myers, W.D. (1985). In vivo caries removal utilizing the YAG laser. *J. Mich. Dent. Assoc. 68*: 66–69.

Nakayama, Y. and Matsuda, T. (1995). Surface microarchitectural design in biomedical applications: preparation of microporous polymer surfaces by an excimer laser ablation technique. *J. Biomed. Mater. Res. 29* (10): 1295–1301.

Nather, A., Sim, Y.E., Chew, L., and Neo, S.H. (2007). Anodyne therapy for recalcitrant diabetic foot ulcers: a report of four cases. *J. Orthop. Surg. (Hong Kong) 15*: 361–364.

Nelson, J.S., Orenstein, A., Liaw, L.H. et al. (1989 Jun 15). Ultraviolet 308-nm excimer laser ablation of bone: an acute and chronic study. *Appl Opt. 28* (12): 2350–2357.

Niemz, M.H. (2019). *Laser-Tissue Interactions: Fundamentals and Applications*, 4e. Berlin: Springer.

Nishioka, N.S., Domankevitz, Y., Flotte, T.J., and Anderson, R.R. (1989). Ablation of rabbit liver, stomach, and colon with a pulsed holmium laser. *Gastroenterology 96*: 831–837.

Nuzzo, V., Savoldelli, M., Legeais, J.M., and Plamann, K. (2010). Self-focusing and spherical aberrations in corneal tissue during photodisruption by femtosecond laser. *J. Biomed. Opt. 15* (3): 038003. https://doi.org/10.1117/1.3455507.

Oswald, V.H. and Bingham, B.J. (1992). A pilot study of the holmium:YAG laser in nasal turbinate and tonsil surgery. *J. Clin. Med. Surg. 10*: 211–216.

Poetke, M., Philipp, C., and Berlien, H.P. (1996). Die Laserbehandlung von Hämangiomen und vaskulären Malformationen - Indikationen, Applikationstechniken und Parameter. *Zbl. Kinderchir. 5*: 138–150. (German).

Ponder, E. (1962). The coefficient of thermal conductivity of blood and of various tissues. *J. Gen. Physiol. 45*: 545–551.

Powell, G.L., Kelsey, W.P., Blankenau, R.J., and Barkmeier, W.W. (1989). The use of an argon laser for polymerization of composite resin. *J. Esthet. Restor. Dent. 1*: 34–37.

Powell, G.L., Ellis, R., Blankenau, R.J., and Schouten, J.R. (1995). Evaluation of argon laser and conventional light-cured composites. *J. Clin. Laser Med. Surg. 13*: 315–317.

Preissig, J., Hamilton, K., and Markus, R. (2012). Current laser resurfacing technologies: a review that delves beneath the surface. *Semin. Plast. Surg. 26* (3): 109–116.

Reichelt, J., Winter, J., Meister, J. et al. (2017). A novel blue light laser system for surgical applications in dentistry: evaluation of specific laser-tissue interactions in monolayer cultures. *Clin. Oral Investig. 21* (4): 985–994.

Renner, A.T., Bobek, J., Ostermann, H. et al. (2015). A cost/benefit analysis of self-care initiatives in the European Union: who gains, who loses? *J. Pharm. Policy Pract. 8*: O5.

Romanos, G.E. (1994). Clinical applications of the Nd:YAG laser in oral soft tissue surgery and periodontology. *J. Clin. Laser Med. Surg. 12*: 103–108.

Romanos, G.E., Gladkova, N.D., Feldchtein, F.I. et al. (2013). Oral mucosa response to laser patterned microcoagulation (LPM) treatment. An animal study. *Lasers Med. Sci. 28*: 25–31.

Rosenberg, C., Tadir, Y., Braslavsky, D. et al. (1990). Endometrial laser ablation in rabbits: a comparative study of three laser types. *Laser Surg. Med. 10*: 66–73.

Rossi, M., Di Censo, F., Di Censo, M., and Oum, M.A. (2015). Changes in aqueous humor pH after femtosecond laser-assisted cataract surgery. *J. Refract. Surg. 31* (7): 462–465.

Rubio, P.A. (1991). Endoscopic cholecystectomy with Ho:YAG laser: a preliminary report. *J. Clin. Laser Med. Surg. 9*: 127–128.

Sacks, Z.S., Kurtz, R.M., Juhasz, T. et al. (2003). Subsurface photodisruption in human sclera: wavelength dependence. *Ophthalmic Surg. Lasers Imaging 34* (2): 104–113.

Sarp, A.S. and Gülsoy, M. (2011). Ceramic bracket debonding with ytterbium fiber laser. *Lasers Med. Sci. 26* (5): 577–584.

Serra, C. and Silveira, L. (2019 May 6). Near-infrared irradiation of the thyroid area: effects on weight development and thyroid and parathyroid secretory patterns. *Lasers Med. Sci.* https://doi.org/10.1007/s10103-019-02800-w. [Epub *ahead* of print].

Severin, C. and Maquin, M. (1989). Argon laser beam as composite resin light curing agent. *Lasers Dent. 1*: 241–246.

Shapshay, S.M., Aretz, H.T., and Setzer, S.E. (1990). Soft tissue effects of the holmium:YSGG laser in the canine trachea. *Otolaryngol. Head Neck Surg. 102*: 251–256.

Shi, W., Vari, S.G., van der Veen, M.J. et al. (1993). Effect of varying laser parameters on pulsed Ho:YAG ablation of bovine knee joint tissues. *Arthroscopy 9* (1): 96–102.

Srinivasan, R. and Leigh, W.J. (1982). Ablative photodecomposition: action of far-ultraviolet (193 nm) laser radiation on poly-(ethyleneterephtalate) films. *J. Am. Chem. Soc. 104*: 6784–6785.

Stern, R.H., Vahl, J., and Sognnaes, R.F. (1972). Laser enamel: ultrastructural observations of pulsed carbon dioxide laser effects. *J. Dent. Res. 51*: 455–460.

Stevens, B.H., Trowbridge, H.O., Harrison, G., and Silverton, S.F. (1994). Dentin ablation by Ho:YAG laser: correlation of energy versus volume using stereophotogrammetry. *J. Endod. 20*: 246–249.

Stewart, L., Powell, G.L., and Wright, S. (1985). Hydroxyapatite attached by laser: a potential sealant for pits and fissures. *Oper. Dent. 10*: 2–5.

Sun, F., Han, B., Cui, D. et al. (2015). Long-term results of thulium laser resection of the prostate: a prospective study at multiple centers. *World J. Urol. 33* (4): 503–508.

Takasaki, A.A., Mizutani, K., Schwarz, F. et al. (2009). Application of antimicrobial photodynamic therapy in periodontal and peri-implant diseases. *Periodontol. 51*: 109–140.

Tang, J., Godlewski, G., Rouy, S. et al. (1994). Microarterial anastomosis using a noncontact diode laser versus a control study. *Lasers Surg. Med. 14*: 229–237.

Tappenier, H. and Jesionek, A. (1903). Therapeutische Versuche mit fluoreszierenden Stoffen. *Münch. Med. Wschr. 1*: 2042. (German).

Thomsen, S. and Pearce, J.A. (2011). Thermal damage and rate processes in biologic tissues. In: *Optical-Thermal Response of Laser-Irradiated Tissue*, 2e (eds. A.J. Welch and M.J.C. Van Gemert), 487–498. Springer.

Townes, C.H. (1964). Production of coherent radiation by atoms and molecules. *Science (New York, N.Y.) 149*: 831–841.

Trauner, K., Nishioka, N., and Patel, D. (1990). Pulsed Ho:YAG laser ablation of fibrocartilage and articular cartilage. *Am. J. Sports Med. 18*: 316–321.

Traxer, O. and Keller, E.X. (2019 Feb 6). Thulium fiber laser: the new player for kidney stone treatment? A comparison with Ho:YAG laser. *World J. Urol.* https://doi.org/10.1007/s00345-019-02654-5. [Epub ahead of print.

Unal, S.M., Nigiz, R., Polat, Z.S., and Usumez, A. (2015). Effect of ultrashort pulsed laser on bond strength of Y-TZP zirconia ceramic to tooth surfaces. *Dent. Mater. J. 34* (3): 351–357.

Valvano, J. (2011). Tissue thermal properties and perfusion. In: *Optical-Thermal Response of Laser-Irradiated Tissue*, 2e (eds. A.J. Welch and V.G. MJC), 455–485. Springer.

Vogel, A., Capon, M.R., Asiyo-Vogel, M.N., and Birngruber, R. (1994). Intraocular photodisruption with picosecond and nanosecond laser pulses: tissue effects in cornea, lens, and retina. *Invest. Ophthalmol. Vis. Sci.* *35* (7): 3032–3044.

Ward, P.D. and Baker, S.R. (2008). Long-term results of carbon dioxide laser resurfacing of the face. *Arch. Facial Plast. Surg. 10* (4): 238–243. discussion 244-5.

White, J.M., Goodis, H.E., and Marshall, S.J. (1993). Identification of the physical modification threshold of dentin induced by neodymium and holmium:YAG lasers using scanning electron microscopy. *Scanning Microsc. 7*: 239–246.

Wilson, S.W. (2014). Medical and aesthetic lasers: semiconductor diode laser advances enable medical applications. *BioOpt. World 7*: 21–25.

Xu, X.G., Gao, X.H., Li, Y.H., and Chen, H.D. (2013). Ultrapulse-mode versus superpulse-mode fractional carbon dioxide laser on normal back skin. *Dermatol. Surg. 39* (7): 1047–1055.

2

Lasers and Wound Healing

Georgios E. Romanos

Stony Brook University, School of Dental Medicine, Stony Brook, NY, USA

2.1 Introduction

The alterations of living tissue after the use of laser irradiation are of particular importance for the surgically active clinician. Various investigations still try today to explain the influence of the laser light on wound healing. The use of low-level-therapy (low intensity) lasers (soft lasers) possibly provides biostimulatory effects in the tissues (biomodulation), while the various wavelengths and features of surgical lasers (hard lasers) influence wound healing directly or indirectly.

A less well-known clinical application is the therapeutic use of low-dose biophotonics, termed photobiomodulation (PBM) therapy, which is aimed at alleviating pain and inflammation, modulating immune responses, and promoting wound healing and tissue regeneration. There are potential paths for clinical translation with PBM therapy with an emphasis on craniofacial wound healing and a novel opportunity to examine fundamental nonvisual photobiological processes as well as develop innovative clinical therapies in order to control or eliminate conventional invasive procedures (Arany 2016). Although, expert opinions based on ongoing research studies and reported literature are offered, and noninvasive, economical, and multipurpose light devices are attractive tools for wound management, there is an urgent need in the wound care community to develop optimal clinical protocols for use based on well-designed, rigorous clinical research studies (Mosca et al. 2019).

Dependent on the laser wavelength, power settings, irradiation period, fluence, and the application technique, the light will absorb or scatter within the tissue accelerating or delaying wound healing, and based on the host response, the heat transfer will create positive of negative effects on the target tissues. All these parameters can have an impact on the final clinical outcome.

More specifically, soft biological tissues contain cells in attachment with the matrix. The water content, in most soft tissues, is approximately 55–99% and collagen 0–35%, dependent on location and functional ability. These mechanical properties and structural characteristics of the tissues determine the thermal conductivity and heat transfer during laser irradiation. Water or collagen are the main tissue constituents absorbing the radiation. The thermal denaturation of the collagenous matrix depends on the molecular structures of the collagen fibrils. Older tissues, i.e. in aging, contain more dense collagen fibers and cross-linking, which provides increased thermal stability and further increased temperature to allow tissue shrinkage and stress relaxation. Collagen is in general a good thermal insulator. Therefore, tissues with more collagen have lower thermal conductivity; therefore, cannot be excised easily with laser.

In general, collagen becomes denatured in a temperature of approximately 60 °C, and this temperature may be higher in older tissues with higher collagen density, where no stress relaxation was observed in temperatures higher than 100 °C for several minutes (Le Lous et al. 1982).

These phenomena of stress relaxation and tissue shrinkage occur faster when the structural integrity in the tissue is less dense or when microfibrillar collagenous structures are present. For instance, the presence of the fibrillar collagen type V, which is predominant in the granulation and inflamed tissues, has an impact to the mechanical instability even after short periods of irradiation.

When longer wavelengths (far-infrared spectral region) are applied, the water absorption peaks up, and therefore absorption dominates over scattering. In contrast to this effect, the optical absorption properties in pigmented and highly vascularized tissues are predominant in the red and near infrared spectrum, due to the presence of the biomolecules hemoglobin (Hb) and oxyhemoglobin (HbO$_2$) in those tissues.

> In order to accomplish the maximum of opportunities providing to the tissues from the laser irradiation, the absorption should dominate the scattering.

2.2 Wound Healing and Low Power Lasers

The first studies on low power lasers came from the group of Mester et al. (1969, 1971). They observed a biostimulatory effect on the skin of mice after the use of a ruby laser. The same effect was also achieved in dogs and pigs with a GaAs laser (Cho and Cho 1986; Sapeira et al. 1986). Studies of rat skin showed a raised tensile strength and quicker healing of wounds. The exact mechanism of function is still not yet clear.

Recently, many studies showed that low-level laser therapy (LLLT) can accelerate the repair of different tissues in the body, leading to inflammatory, immunological, and metabolic effects (Sun and Tunér 2004; Nussbaum et al. 2009; Demir et al. 2010). Low power lasers do not have such effects but act on the tissue thermally to increase the rate of repair of the injured tissue (Yu et al. 1996).

Abergel et al. (1984) researched the effect of the Nd:YAG laser and Kana et al. (1981) of the argon laser on wound healing. In the current literature one finds mostly positive information about the biostimulatory effect of the laser light (Table 2.1) after use of He:Ne lasers (Kovacs et al. 1974; Mester et al. 1974; Sapeira et al. 1986; Abergel et al. 1987; Lyons et al. 1987; Braverman et al. 1989; Hans et al. 1992) or of GaAs lasers (Abergel et al. 1984; Cho and Cho 1986; Anneroth et al. 1988; Asencis-Arana and Martinez-Soriano 1988; Takeda 1988a; Braverman et al. 1989). Most studies are in vitro experiments (e.g. with cell cultures, biochemical measurements, like identification of type I and type III pro-collagen, RNA analysis, collagen synthesis, etc.) or animal studies.

The dental studies of Takeda (1988a) gave the histological proof of a higher fibroblast proliferation and quicker osseous healing after GaAs-irradiation of fresh extraction sockets of rats. Directly after tooth extraction, the wounds were irradiated for five minutes with a GaAs laser (904 nm and light intensity of 25 mW/cm^2). This irradiation was continued the next day. In another study Takeda (1988b) ascertained a raised salivary gland function after use of light with a wavelength of 904 nm.

Trelles and Mayayo (1987) carried out studies about the osseous healing of mice. Fractured bones were irradiated for 21 days with a He:Ne laser (total dose: 2.4 J every other day). The study showed a clear increase of vascularization and osseous density in the fracture region.

After a He:Ne-irradiation of dentin surfaces at *in vivo* investigations of monkeys (Matsumoto et al. 1985, 1988) or human wisdom teeth (Kondo et al. 1988), no histological changes of the pulp were observed. Other studies showed a reduction of pain at the orofacial area after use of such lasers (Bezuur et al. 1988), as well as of the cervical tooth sensitivity (Renton-Harper and Midda 1992).

In the literature, there is a partly controversial discussion about the effect of laser light on wound healing (Table 2.1). The studies of Brunner et al. (1984) could not confirm a positive effect of the krypton laser light on epidermis regeneration. Also Colver and Priestley (1989) could prove no stimulatory effects of the He:Ne on epithelial cells, fibroblasts, and collagen synthesis. Other studies with different tissues showed contradictory effects of the soft lasers on wound healing or a dependence on the applied energy settings and the chosen wavelengths.

Recent studies by Fekrazad et al. (2015) showed the impact of different color lasers (blue, green, and red) on the healing of oral wounds in diabetic rats. The investigators compared the effects of red, green, and blue lasers in terms of accelerating oral wound healing in diabetic rats. The findings suggested that wound healing occurs faster with a red (630 nm) laser compared to blue (425 nm) and green (532 nm) lasers. The energy density was 2 J/cm^2 with a treatment schedule of 3 times/week for 10 days. A faster and more organized reepithelialization and tissue healing of the oral mucosa were achieved with an energy density of 4 J/cm^2 in comparison to 20 J/cm^2 (Wagner et al. 2013).

Other studies (Rupel et al. 2018) also showed that various wavelengths differentially modulate reactive oxygen species (ROS) production. In particular, the 660 nm laser light increases ROS production when applied either before or after an oxidative stimulus. The 970 nm laser light exerted a moderate antioxidant activity in the saliva of cancer patients with oral mucositis (OM) who receive chemotherapy or radiotherapy. The most marked reduction in the levels of ROS was detected in cells exposed either to the 800 nm laser light or to the combination of the three wavelengths. Overall, the study demonstrates that PBM exerts different effects on the redox state of both PMNs and keratinocytes depending on the used wavelength and prompts the validation of a multiwavelength protocol in clinical settings.

Table 2.1 Wound healing effects of the low-power lasers.

Study	Laser type	Tissue	Examined parameters	Results
Mester et al. (1969)	Rubin	skin (mouse)	macroscopy /histology	+
Mester et al. (1971)	Rubin	skin (mouse)	macroscopy / histology	+
Kovacs et al. (1974)	He:Ne	skin (rat)	tensile strength	+
Mester et al. (1974)	Rubin	skin tumors (human)	macroscopy electron microscopy	+
Hutschenreiter et al. (1980)	He:Ne	skin (rat)	tensile strength macroscopy histomorphometry	no differences
Haina et al. (1981)	He:Ne	skin (rat)	granulation tissue	+
Kana et al. (1981)	Ar, He:Ne	skin (rat)	collagen synthesis macroscopy	+
Abergel et al. (1984)	Nd:YAG, He:Ne, Ar	fibroblast culture	collagen synthesis	+
Brunner et al. (1984)	Kr	skin (human)	epidermis regeneration	no differences
Matsumoto et al. (1985)	GaAlAs	dentin (monkey) (monkey)	pulp	no differences
Cho and Cho (1986)	Ga-As	oral mucosa (dog)	histology	+
Sapeira et al. (1986)	He:Ne	skin (pig)	biochemistry	+
Abergel et al. (1987)	He:Ne	fibroblast culture	collagen synthesis	+
Lyons et al. (1987)	He:Ne	skin (mouse)	tensile strength collagen synthesis	+
Trelles and Mayayo (1987)	He:Ne	bone mouse	vascularization bone density	+
				+
Anneroth et al. (1988)	Ga-As	skin (rat)	macroscopy histology	no differences
Asencis-Arana and Martinez-Soriano (1988)	He:Ne	colon (rat)	tensile strength	+
Kondo et al. (1988)	He:Ne	dentin (human)	pulp histology	no differences
Matsumoto et al. (1988)	He:Ne	dentin (monkey) pulp	no differences	
Takeda (1988a)	Ga-As	bone (rat)	histology	+
Takeda (1988b)	Ga-As	salivary gland (rat)	function salivary flow	+
				+
Braverman et al. (1989)	Ga-As, He:Ne	skin (rabbits)	tensile strength histology	no differences
Colver u. and Priestley (1989)	He:Ne	fibroblast-culture	collagen synthesis	no differences
Hans et al. (1992)	He:Ne	fibroblast culture	collagen synthesis	+
Smith et al. (1992)	He:Ne	skin (pig and rat)	macroscopy	scar tissue formation

+ positive result.
– delayed wound healing.

In contrast to wound healing in the oral mucosa, systematic reviews were able to evaluate the efficacy of laser therapy to improve alveolar healing after tooth extractions. The current available evidence in the literature showed that laser therapy improved the wound healing process, but these findings were limited to the type of laser applied and its specific settings. The most widespread organized bone formation in the extraction socket was observed in the gallium-aluminum-arsenide laser group with the energy dose of $10 \, J/cm^2$ (Cirak et al. 2018).

Further well-designed and randomized controlled trials are needed to support a beneficial effect of using laser therapy after tooth extraction (Lemes et al. 2019). Because there are currently still no reproductive results given, the effects of these lasers on wound healing should be evaluated critically.

2.3 Wound Healing and High-Power Lasers

Hard lasers or the so-called "optical scalpels" are applied in oral surgical procedures. Depending on the wavelength, there is a different influence on the wound healing process. A large number of clinical observations exists in the literature, which show the effects of laser irradiation on the tissues using histological, immunohistochemical, and electron-microscopic methods (Table 2.2).

This part of the present chapter is focused on the typical changes of the tissues during wound healing and an overview about the wound healing processes after laser use.

During laser irradiation, light energy will be absorbed and transformed into heat. Heating of cells and tissues can produce reversible injury that can be repaired by host and cellular mechanisms. When energy is higher, irreversible damage leads to tissue death immediately or after the irradiation.

Incisions have different qualities and are associated with the laser wavelength, the power settings, and the laser-tissue interactions. The cutting efficiency seems to be better for the CO_2 and Er,Cr:YSGG lasers compared to Er:YAG or a 980 nm diode laser with noninitiated tip (Figure 2.1). Temperature increase of the tissue during laser irradiation is always fundamental in order to avoid complications and nonreversible tissue damages. The lowest temperature increase occurs using an Er,Cr:YSGG laser (Figure 2.2).

2.3.1 Wound Healing and CO_2 Laser

Three different laser systems (CO_2, Nd:YAG, and argon) were used in animals to compare histologically the wound healing of tissues. Only the CO_2 laser produced a good incision quality; however, wound healing was delayed for approximately four to five days compared to the scalpel. A delay of wound healing (up to 11 days) was also shown by Luomanen (1987) performing incisions on rat mucosa. The study showed an increased infiltration of the connective tissue and delay of wound healing due to the effect of the lateral heat transfer during the CO_2 laser incision (Howard et al. 1997). Another immunohistochemical study of the connective tissue showed remarkable, resistant (extracellular) matrix formation after laser irradiation (Luomanen et al. 1987). The foreign body reaction of the laser-induced wounds was more distinctive (Filmar et al. 1989). In comparison to the scalpel incision, a delayed wound healing took place on pigs after use of the CO_2 laser and the electrosurgery (Arashiro et al. 1996). The tensile strength of these wounds was decreased (Ben-Baruch et al. 1988; Hambley et al. 1988).

Positive results of wound healing after laser use have been proven by Pogrel et al. (1990), with a distinct acceleration of the epithelialization in comparison to cryosurgical and conventional scalpel incisions. Gaspar et al. (1991) histologically confirmed the excellent hemostatic effect of the CO_2 laser as well as the extremely low thermal damage of the tissue in comparison to electrosurgery.

Of great importance is also the removal of pathological alterations with the CO_2 laser in esthetically critical regions, because no scarring could be observed (Gaspar and Toth 1990). On the other hand, Kardos and Ferguson (1991) have not observed any clear differences between laser incisions and cryosurgery with regard to the wound healing process. Wound healing after CO_2 laser induced incisions was compared to scalpel incisions on beagle dogs (Fisher et al. 1983). The healing of the laser wounds developed without damage to the adjacent tissues. Initially, a coagulum of denatured protein formed on the surface; the inflammatory reaction was less; fewer myofibroblasts were present and there was little wound contraction; less collagen was formed and epithelial regeneration was delayed and more irregular.

Previous studies also from our group showed that healing in oral wounds after incisions in the soft tissue in the palate of monkeys is delayed when a CO_2 laser was used. The tissue heals delayed and the healing process is slower when the power settings are relatively high. Specifically, the healing was examined after irradiation of the tissue using a noncontact CO_2 laser and 2 W, 4 W, and 6 W continuous wave (CW) power in comparison with the scalpel incision. In general, the study showed that the healing was similar with the conventional scalpel incision but only delayed (Romanos et al. 1999).

Table 2.2 Wound healing effects of the high-power lasers.

Study	Laser type	Tissue	Examined parameters	Results
Verschueren and Oldhoff (1975)	CO_2	bone	histology	−
Clayman et al. (1978)	CO_2	bone	histology	−
Horch and Rehrmann (1978)	CO_2, Nd:YAG, Ar	mucosa (rabbit)	cutting effect	+
				−
Small et al. (1979)	CO_2	bone (rabbit)	histology	−
Horch and Keiditsch (1980)	CO_2	bone (dog)	histology	−
Gertzbein et al. (1981)	CO_2	bone	histology	−
Pao-Chang et al. (1981)	CO_2	bone	histology	−
Fisher et al. (1983)	CO_2	mucosa (dog)	histology	+
Luomanen (1987)	CO_2	tongue (rat)	histology	−
Luomanen et al. (1987)	CO_2	tongue (rat)	immunohistochemistry	resistance in the matrix
Ben-Baruch et al. (1988)	CO_2	skin (pig)	tensile strength	−
Hambley et al. (1988)	CO_2	skin (pig)	tensile strength histology	−
Nuss et al. (1988)	Ho:YAG	bone ablation	histology	
Tawakol et al. (1988)	Nd:YAG	skin (rabbit)	tensile strength	no differences
Filmar et al. (1989)	CO_2	uterus (rat)	histology	−
Myers et al. (1989)	Nd:YAG	skin (rat)	cutting effect	+
Nelson et al. (1989a)	Er:YAG	bone rabbit	histology	−
Schmelzeisen et al. (1989)	Nd:YAG	mucosa (rabbit)	histology	+
Walsh and Deutsch (1989)	Er:YAG	bone cartilage	histology	+
Gaspar and Toth (1990)	CO_2	mucosa (rat)	histology	no scar
Gonzales et al. (1990)	Er:YAG	bone ablation, cartilage	histology	
Pogrel et al. (1990)	CO_2	skin (rat)	histology	+
Stein et al. (1990)	Ho:YAG	bone ablation	histology	
Dressel et al. (1991)	XeCl	bone (rabbit)	histology	no differences
Gaspar et al. (1991)	CO_2	mucosa (rat)	histology	+
Kahle et al. (1991)	Er:YAG	cornea (monkey)	immunohistochemistry	+
Kardos and Ferguson (1991)	CO_2	tongue (sheep)	histology	no differences
Keller et al. (1991)	Er:YAG	bone (dog)	histology	+
White et al. (1991)	Nd:YAG	mucosa (human)	cutting effect	+
Hendler et al. (1992)	Ho:YAG	TMJ	arthroscopy	+
Kautzky et al. (1992)	Ho:YAG	tongue (rat)	histology	no differences
Lustmann et al. (1992)	ArF	bone (rat)	histology	−
Forrer et al. (1993)	CO_2	bone	histology	−
Koslin and Martin (1993)	Ho:YAG	TMJ	arthroscopy	+
Romano et al. (1994)	Ho:YAG, Er:YAG	bone	histology	better with Er:YAG

(Continued)

Table 2.2 (Continued)

Study	Laser type	Tissue	Examined parameters	Results
Moritz et al. (1995)	Er:YAG	TMJ ablation	histology	
Romanos et al. (1995a, b, c)	Nd:YAG	skin (rat)	histology macroscopy Immunohistochemistry	similar to scalpel scar stable matrix
Arashiro et al. (1996)	CO_2	skin (pig)	histology	–
Howard et al. (1997)	CO_2	skin (rat)	histology	–
Romanos et al. (1999)	CO_2	palate (monkey)	histology	delayed healing compared to scalpel

+ accelerated wound healing.
− delayed wound healing.

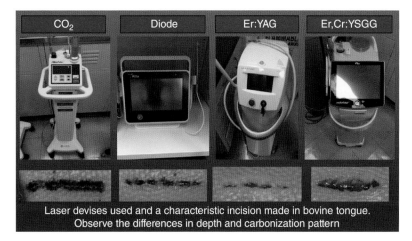

Figure 2.1 Incision quality during laser irradiation of the bovine mucosa showing different penetration depths and carbonization zones. The best incisions occurred using an Er,Cr:YSGG or CO_2 laser. The diode laser incision was performed without initiated tip. *Source:* Dr. Georgios E Romanos.

Laser	Temperature Increase (°C)	Standard Deviation	Range of Temperature change (°C)
CO_2 (10,600nm)	1.58	0.21	1.2 – 1.7
Diode (975nm)	3.68	2.81	0.6 – 7.1
Er:YAG	1.62	0.87	0.6 – 2.6
Er,CR:YSGG	1.04	1.03	0.1 – 2.3

Temperature increase, standard deviation and range of temperature change during laser irradiation on bovine tongue (ex vivo).

Figure 2.2 Temperature changes of the tissue during laser irradiation. The lowest temperature increase occurs using an Er,Cr:YSGG laser (unpublished data provided from incisions in the bovine tongue).

Incisions created by the scalpel, electrocautery, CO_2 laser, and potassium titanyl phosphate (KTP) laser in rat tongues were evaluated in terms of wound healing (Carew et al. 1998). The study showed that oral intake, indirectly assessed by postoperative weight loss, by the third postoperative day was significantly decreased in the electrocautery, CO_2 laser, and KTP laser groups as compared with the scalpel group. The depth of wound healing, as assessed by histologic examination, was successively greater for the scalpel ($75 \pm 13 \mu m$), electrocautery ($110 \pm 10 \mu m$), CO_2 laser ($145 \pm 10 \mu m$), and KTP laser ($195 \pm 23 \mu m$) groups. Wounds created by the KTP laser had the lowest strength ($76.5 \pm 6.9 kPa$) as compared with the CO_2 laser ($156 \pm 28.4 kPa$), electrocautery ($153 \pm 15.7 kPa$), and scalpel groups ($249 \pm 61.8 kPa$).

Also, clinical studies were conducted in order to compare clinical and histopathological outcomes for excisional biopsies when using pulsed CO_2 laser versus Er,Cr:YSGG laser. Patients with a fibrous hyperplasia in the buccal mucosa were randomly allocated to the CO_2 or the Er:YAG laser group. Intraoperative bleeding occurred in 100% of the excisions with Er:YAG and 56% with CO_2 laser. The median thermal damage zone was $74.9 \mu m$ for CO_2 and $34.0 \mu m$ for Er:YAG laser. It was concluded that for excision of oral soft tissue lesions, CO_2 and Er:YAG lasers are both valuable tools with a short time of intervention and postoperative low pain. More postoperative bleeding occurs with the Er:YAG than CO_2 laser, but the lower thermal effect of the Er:YAG laser seems advantageous for histopathological evaluation (Suter et al. 2017).

A previous study investigated and compared the clinical and histopathologic characteristics of CW and pulsed CO_2 laser modes for excisional biopsies. No statistically significant differences in the duration of the laser excision were found between laser modes. The width of the thermal damage zone (micrometers) was expected to be smaller for the pulsed CO_2 laser mode (CF group), but there was no statistically significant difference in the widths of thermal damage zones between the CW and CF groups (Suter et al. 2012).

In contrast to this study, other authors presented that heat, sufficient to damage tissue, was conducted to adjacent tissue during laser pulses of $100 \mu s$ and longer, like in the conventional surgical CO_2 lasers for soft tissue excisions. However, surgical CO_2 lasers with short pulses of approximately $60 \mu s$ or less could offer more prompt wound healing, while maintaining the advantages of a 10 600 nm wavelength (Fortune et al. 1998).

Similarly, Sanders and Reinisch (2000) compared the thermal damage and wound healing of a $7.5 \mu s$-pulsed CO_2 laser with scalpel and CW CO_2 laser incisions.

Specifically, incisions on the dorsal pelts of rats with a $7.5 \mu s$ pulsed CO_2 laser at a 5-, 10-, or 15-Hz repetition rate were compared with a conventional CW laser, or scalpel. Using a $7.5-\mu s$ pulse duration, CO_2 laser incisions healed at a rate similar to scalpel incisions and reduced the wound healing process, which was delayed with typical surgical CO_2 lasers.

Therefore, CO_2 lasers and tissue healing are associated with the application mode and the manufacturer device features, which may be fundamental in order to control heat transfer to the tissues and lateral coagulation zone in order to accelerate the wound healing process.

2.3.2 Wound Healing and the Nd:YAG Laser

Various studies were also carried out to clarify the effect of the wavelength of the Nd:YAG laser on wound healing (Table 2.2). Schmelzeisen et al. (1989) have observed on rabbits after laser incisions and three weeks of healing a complete reepithelialization in comparison to cryosurgical incisions. Wound healing was clearly accelerated, while the tensile strength was low.

With the use of a pulsed Nd:YAG laser, a strong coagulation took place in the area of the incision. A minimal injured zone was histologically proved on rats. White et al. (1991) also showed a low thermal damage in the incision borders on the oral mucosa.

Studies confirmed the positive effect of the laser use by animal-experimental studies on the skin of rats. Scarring was not present in comparison to the conventional scalpel incisions. Wound healing after the use of a Nd:YAG laser, set at low power, appeared not only clinically and histologically (Romanos et al. 1995a, b) but also immunohistochemically (Romanos et al. 1995a, c) to succeed, and similarly to the scalpel incision (Figures 2.3–2.5) and the extracellular matrix of the connective tissue, remains imperishable and stable (Romanos et al. 1991). If the power of the beam is high, wound healing is delayed, and it can be compared to wound healing after electrosurgery (Romanos 1997) (Figures 2.3–2.5). Synoptically, the results of the wound healing that were observed on rat skin four weeks after Nd:YAG laser use are shown in the Table 2.3.

Full thickness incisions were made in rat skin using a diode laser (805 nm, 10 W, contact mode), a Nd:YAG laser (1064 nm, 10 W, contact mode), and a stainless steel scalpel blade (control). Wound breaking strength measurements were obtained at 7, 14, and 21 days using a specially designed tensiometer. The study showed that there was no significant difference in the breaking strengths (group 1) or tensile strengths (groups 2 and 3) of the diode and Nd:YAG

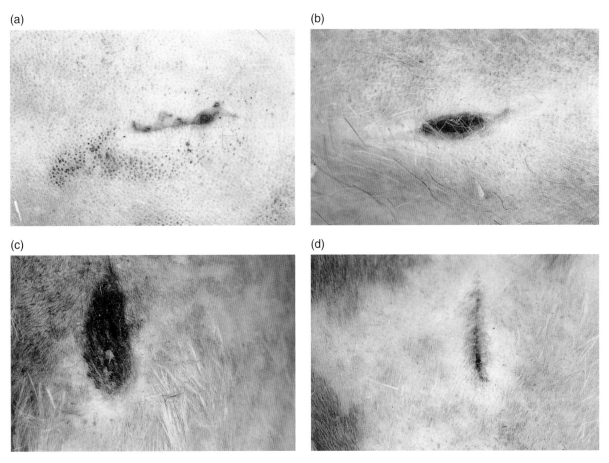

Figure 2.3 Wound healing after scalpel incision (a); 1.75 W power Nd:YAG (b); 3 W power Nd:YAG (c); or after electrosurgery (d); four days after surgery. *Source:* Dr. Georgios E Romanos.

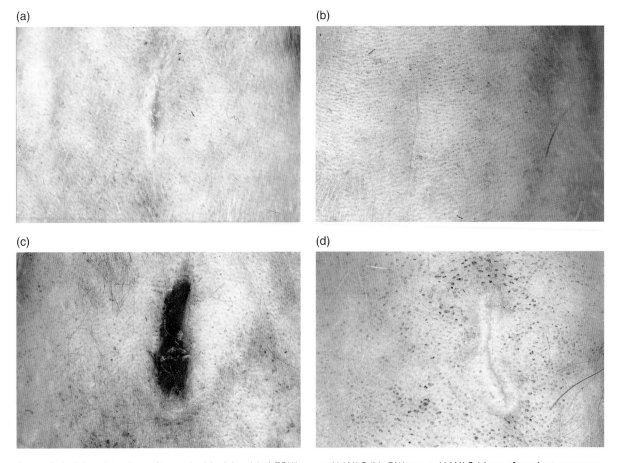

Figure 2.4 Wound healing after scalpel incision (a); 1.75 W power Nd:YAG (b); 3 W power Nd:YAG (c); or after electrosurgery (d); two weeks after surgery. *Source:* Dr. Georgios E Romanos.

(a) (b) (c) (d)

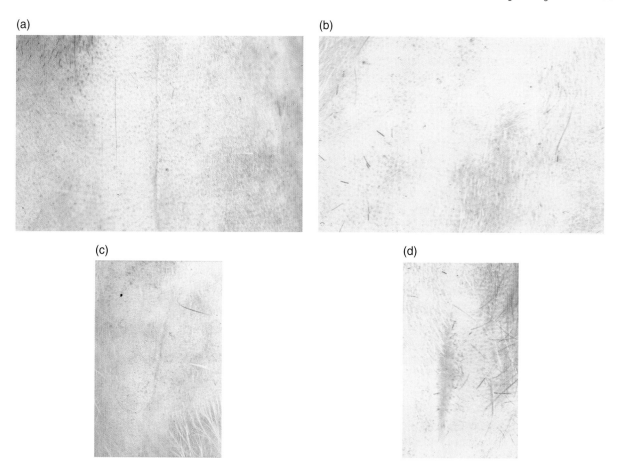

Figure 2.5 Wound healing after scalpel incision (a); 1.75 W power Nd:YAG (b); 3 W power Nd:YAG (c); or after electrosurgery (d); four weeks after surgery. The low power Nd:YAG laser wound does not demonstrate any signs of tissue discoloration (b) compared to the scalpel incision (a). *Source:* Dr. Georgios E Romanos.

Table 2.3 Wound healing in the rat skin, four weeks after Nd:YAG laser irradiation.

	low power (1.75W) Nd:YAG Laser	scalpel	electrosurgery	high power (3W) Nd:YAG Laser
pigmentation	−	+	+	+
scar	−	−	+	+
wound healing process delayed	++	++	+	+
granulation tissue formation	+++	+++	++	+
stable and collagen resistant matrix	+++	++	+	+
necrosis	+	++	++	+++

laser incisions. As predicted, breaking strengths and tensile strengths of scalpel blade incisions were significantly greater than those of incisions made with laser energy. Histopathologic evaluation revealed that through day 14, the degree of inflammation and collagen production was similar for diode and Nd:YAG laser incisions. Laser incisions had greater inflammation and a lag in fibroblast invasion and collagen production compared with scalpel incisions. By day 21, all incisions were similar in fibroblast population and collagen production, but laser incisions had slightly more inflammation than scalpel incisions. The authors concluded that in the primary wound healing model described, the tissue effect, cellular response, and development of wound strength were essentially the same for the high-power diode laser at 10 W and the Nd:YAG laser at 10 W (Taylor et al. 1997).

A recent study aimed to investigate the capacity of bone repair using a high-power, Q-switched, pulsed, Nd:YAG laser, using bilateral calvarial defect animal models, with noncritical sized 5 mm (rat) or 8 mm (rabbit) diameter (Kim et al. 2015). Laser irradiation significantly increased new bone formation by approximately 45%, not only in the sponge-filled defects of rats but also when the defects were left empty, compared to the non-irradiated group. Consistently, both doses of output power (0.75 and 3 W) enhanced new bone formation, but there was no significant difference between the two doses. This study is one of the first to demonstrate the beneficial effect of Nd:YAG lasers on the regeneration of bone defects which were left empty or filled with collagen sponge, suggesting its great potential in postoperative treatment targeting local bone healing.

The fact that there are various results described in the literature for the use of laser is presumably caused by several factors, e.g. the wavelength and power setting used in each case, as well as the kind of the irradiated tissue and species. Therefore, a critical judgment of the results by the active clinician is of utmost importance.

2.3.3 Wound Healing and Other Laser Wavelengths

Wound healing studies evaluate the use of different laser wavelengths with specific power settings and application parameters in comparison with other conventional methods or application of different incisions.

Previous studies performed in monkeys' corneas after the use of Er:YAG and excimer lasers (ArF). The healing with the excimer laser appeared to be worse, compared to the Er:YAG laser, although with this laser type the thermal damage was lower (Kahle et al. 1991). Other studies with excimer (XeCl, 308 nm) and pulsed Ho:YAG laser were

carried out on the tongue mucosa of rats. The Ho:YAG laser showed an impressive hemostasis. The wound healing process was similar, even though the temperature of the irradiated tissue during the use of the Ho:YAG laser was higher (Kautzky et al. 1992).

Unpublished data from our group showed that, in palatal incisions in monkeys, the impact of a diode 980 nm laser is similar to scalpel wound healing, when noninitiated tips are used in contact with the oral mucosa. Specifically, a 5-W diode laser demonstrates a complete wound closure after three days with reepithelialization, formation of long rete pegs, and complete organization of the epithelial layer (Figure 2.6, unpublished data).

In contrast, a wound healing delay was found when the power was higher, such as 10 W, demonstrating the closure of the wound with a pseudo-membranous epithelial coverage (Figure 2.7, unpublished data). High power of 15 W was associated with high temperature changes and showed a delayed wound healing after two weeks but without tissue necrosis. Specifically, exudation, microhemorrhage, and blistering (vacuole formation) due to the high heat transfer were observed in palatal wounds (Figure 2.8, unpublished data).

Compared to the traditional scalpel, the incision of the Er:YAG laser provides a smaller inflammatory reaction, more pseudomembranous formation, and minimal damage of the tissue in palatal mucosa of rats (Qu et al. 2018).

In contrast to the previous laser systems, recent studies evaluated the 445 nm semiconductor laser (blue light) for tissue incision and demonstrated an effective cut as expected due to the special absorption properties of blue laser light in soft tissues. Forty soft tissue specimens were obtained from pork oral mucosa and mounted on a motorized linear translation stage. The handpiece of a high-frequency surgery device, a 970 nm

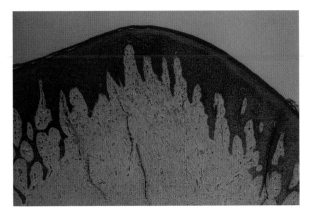

Figure 2.6 Incision area three days after 5 W diode laser (980 nm) incision presenting complete wound closure with normal epithelium layers and long rete pegs.
Source: Dr. Georgios E Romanos.

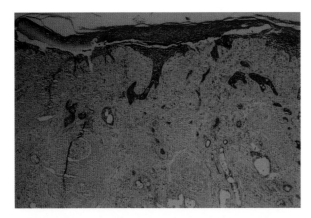

Figure 2.7 Incision area 14 days after 10 W diode laser (980 nm) presenting complete wound closure with pseudomembrane on the epithelial surface. This provides evidence about the delayed wound healing using this power setting. *Source:* Dr. Georgios E Romanos.

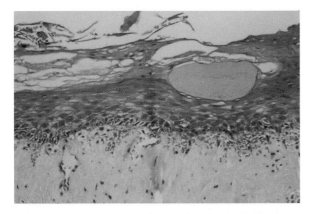

Figure 2.8 Incision area 14 days after 15 W diode (980 nm) laser presenting microhemorrhage and blistering due to the high heat transfer to the tissue especially in the subepithelial layer. *Source:* Dr. Georgios E Romanos.

semiconductor laser (with initiated fiber, contact mode at 3 W CW), a 445 nm semiconductor laser with noninitiated fiber tip, and a high-frequency surgery device with straight working tip were used to make incisions.

The highest incision depth was achieved with the 445 nm laser contact mode demonstrating the lowest amount of soft tissue denaturation. The lowest incision depth was measured for the high-frequency surgical device. Using a 445 nm semiconductor laser, a higher cutting efficiency can be expected when compared with a 970 nm diode laser and high-frequency surgery. Even the 445 nm laser application in noncontact mode shows clinically acceptable incision depths without signs of extensive soft tissue denaturation (Braun et al. 2018).

A recent report compared the efficacy and precision of femtosecond laser ablation with conventional surgical laser devices. Femtosecond lasers do not provide collateral ther-

mal damage and therefore there are increased applications in number and diversity of these lasers. Future innovations in laser design will make them more accessible, facilitating clinical and research applications (Chung and Mazur 2009).

2.4 Lasers and Bone Healing

Osteotomies with lasers were carried out for the first time during the 1970s (Goldman et al. 1970); however, such procedures were not routinely applicable until recently in private practice (see Chapter 4). Collateral thermal damage and residual char formation have severely limited the use of conventional lasers in the surgical preparation of bony tissue. This thermal damage from lasers can be controlled using specific laser wavelengths that are strongly absorbed by the bone and by reducing laser pulse durations.

Morphologic and chemical changes were induced in the near-surface region of bone following exposure to the free electron laser (FEL) at 3.0, 6.1, and 6.45 μm wavelengths. The selected wavelengths coincide with the vibrational modes of proteins and water within bone. Laser parameters included 22.5 ± 2.5 mJ/pulse delivered in individual 4 μs macropulses at a repetition rate of 30 Hz, focused to 200 and 500 μm spot sizes.

The light microscopy sections of the ablation defects created at the differing wavelengths showed similar features, i.e. two zones of collateral damage: a zone generally <10 mm of extensive thermal damage and a wider zone of empty lacunae (Spencer et al. 1999). The spectroscopic results suggested that the char layer is limited to an area less than approximately 6 μm from the surface.

Thermal damage and two to three weeks delay of wound healing were presented earlier (Schmelzeisen et al. 1989). Studies with the pulsed excimer laser on the shinbone of rats (Lustmann et al. 1992) and with the Er:YAG laser on rabbits (Nelson et al. 1989a, b) led to similar results. Most studies of laser-induced CO_2 osteotomies showed a delayed wound healing because of the increased temperature increase leading to thermal damage of the bone (Verschueren and Oldhoff 1975; Clayman et al. 1978; Gertzbein et al. 1981; Pao-Chang et al. 1981; Forrer et al. 1993). Forrer et al. (1993) confirmed with their studies that the pulse rate and the energy setting are closely related to an osseous necrosis and, hence, short pulse duration is recommended to obtain controlled tissue damage.

In contrast, no differences in the osseous healing could be ascertained after the osteotomy with an excimer (XeCl) laser or with custom surgical bone-cutting burs (Dressel et al. 1991).

Comparative studies evaluated the healing of bone in rat tibial osteotomy defects created by a dental bur, a CO_2 laser with and without removal of the char layer, and a Nd:YAG laser with char layer removed and with and without use of an air/water surface cooling-spray (Friesen et al. 1999). Tibial osteotomy defects were created in four groups of rats each using the following: (i) #6 round bur with simultaneous saline irrigation; (ii) CO_2 laser with char layer intact; (iii) CO_2 laser with char layer removed; (iv) Nd:YAG laser with air/water surface cooling and char layer intact; (v) Nd:YAG laser with air/water surface cooling and char layer removed; and (vi) Nd:YAG laser without air/water surface cooling and char layer removed. Both laser types were used at energy densities typically utilized for oral soft tissue surgery. Laser-induced osteotomy defects, when compared to those prepared by rotary bur, exhibited a delayed healing response that appeared to be related to the presence of residual char in the osseous defect.

Also, other studies compared the effect of CO_2 and Nd:YAG laser on the bone. Specifically, the studies were focused on the long-term effects of laser irradiation after 21, 35, and 63 days posttreatment: (i) a negative control (no treatment); (ii) a positive control (bur osteotomy); (iii) a CO_2 laser at 5 W ($860 J/cm^2$); (iv) a CO_2 laser at 6 W ($1,032 J/cm^2$); (v) a Nd:YAG laser at 5 W ($714 J/cm^2$); and (vi) a Nd:YAG laser at 7 W ($1,000 J/cm^2$). All laser irradiation was delivered in the presence of a surface coolant consisting of air and sterile water. Under the conditions of this study, the healing was severely delayed in all laser-treated sites compared to positive control sites. Of the laser-treated sites, those irradiated by the CO_2 laser at 5 W exhibited the greater amount of bone regeneration. In general, the osseous healing response was severely delayed by CO_2 and Nd:YAG laser irradiation of bone, even in the presence of a surface cooling spray of air/water (McDavid et al. 2001).

The healing of beagle dogs was also the same after the use of a Er:YAG laser (Keller et al. 1991). The Er:YAG laser allows ablation of bone, as well as cartilage (Tawakol et al. 1988; Nelson et al. 1989a; Gonzales et al. 1990) and, therefore, is used today, at least experimentally, in the surgery of the temporomandibular joint (Moritz et al. 1995). The thermal damage of an Er:YAG laser–osteotomized bone is lower than with the Ho:YAG laser (Romano et al. 1994). Currently, only the Er:YAG laser is the most suitable in orthopedics and experimentally qualified in arthroscopy.

Bone healing in an inferior border defect of the rat mandible was examined using either an Er:YAG laser or a mechanical bur for drilling (Lewandrowski et al. 1996). The histologic evaluation demonstrated no difference in the amount of newly formed woven bone at the osteotomy site or screw holes made by either the Er:YAG laser or the drill. The extent of thermal damage at the osteotomy sites was comparable in laser and mechanically cut bone fragments. Based on this study, the Er:YAG laser can be used clinically in thin, fragile bones in the maxillofacial region.

De Oliveira et al. (2016) showed in recent studies the impact of the application of Er:YAG and Er,Cr:YSGG lasers during osteotomy on bovine bone blocks. A conventional bur was compared with an Er:YAG laser and Er,Cr:YSGG laser. Even though the bur was the instrument that performed the osteotomy in the shortest amount of time, all instruments caused thermal damage; however, the Er,Cr:YSGG laser was the only type that induced carbonization, and the Er:YAG laser induced the lowest degree of thermal damage in bone tissue after osteotomy.

> The thermal damage of the surrounding osseous tissue currently limits the use of the various laser systems in clinical osseous treatment. In this field, more research is necessary in the future. However, the Er:YAG and the Er,Cr:YSGG lasers are the only laser wavelengths today which can provide some evidence of the benefits of laser-assisted osteotomy procedures.

References

Abergel, R.P., Meeker, C.A., Lam, T.S. et al. (1984). Control of connective tissue metabolism by lasers: recent developments and future prospects. *J. Am. Acad. Dermatol.* 11: 1142–1150.

Abergel, R.P., Lyons, R.F., Castel, J.C. et al. (1987). Biostimulation of wound healing by lasers experimental approaches in animal models and in fibroblast cultures. *J. Dermatol. Surg. Oncol.* 13: 127–133.

Anneroth, G., Hall, G., Ryden, H., and Zetterqvist, L. (1988). The effect of low-energy infra-red laser irradiation on wound healing in rats. *Br. J. Oral Maxillofac. Surg.* 26: 12–17.

Arany, P.R. (2016). Craniofacial wound healing with photobiomodulation therapy: new insights and current challenges. *J. Dent. Res.* 95: 977–984.

Arashiro, D.S., Rapley, J.W., Cobb, C.M., and Killoy, W.J. (1996). Histologische Untersuchung von CO_2-Laser,

Elektrochirurgie- und Skalpell-Schweinehautinzisionen. *Int. J. Periodontics Restorative Dent.* 16: 455–467. (German).

Asencis-Arana, F. and Martinez-Soriano, F. (1988). Stimulation of the healing in experimental colon anastomoses by low power lasers. *Br. J. Surg.* 75: 125–127.

Ben-Baruch, G., Fidler, J.P., Wessler, T. et al. (1988). Comparison of wound healing between chopped mode-superpulse mode CO_2-laser and steel knife incision. *Lasers Surg. Med.* 8: 596–599.

Bezuur, N.J., Habets, L.L., and Hansson, T.L. (1988). The effect of therapeutic laser treatment in patients with craniomandibular disorders. *J. Craniomandib. Disord.* 2: 83–86.

Braun, A., Kettner, M., Berthold, M. et al. (2018). Efficiency of soft tissue incision with a novel 445-nm semiconductor laser. *Lasers Med. Sci.* 33: 27–33.

Braverman, B., McCarthy, R.J., Ivankovich, A.D. et al. (1989). Effect of helium-neon and infrared laser irradiation on wound healing in rabbits. *Lasers Surg. Med.* 9: 50–58.

Brunner, R., Landthaler, M., Haina, M. et al. (1984). Experimentelle Untersuchungen zum Einfluß von Laserlicht niedriger Leistungsdichte auf die Epidermisregeneration. In: Optoelektronik in der Medizin. Laser 83. (ed. W. Waidelich), 181–186. Berlin: Springer 10 (German).

Carew, J.F., Ward, R.F., LaBruna, A. et al. (1998). Effects of scalpel, electrocautery, and CO_2 and KTP lasers on wound healing in rat tongues. *Laryngoscope* 108: 373–380.

Cho, B.Y. and Cho, J.O. (1986). Experimental study of the effect of the laser irradiation in treating oral soft tissue damage. *J. Dent. Res.* 65: 600. (Abstract No. 34).

Chung, S.H. and Mazur, E. (2009). Surgical applications of femtosecond lasers. *J. Biophotonics* 10: 557–572.

Cirak, E., Özyurt, A., Peker, T. et al. (2018). Comparative evaluation of various low-level laser therapies on bone healing following tooth extraction: an experimental animal study. *J. Craniomaxillofac. Surg.* 46: 1147–1152.

Clayman, L., Fuller, T., and Beckman, H. (1978). Healing of continuous-wave and rapid superpulsed carbon dioxide laser-induced bone defects. *J. Oral Maxillofac. Surg.* 36: 932–937.

Colver, G.B. and Priestley, G.C. (1989). Failure of a helium-neon laser to affect components of wound healing in vitro. *Br. J. Dermatol.* 121: 179–186.

Demir, T., Kara, C., Ozbek, E., and Kalkan, Y. (2010). Evaluation of neodymium-doped yttrium aluminum garnet laser, scalpel incision wounds, and low-level laser therapy for wound healing in rabbit oral mucosa: a pilot study. *Photomed. Laser Surg.* 28: 31–37.

de Oliveira, G.J., Rodrigues, C.N., Perussi, L.R. et al. (2016). Effects on bone tissue after osteotomy with different high-energy lasers: an ex vivo study. *Photomed. Laser Surg.* 34: 291–296.

Dressel, M., Jahn, R., Neu, W., and Jungluth, K.H. (1991). Studies in fiber guided excimer laser surgery for cutting and drilling bone and meniscus. *Lasers Surg. Med.* 11: 569–579.

Fekrazad, R., Mirmoezzi, A., Kalhori, K.A., and Arany, P. (2015). The effect of red, green and blue lasers on healing of oral wounds in diabetic rats. *J. Photochem. Photobiol. B* 148: 242–245.

Filmar, S., Jetha, N., McComb, P., and Gomel, V. (1989). A comparative histologic study on the healing process after tissue transection. II. Carbon dioxide laser and surgical microscissors. *Am. J. Obstet. Gynecol.* 160: 1068–1072.

Fisher, S.E., Frame, J.W., Browne, R.M., and Tranter, R.M. (1983). A comparative histological study of wound healing following CO_2 laser and conventional surgical excision of the buccal mucosa. *Arch. Oral Biol.* 28: 287–291.

Forrer, M., Frenz, M., Romano, V. et al. (1993). Bone-ablation mechanism using CO_2 lasers of different pulse duration and wavelength. *Appl. Phys.* B56: 104–112.

Fortune, D.S., Haung, S., Soto, J. et al. (1998). Effect of pulse duration on wound healing using a CO_2 laser. *Laryngoscope* 108: 843–848.

Friesen, L.R., Cobb, C.M., Rapley, J.W. et al. (1999). Laser irradiation of bone: II. Healing response following treatment by CO_2 and Nd:YAG lasers. *J. Periodontol.* 70: 75–83.

Gaspar, L. and Toth, J. (1990). Comparative experimental study on wound healing of incisions made with scalpel, electrocautery and CO_2 laser in the oral cavity. *J. Clin. Laser Med. Surg.* 8: 35–38.

Gaspar, L., Sudar, F., Toth, J., and Madarasz, B. (1991). Oral lesions induced by scalpel, electrocautery and CO_2 laser compared with light, scanning and electron microscopy. *J. Clin. Laser Med. Surg.* 9: 349–353.

Gertzbein, S.D., de Demeter, D., Cruickshank, B., and Kapasouri, A. (1981). The effect of laser-osteotomy on bone healing. *Lasers Surg. Med.* 1: 361–373.

Goldman, L., Rockwell, R.J., Naprstek, Z. et al. (1970). Some parameter of high output CO_2 laser experimental surgery. *Nature* 228: 1344–1345.

Gonzales, C., van de Merwe, W.P., Smith, M., and Reinisch, L. (1990). Comparison of the erbium-yttrium aluminium garnet and carbon dioxide lasers for in vitro bone and cartilage ablation. *Laryngoscope* 100: 14–17.

Haina, D., Brunner, P., Landhaler, M. et al. (1981). Stimulierung der Wundheilung mit Laserlicht - klinische und tierexperimentelle Untersuchungen. *Hautarzt* 32: 429–432. (German).

Hambley, R., Hebda, P.A., Abell, E. et al. (1988). Wound healing of skin incisions produced by ultrasonically vibrating knife scalpel, electrosurgery, and carbon dioxide laser. *J. Dermatol. Surg. Oncol.* 14: 1213–1217.

Hans, H.F.I., Breugel, V., and Bar, D. (1992). Power density and exposure time of He-Ne laser irradiation are more important than total energy dose in photo-biostimulation of human fibroblasts in vitro. *Lasers Surg. Med.* 12: 528–537.

Hendler, B.H., Gateno, J., Moar, P., and Sherk, H.H. (1992). Holmium:YAG laser arthroscopy of the temporomandibular joint. *J. Oral Maxillofac. Surg.* 50: 931–934.

Horch, H.H. and Keiditsch, E. (1980). Morphologische Befunde über die Gewebeschädigung und Knochenregeneration nach Laser-Osteotomie. *Dtsch. Zahnärztl. Z.* 35: 22–24. (German).

Horch, H.H. and Rehrmann, A. (1978). Tierexperimentelle Studien zur oralen Laserchirurgie der Weichteile. *Dtsch. Z. Mund Kiefer Gesichtschir.* 2: 67–71. (German).

Howard, J., Arango, P., Ossoff, J. et al. (1997). Healing of laser incisions in rat dermis: comparisons of the carbon dioxide laser under manual and computer control and the scalpel. *Lasers Surg. Med.* 20: 90–96.

Hutschenreiter, G., Haina, D., Paulini, K., and Schumacher, G. (1980). Wundheilung nach Laser- und Rotlichtbestrahlung. *Z Exp Chir.* 13: 75–85.

Kahle, G., Daqun, X., Seiler, T. et al. (1991). Wundheilung der Kornea von Neuweltaffen nach flächiger Keratektomie: Er:YAG-Excimer-Laser. *Fortschr. Ophthalmol.* 88: 380–385. (German).

Kana, J.S.S., Hutschenreiter, G., and Haina, D. (1981). The effect of low power density laser irradiation on the healing of open skin wounds in rats. *Arch. Surg.* 116: 293–296.

Kardos, T.B. and Ferguson, M.M. (1991). Comparison of cryosurgery and the carbon dioxide laser in mucosal healing. *Int. J. Oral Maxillofac. Surg.* 20: 108–111.

Kautzky, M., Susani, M., and Schenk, P. (1992). Holmium:YAG Infrarot Laser- und UV-Excimer. Laser-Effekte auf orale Schleimhautgewebe. *Laryngol. Rhinol. Otol.* 71: 347–352.

Keller, U., Hibst, R., and Mohr, W. (1991). Tierexperimentelle Untersuchungen zur Laserosteotomie mit dem Erbium:YAG-Laser. *Dtsch. Z. Mund Kiefer Gesichtschir.* 15: 197–199. (German).

Kim, K., Kim, I.S., Cho, T.H. et al. (2015). High-intensity Nd:YAG laser accelerates bone regeneration in calvarial defect models. *J. Tissue Eng. Regen. Med.* 9: 943–951.

Kondo, M., Kamiya, K., Goni, A. et al. (1988). A histological study of the effects of laser irradiation by "soft laser 632" on the oral mucosa, dorsal skin, knee joint, temporomandibular joint of rats and the dental pulp of humans. *Aichi-Gakuin J. Dent. Sci.* 26: 795–804.

Koslin, M.G. and Martin, J.C. (1993). The use of the holmium laser for temporomandibular joint arthroscopic surgery. *J. Oral Maxillofac. Surg.* 51: 122–123.

Kovacs, I., Mester, E., and Görög, P. (1974). Stimulation of wound healing with laser beam in the rat. *Experimentia* 30: 1275–1276.

Le Lous, M., Flandin, F., Herbage, D., and Allain, J.C. (1982). Influence of collagen denaturation on the chemorheological properties of skin, assessed by differential scanning calorimetry and hydrothermal isometric tension measurement. *Biochim. Biophys. Acta* 717: 295–300.

Lemes, C.H.J., da Rosa, W.L.O., Sonego, C.L. et al. (2019). Does laser therapy improve the wound healing process after tooth extraction? A systematic review. *Wound Repair Regen.* 27: 102–113.

Lewandrowski, K.U., Lorente, C., Schomacker, K.T. et al. (1996). Use of the Er:YAG laser for improved plating in maxillofacial surgery: comparison of bone healing in laser and drill osteotomies. *Lasers Surg. Med.* 19: 40–45.

Luomanen, M. (1987). A comparative study of healing of laser and scalpel incision wounds in rat oral mucosa. *Scand. J. Dent. Res.* 95: 65–73.

Luomanen, M., Meurman, J.H., and Lehro, V.P. (1987). Extracellular matrix in healing CO_2 laser incision wound. *J. Oral Pathol.* 16: 322–331.

Lustmann, J., Ulmansky, M., Fuxbrunner, A., and Lewis, A. (1992). Photocaustic injury and bone healing following 193nm excimer laser ablation. *Lasers Surg. Med.* 12: 390–396.

Lyons, R.F., Abergel, R.P., White, R.A. et al. (1987). Biostimulation of wound healing in vivo by helium-neon laser. *Am. J. Pathol.* 18: 47–50.

Matsumoto, K., Wakabayashi, H., and Funato, A.T. (1985). Pathohistologic findings of dental pulp irradiated by GaAlAs laser diode. *Jap. J. Conserv. Dent.* 28: 1361–1365.

Matsumoto, K., Wakabayashi, H., Funato, A. et al. (1988). Pathohistologic findings of dental pulp irradiated by He-Ne gas laser. *J. Conserv. Dent.* 31: 63–64.

McDavid, V.G., Cobb, C.M., Rapley, J.W. et al. (2001). Laser irradiation of bone: III. Long-term healing following treatment by CO_2 and Nd:YAG lasers. *J. Periodontol.* 72: 174–182.

Mester, E., Gynes, C., and Tota, J.G. (1969). Experimentelle Untersuchungen über die Wirkung der Laserstrahlen auf die Wundheilung. *Z. Exp. Chir.* 2: 94–101. (German).

Mester, E., Spiry, T., Szende, B., and Tota, J.G. (1971). Effect of laser rays on wound healing. *Am. J. Surg.* 122: 532–535.

Mester, E., Korenyi-Bothz, A., Spiry, T. et al. (1974). Neuere Untersuchungen über die Wirkung der Laserstrahlen auf die Wundheilung (klinische und elektronenoptische Erfahrungen). *Z. Exp. Chir.* 7: 9–17. (German).

Moritz, M., Niederdellmann, H., Deuerling, C. et al. (1995). In vitro light and scanning electron microscopic study involving erbium:YAG laser irradiation of temporomandibular joint tissue. *J. Clin. Laser Med. Surg.* 13: 23–26.

Mosca, R.C., Ong, A.A., Albasha, O. et al. (2019). Photobiomodulation therapy for wound care: a potent, noninvasive, photoceutical approach. *Adv. Skin Wound Care* 32: 157–167.

Myers, T.D., Myers, D., and Stone, R.M. (1989). First soft tissue study utilizing a pulsed Nd:YAG dental laser. *Northwest Dent.* 68: 14–17.

Nelson, J.S., Orenstein, A., Liaw, L.H.L., and Berns, M.W. (1989a). Mid-infrared erbium:YAG laser ablation of bone: the effect of laser osteotomy on bone healing. *Lasers Surg. Med.* 9: 362–374.

Nelson, J.S., Orenstein, A., Liaw, L.H.L. et al. (1989b). Ultraviolet 308-nm excimer laser ablation of bone: an acute and chronic study. *Appl. Opt.* 28: 2350–2357.

Nuss, R.C., Fabian, R.L., Sarkar, R., and Puliafito, C.A. (1988). Infrared laser bone ablation. *Lasers Surg. Med.* 8: 381–392.

Nussbaum, E.L., Mazzulli, T., Pritzker, K.P. et al. (2009). Effects of low intensity laser irradiation during healing of skin lesions in the rat. *Lasers Surg. Med.* 41: 372–381.

Pao-Chang, M., Xiou-Qui, X., Hui, Z. et al. (1981). Preliminary report on the application of CO_2 laser scalpel for operations on the maxillo-facial bones. *Lasers Surg. Med.* 1: 375–384.

Pogrel, M.A., Yen, C.K., and Hansen, L.S. (1990). A comparison of carbon dioxide laser, liquid nitrogen cryosurgery, and scalpel wounds in healing. *Oral. Surg. Oral. Med. Oral. Pathol.* 69: 269–273.

Qu, W., Shang, J., Liu, L. et al. (2018). Comparative study on the incision healing of the palatal mucosa by using Er:YAG laser or traditional scalpel in the SD rats. *Lasers Med. Sci.* 33: 1019–1024.

Renton-Harper, P. and Midda, M. (1992). Nd:YAG laser treatment of dentinal hypersensitivity. *Br. Dent. J.* 172: 13–16.

Romano, V., Rodriguez, R., Altermatt, H.J. et al. (1994). Bone microsurgery with IR-lasers: a comparative study of the thermal action at different wavelengths. *Proc. SPIE* 2077: 87–97.

Romanos, G.E. (1997). Der Wundheilungsverlauf nach Anwendung von Skalpell, Nd:YAG-Laser und Elektrotom. Klinische, histologische und immunhistochemische Untersuchungen an der Rattenhaut. In: Angewandte Laserzahnheilkunde (eds. G. Müller and T. Ertl). Ecomed Verlag (German).

Romanos, G.E., Schröter-Kermani, C.C., Hinz, N., and Bernimoulin, J.P. (1991). Immunohistochemical distribution of the collagen types IV, V, VI and glycoprotein laminin in the healthy rat, marmoset (Callithrix jacchus) and human gingivae. *Matrix* 11: 125–132.

Romanos, G.E., Pelekanos, S., and Strub, J.R. (1995a). Effects of Nd:YAG laser on wound healing processes. Clinical and immunohistochemical findings in rat skin. *Lasers Surg. Med.* 16: 368–379.

Romanos, G.E., Pelekanos, S., and Strub, J.R. (1995b). A comparative histological study of wound healing following Nd:YAG laser with different energy parameters and conventional surgical incision in rat skin. *J. Clin. Laser Med. Surg.* 13: 11–16.

Romanos, G.E., Pelekanos, S., and Strub, J.R. (1995c). Histological and immunohistochemical observations of the wound healing processes after the use of the Nd:YAG laser in rat skin: distribution of collagen types IV, V and VII in connective tissue. *J. Clin. Laser Med. Surg.* 13: 87–95.

Romanos, G., Siar, C.H., Ng, K., and Toh, C.G. (1999). A preliminary study of healing of superpulsed carbon dioxide laser incisions in the hard palate of monkeys. *Lasers Surg. Med.* 24 (5): 368–374.

Rupel, K., Zupin, L., Colliva, A. et al. (2018). Photobiomodulation at multiple wavelengths differentially modulates oxidative stress in vitro and in vivo. *Oxidative Med. Cell. Longev.* 11: 6510159.

Sanders, D.L. and Reinisch, L. (2000). Wound healing and collagen thermal damage in 7.5-microsec pulsed CO_2 laser skin incisions. *Lasers Surg. Med.* 26: 22–32.

Sapeira, D., Glassberg, E., Lyons, R.F. et al. (1986). Demonstration of elevated type I and type III pro collagen mRNA levels in cutaneous wounds treated with helium-neon laser. Proposed mechanism for enhanced wound healing. *Biochem. Biophys. Res. Commun.* 138: 1123–1128.

Schmelzeisen, R., Stauch, G., and Hessel, S. (1989). Effects of Nd:YAG laser and cryosurgery on the oral mucosa of rabbits. *Int. J. Oral Maxillofac. Surg.* 18: 114–116.

Small, I.A., Osborn, T.P., Fuller, I. et al. (1979). Observations of carbon dioxide laser and bone bur in the osteotomy of the rabbit tibia. *J. Oral Surg.* 37: 159–166.

Smith, R.J., Birndorf, M., Gluck, G. et al. (1992). The effect of low-energy laser on skin-flap survival in the rat and porcine animal models. *Plast. Reconstr. Surg.* 89: 306–310.

Spencer, P., Payne, J.M., Cobb, C.M. et al. (1999). Effective laser ablation of bone based on the absorption characteristics of water and proteins. *J. Periodontol.* 70: 68–74.

Stein, E., Sedlacek, T., Fabian, R.L., and Nishioka, N.S. (1990). Acute and chronic effects of bone ablation with a pulsed holmium laser. *Lasers Surg. Med.* 10: 384–388.

Sun, G. and Tunér, J. (2004). Low-level laser therapy in dentistry. *Dent. Clin. N. Am.* 48: 1061–1076.

Suter, V.G., Altermatt, H.J., Dietrich, T. et al. (2012). Does a pulsed mode offer advantages over a continuous wave mode for excisional biopsies performed using a carbon dioxide laser? *J. Oral Maxillofac. Surg.* 70: 1781–1788.

Suter, V.G., Altermatt, H.J., and Bornstein, M.M. (2017). A randomized controlled clinical and histopathological trial comparing excisional biopsies of oral fibrous hyperplasias using CO_2 and Er:YAG laser. *Lasers Med. Sci.* 32: 573–581.

Takeda, Y. (1988a). Irradiation effect of low-energy laser on alveolar bone after tooth extraction. *Int. J. Oral Maxillofac. Surg.* 17: 388–389.

Takeda, Y. (1988b). Irradiation effect of low-energy laser on rat submandibular salivary gland. *J. Oral Pathol.* 17: 91–94.

Tawakol, M., Peyman, G., and Abou-Streit, M. (1988). Wound healing strength: a comparative study of stainless steel blade excisions and contact Nd:YAG laser excisions. *Int. Ophthalmol.* 12: 147–149.

Taylor, D.L., Schafer, S.A., Nordquist, R. et al. (1997). Comparison of a high power diode laser with the Nd:YAG laser using in situ wound strength analysis of healing cutaneous incisions. *Lasers Surg. Med.* 21: 248–254.

Trelles, M.A. and Mayayo, E. (1987). Bone fracture consolidates faster with low-power laser. *Lasers Surg. Med.* 7: 36–45.

Verschueren, R.C.J. and Oldhoff, J. (1975). The carbon dioxide laser, a new surgical tool. *Arch. Chir. Neerl.* 27: 199–207.

Wagner, V.P., Meurer, L., Martins, M.A. et al. (2013). Influence of different energy densities of laser phototherapy on oral wound healing. *J. Biomed. Opt.* 18 (12): 128002.

Walsh, J.T. and Deutsch, T.F. (1989). Er:YAG laser ablation of tissue: measurement of ablation rates. *Lasers Surg. Med.* 9: 327–337.

White, J.M., Goodis, H.E., and Rose, C.L. (1991). Use of pulsed Nd:YAG laser for intraoral soft tissue surgery. *Lasers Surg. Med.* 11: 455–461.

Yu, H.S., Chang, K.L., Yu, C.L. et al. (1996). Low-energy He–Ne laser irradiation stimulates. *J. Invest. Dermatol.* 107: 593–596.

3

Lasers in Oral Surgery
Georgios E. Romanos

Stony Brook University, School of Dental Medicine, Stony Brook, NY, USA

3.1 Introduction

The application of the laser as a surgical method is comparable to that of the scalpel, and it has become an important component of modern clinical dentistry. The different effects of certain laser systems can apply for the removal of soft tissue tumors, soft tissue cysts, and precancerous lesions, such as leukoplakia. Frenectomies, pre-prosthetic surgical procedures, like vestibuloplasties, treatment of gingival hyperplasia, and removal of vascular benign tumors or malformations are other clinical indications.

Exact knowledge of the benefits of the laser light and the effects of the respective wavelength on biological structures are essential for the achievement of an optimum effect (see also Chapter 1). Only under these requirements is it possible to achieve a positive effect of the laser beam on the tissue and to accomplish excellent wound healing without complications.

The indications of the lasers in oral surgery vary from the common excision, biopsies, and coagulation of blood vessels to the complicated therapy of the removal of precancerous lesions and the treatment of vascular tumors and peri-implantitis, which indeed seems to be very promising for the future (see also Chapter 6).

This chapter intends to provide an overview about the application of various laser wavelengths with different clinical indications for the surgically oriented clinician.

In oral soft tissue surgery, the most used and accepted laser systems at the moment are the CO_2, the Nd:YAG, and the diode lasers. The argon ion, the Ho:YAG and the Er:YAG lasers can be also applied under special circumstances and depending on the clinical indication.

3.2 Basic Principles

The power and energy density in laser therapy must be defined precisely. A vaporized, a necrotic zone, and a zone of reversible thermal changes may be generated by the effect of the laser beam on the tissues.

In comparison to Nd:YAG, diode, or argon lasers, there is a stronger absorption of CO_2 laser beams from fair and slightly inflamed tissues. Due to the effect that granulation tissue contains a high number of blood vessels and capillaries, the high hemoglobin tissue content leads to a higher absorption of the Nd:YAG laser beam.

This means that with the same beam's energy, on the one hand we achieve quicker surgical excision in the inflamed area, and on the other hand, we have less risk of a pronounced tissue necrosis and/or bone dehiscence in cases of incautious or uncontrolled work using this laser wavelength. From the physical point of view, a slow application will result in a drastic increase of the respective energy density, which is dependent on the entire irradiation period and must be controlled at every surgical intervention.

> Exact knowledge of the different tissue morphology, the physical properties of the laser beam, and the indications of each type of laser are basic requirements for a successful and complication-free surgical therapy.

3.3 Excision Biopsies

Several laser systems are used today in order to excise biopsies, especially the CO_2, the diode, and/or the Nd:YAG pulsed laser. The incision occurs according to the surgical principles considering that thermal effects occur in variable degree in each case. A focus diameter of 0.2 mm generates a zone of thermal impact, which amounts to 50–200 µm with the CO_2, and 500 µm–3 mm with the Nd:YAG laser (deep penetration into the tissue for the Nd:YAG laser) (Figure 3.1).

When the handpiece is focused and vertically applied on the tissue, a distinct marking appears, due to thermal damage (carbonization). This represents the "incision line." The tissue elevation starts from the peripheral area of this marking and is directed in the depth of the lesion, until the tissue can be lifted easily from its base (Figure 3.2).

At this point, the handpiece is held perpendicular or in a slightly tilted direction to the tissue in order to separate the pathological tissue from the healthy basis. In cases of use of a diode laser, initiation of the fiber before surgery using an articulated paper (black or blue color) or a cork concentrating the maximum energy in the fiber tip is fundamental to control the peripheral thermal damage. The simultaneous coagulation allows a bloodless incision and excision (Table 3.1).

The lesion after removal with the laser must be referred to an oral, maxillofacial pathologist with the explanation of "laser excision," in order to better illustrate the potential thermal effects and to avoid misdiagnosis. Only after histopathological confirmation of the diagnosis, can the complete excision of the lesion

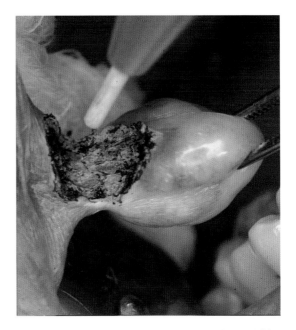

Figure 3.2 Perpendicular irradiation using a focused CO_2 laser (noncontact) allows a clean separation of the pathologic tissue from the surrounding tissues. *Source:* Dr. Georgios E Romanos.

be performed, dependent on the laser wavelength and the type of lesion using a focused or defocused mode. The decrease of the distance between handpiece and tissue under constant power changes modifies the focus and therefore the power density, influencing cutting depth. In contrast to that, the increase of the distance of the handpiece decreases the power density and provides as a result the tissue ablation, so-called vaporization, without distinctive thermal damage.

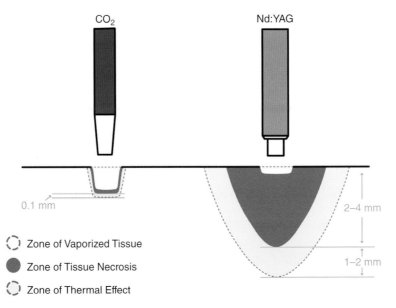

Figure 3.1 Differences in penetration depths between CO_2 laser and Nd:YAG laser (the penetration of the light using the Nd:YAG laser is 10 times higher than CO_2 laser with a high absorption of the connective tissue (chromophores, hemoglobin, etc.).

Table 3.1 Operation mode and clinical procedure.

Type of Procedure	Mode of Operation	Operative Mode	Applicator
Excision/incision	Focused beam	CW or pulsed	Angled
Ablation	Defocused beam	CW or pulsed	90°
Coagulation	Defocused beam	Pulsed	90°

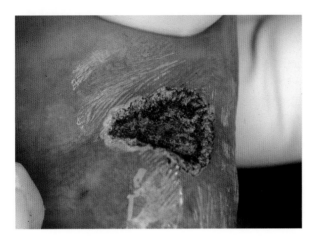

Figure 3.3 Superficial irradiation of the tissue after excision to create a small, coagulated zone. This may control the postoperative pain and provide an excellent wound dressing. *Source:* Dr. Georgios E Romanos.

This is of clinical significance in the removal of wide lesions, such as leukoplakia, lichen planus, or other pathological lesions.

Suturing and special postoperative surgical measures are usually not necessary. Directly after excision of a lesion with the CO_2 laser, a superficial irradiation of the tissue to create a small, coagulated zone (using the defocused beam) is clinically recommended (Figure 3.3) because this may significantly reduce postoperative pain and protect the wound from infection (wound dressing).

3.4 Removal of Benign Soft Tissue Tumors

In clinical practice, the surgically oriented dentist and/or specialist is confronted with small or big, stalked and superficial soft tissue tumors. The most frequent benign tumors of the oral cavity are the following:

- fibromas
- papillomas
- lipomas
- pyogenic granulomas

The most frequent wide tumors or soft tissue pathologies of the oral cavity are papillomatosis (especially in the palate), symmetric fibromas, vascular lesions and malformations, precancerous lesions (i.e. leukoplakia as well as oral lichen planus) (see also Figure 3.4). The surgical removal of papillomatosis of the palate, as well as the symmetrical fibromas and denture-related fibromas, is often indicated in oral surgery from the preprosthetic perspective. In comparison to the scalpel, the surgical laser permits the removal of such abnormalities with particular advantages for patients and surgeons.

3.4.1 Surgical Protocol for Removal of Small Tumors

In general, the incision design is similar to the conventional surgical method, but in comparison to that, there is only a small number of instruments necessary (Figure 3.5).

Clinical Cases

Excision Biopsy of a White Lesion (Leukoplakia)

A 65-year-old patient was referred with the request of diagnostic clarification of the white pathological lesion at her oral mucosa in areas # 22 and 27 (Figure 3.4a). After topical anesthesia with xylocaine spray 2%, the pathological tissue was excised completely with the noncontact CO_2 laser handpiece and power of 4 W in a continuous mode (Figure 3.4b). The excision succeeded free of blood and without any other intraoperative complications. Directly after the

biopsy, the whole area was ablated, in order to form a distinctive coagulation. Suturing was not necessary. The tissue was examined histopathologically. The diagnosis was a common leukoplakia. There were no complications during the healing period and after three weeks there were no pathological findings (Figure 3.4c). Four years after excision, the mucous membrane was still free from any recurrence (Figure 3.4d).

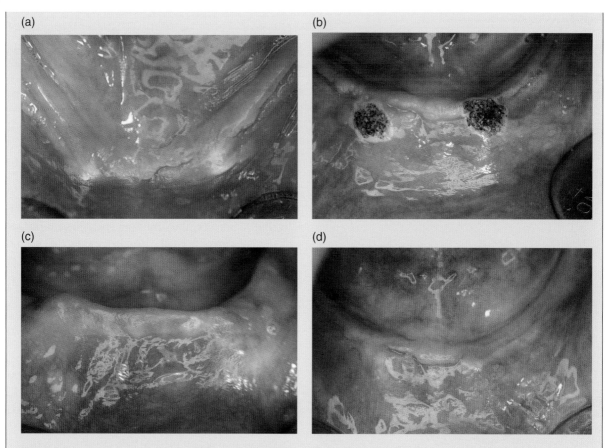

Figure 3.4 Hyperkeratosis of the mandible (a); the pathological tissue was excised with the noncontact CO_2 laser (power: 4 W; continuous mode) (b). The excision succeeded free of blood and without any other intraoperative complications. Directly after the biopsy removal, the whole area was ablated, in order to form a superficial coagulation. The histopathological diagnosis was a common leukoplakia. No complications were observed during the three weeks of postoperative period (c). Four years after excision, the oral mucosa was healthy without any recurrence (d). *Source:* Dr. Georgios E Romanos.

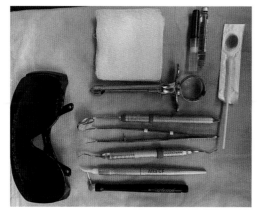

Figure 3.5 Necessary instruments for conventional laser-assisted surgical procedures. *Source:* Dr. Georgios E Romanos.

After a topical or local anesthesia, a wedge-shaped excision will be performed with the laser handpiece. For the removal of the tissue, the handpiece is used in a focused mode. After the removal of a soft tissue tumor, the margins of the adjacent tissues should be ablated in order to achieve smooth excision margins. Afterwards the entire wound should be coagulated using a defocused beam and lower power settings (Table 3.2).

The noncontact CO_2 laser is used with straight or angulated handpieces based on the location of the lesion. The articulated arm with the integrated glass mirror system is associated with some loss of power. This effect may lead to a local overheating at the end of the handpiece, particularly in cases of longer lasting surgical interventions. During surgical procedures under local (or general) anesthesia, there is a small risk of tissue overheating in the adjacent healthy tissues. For this reason, a periodical checking of the fiber condition is absolutely necessary to avoid complications (Figure 3.6).

In case of the Nd:YAG or diode laser application, the blood vessels and/or capillaries will be coagulated with

Table 3.2 Chronological order in laser surgical procedures.

Treatment	Laser
Medical/dental history (update)	
Clinical examination/ informed consent	
Anesthesia (topical and/or local)	
Laser safety measures – test firing	
Excision	Focused beam (CW or pulsed)
Marginal ablation	Defocused beam (CW or pulsed)
Coagulation	Defocused beam (pulsed/low power)
(Histopathological examination)	
Postoperative instructions	
Follow-up	

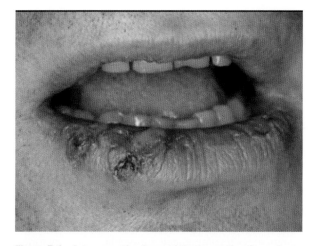

Figure 3.6 Intraoperative burn of the lower lip of a patient during laser-assisted periodontal therapy at the right mandibular teeth. The glass fiber was broken within the handpiece, and the laser was irradiating the wrong area (procedure was performed under block anesthesia). *Source:* Dr. Georgios E Romanos.

a defocused (noncontact) beam. The risk of secondary bleeding, postsurgical discomfort, and edema is in general significantly reduced. The carbonized surface, which is formed directly after surgery can protect against an infection, and after three to four days there are no pathological changes of the mucosa to be observed. After the formation of a temporary thick fibrin layer (Figure 3.7), the healing is completed within three to four weeks.

The use of lasers with glass fibers, like diode and Nd:YAG lasers, provide an easier control of the tissue irradiation, since dentists, in general, feel comfortable having contact with the tissue in routine clinical dentistry.

> A constant pressure with the glass fiber on the tissue must be avoided.

Therefore, excisions can be performed when the glass fiber is in contact with the tissue, compared to other laser wavelengths like the CO_2 laser or the Er:YAG laser, where a noncontact handpiece provides tissue removal.

However, knowledge of the penetration depth of the laser light within the tissue should be considered during incision. When a glass fiber of 300 μm in diameter is applied, a continuous contact with the tissue should be avoided in order to provide possible cooling of the tissue (thermal relaxation effect).

During the surgical procedure with the laser, surgical forceps should hold the soft tissue tumor, which is excised from the base with the laser glass fiber. The blood-free surgical area permits an optically accessible treating of the tissue, whereas carbonization is not so pronounced in comparison to irradiation with the CO_2 laser. Suturing is not necessary, and a soft/liquid diet is recommended for the first two to three postoperative days to avoid removal of the superficial wound layer. Local tissue irritation, as for example by a toothbrush, should be avoided particularly during the first three days (stage of a fibrin layer deposition), so that postoperative bleeding, associated with pain and wound healing problems, is avoided. For preventive antibacterial purposes, rinsing with chlorhexidine or other mouth rinses is advised.

Depending on the clinical indication of laser use, different parameters and power settings are recommended by the manufacturers. Clinical experience shows that a power up to 3.0 W (for the Nd:YAG laser) is good enough for use in private practice. The pulse frequency may vary between 40 and 100 Hz. High power settings or slow movement of the glass fiber under irradiation may lead to wound healing complications resulting in scar tissue formation or necrosis (Figure 3.8).

When the CO_2 laser is used, a continuous beam or pulsed mode with short pulse duration and high-pulse energy is recommended. During excisions, the handpiece is applied without tissue contact, with an average output power of 4–6 W. There is a variety of ceramic or metal tips with different diameters (e.g. 0.4 or 0.8 mm), which can be used in the handpiece for small focal spots in order to create precise incisions and excellent coagulation.

(a)

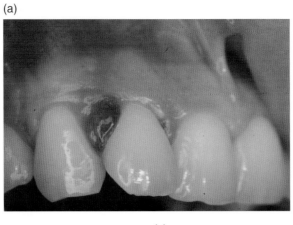

(b)

(c)

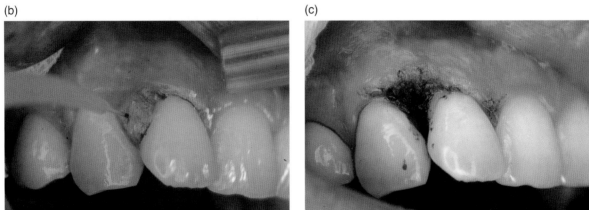

Figure 3.7 Coagulation of the blood vessel tumor in the papilla #6–7 (a) using a noncontact diode laser (pulsed, 4 W) (b) and after conventional scaling and root planing of the site, a gingivoplasty was performed to create normal tissue morphology (c). *Source:* Dr. Georgios E Romanos.

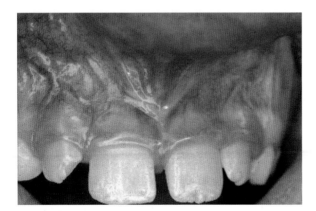

Figure 3.8 Scar tissue formation due to the use of high-power diode laser (980 nm) perpendicular to the soft tissue six weeks after laser surgery. The high power and the 90° angle to the soft tissue during excision should be avoided. *Source:* Dr. Georgios E Romanos.

3.4.2 Surgical Protocol for Removal of Larger Soft Tissue Tumors

The most common larger soft tissue tumors and wide lesions in the oral cavity are fibroepithelial hyperplasia of the palate, and, in general hyperplasia, symmetric fibromas, granulomas, lipomas, hemangiomas, and *last but not least* adenomas. The removal of vascular lesions and malformations as well as precancerous lesions will be separately dealt within this chapter. Depending on the size of the lesion, a combination therapy of tumor excision with a scalpel and subsequent laser coagulation is sometimes recommended. Large fibromas or symmetrical fibromas can be excised today conventionally, and advanced bleeding can be controlled using the laser.

The CO_2 laser in a continuous mode and with no contact to the tissue is mainly used for the treatment of wide (flat) pathologies of the oral soft tissue causing burning symptoms (e.g. oral lichen planus). A power of 6–10 W permits a quick ablation or vaporization of the pathological tissue when the laser is applied in a defocused mode. A small incision biopsy is necessary before the complete tissue is removed in layers (ablation). The decision of whether vaporization or excision of the lesion is indicated will be taken intraoperatively; however, it depends on the size and thickness of the lesion.

Erythematous pathological alterations localized at the palate (the so-called fibroepithelial hyperplasia of the palate) is often associated with a poorly fitting prosthesis and secondary *Candida* superinfection. The tissue can be removed in layers with a CO_2 laser in defocused mode, continuous beam, and a power of approx. 6–10W. A sample incision biopsy of a clinically suspicious area must be carried out before complete ablation. For a better determination of the depth extension of the lesion, the carbonized tissue is continuously wiped away with wet gauze or cotton swabs. After that, a rinsing with hydrogen peroxide solution (3%) is very helpful. The

prosthesis of the patient is then soft relined for the first two to three weeks, and the final relining will be performed at a later time.

Sachs and Borden (1981) were the first who treated such clinical recurrent lesions of the palate using the CO_2 laser without observing any recurrences.

Some clinical applications of the CO_2, diode, and Nd:YAG lasers in surgical treatment of benign soft tissue tumors are demonstrated in the following clinical cases.

Clinical Cases

Removal of a Fibroma of the Maxilla

The 62-year-old patient was referred for removal of a soft tissue tumor in the maxilla in area #8–9 (Figure 3.9a). After local infiltration anesthesia, the tumor was excised with the continuous wave (CW) CO_2 laser, and power of 4W (Figure 3.9b).

The coagulation during the whole surgical area permitted a good view of the surgical site. Possible charring (carbonization) was removed later using wet gauze (Figure 3.9c). After controlling of the smooth margins, the treatment was finished. The specimen was histologically examined (Figure 3.9d) and confirmed the clinical diagnosis of a fibroma of the oral mucosa. Two weeks after surgery, an excellent healing was observed (Figure 3.9e), and there was no reported postoperative pain.

Removal of an Irritation Fibroma

A 74-year-old patient was referred for the removal of a large irritation fibroma before the fabrication of a new complete denture (Figure 3.10a). The tumor was excised under local anesthesia with the noncontact CO_2 laser and a power of 4–5W (CW). The surgical intervention took place under concurrent coagulation and subsequent carbonization of the entire area (Figure 3.10b). The specimen was histologically examined. The diagnosis was an irritation fibroma in the anterior part of the mandible. The denture could be used immediately after surgery. Five days later, a fibrin deposition covering the entire wound area was observed(Figure 3.10c). Three weeks postoperatively excellent wound healing was observed (Figure 3.10d). Postoperative swelling, pain, bleeding, or contraction of the wound with scar tissue formation were not observed.

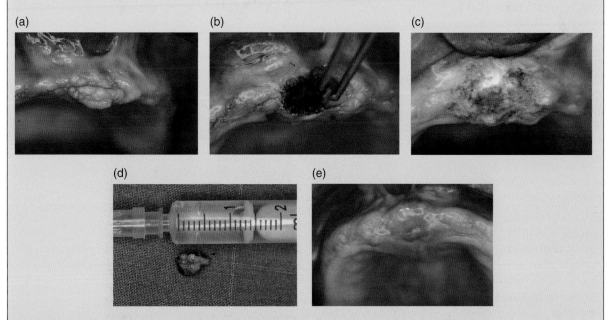

Figure 3.9 Excision of a soft tissue tumor in the maxilla (a) using a continuous wave (CW) CO_2 laser, and power of 4W (b). After removal of charring (carbonization) with a wet gauze (c), the histological examination confirmed the clinical diagnosis (d) of a fibroma. The wound was healed completely in two weeks (e). *Source:* Dr. Georgios E Romanos.

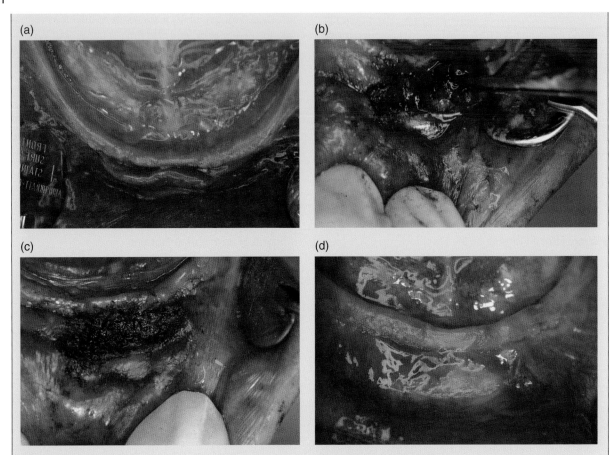

Figure 3.10 Removal of a soft tissue tumor in the vestibule of the anterior mandible (a) using a CO_2 laser; (b) providing sufficient coagulation (c); and no postoperative recurrence (d). *Source:* Dr. Georgios E Romanos.

Removal of an Irritation Fibroma in Combination with a Local Vestibuloplasty

A 68-year-old patient was transferred for the removal of a pedunculus soft tissue tumor (irritation fibroma) in the vestibular fold of the anterior mandible before the treatment of a new full denture (Figure 3.11a). After local anesthesia, the tumor was excised with a power of 4 W (noncontact, continuous CO_2 laser beam). A local extension of the vestibulum depth was performed in this area (secondary intension). The muscle fibers were sharply dissected and separated from the underlying periosteum. The preparation of the tissue occurred without complications, as the blood-free area allowed a good overview of the surgical site. The handpiece of the laser was used in focus, at a distance of approximately 1 cm from the excised tissue in order to remove the fibroma and, later on, in a defocused mode for adequate coagulation.

The working distance or the focus localization of the laser beam was constantly changed depending on the thickness of the tissue to control the power density

so that the periosteum or the underlying bone was not injured. An incorrect application could lead to dehiscence, resorption, or bone necrosis, and possibly other postsurgical complications. The whole surgical area was subsequently superficially coagulated (Figure 3.11b). Four days later, a fibrin layer deposition could be observed (Figure 3.11c). A soft lining of the prosthesis was not necessary. Complications like bleeding, swelling, or pain were not observed. Four weeks after surgery (Figure 3.11d), the clinical condition was unremarkable. A cicatrization or functional difficulties did not occur.

Removal of an Irritation Fibroma in the Mandible

A lingual fibroma (Figure 3.12a) excision was performed with a focused noncontact CO_2 laser and 6 W average power setting (Figure 3.12b) under local anesthesia. The wound was coagulated (defocused beam) in order to reduce the postoperative pain (Figure 3.12c). The specimen (Figure 3.12d) was examined histologically. No postoperative complications were reported.

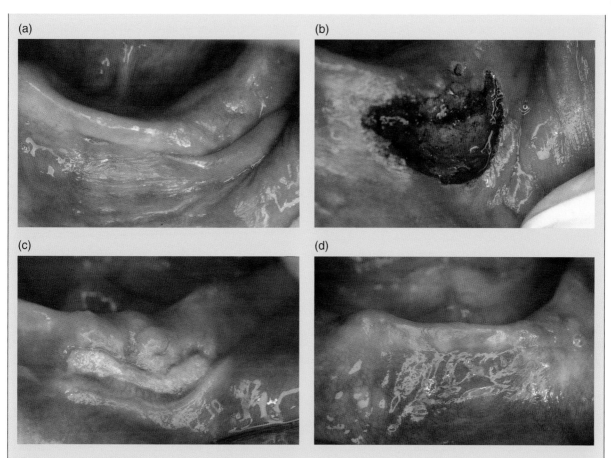

Figure 3.11 Irritation fibroma in the vestibular fold before the laser surgery (a); laser excision with a noncontact (CW) CO_2 laser and power of 4 W (b); fibrin layer wound coverage was observed four days after surgery (c); excellent wound healing four weeks after surgery (d). *Source:* Dr. Georgios E Romanos.

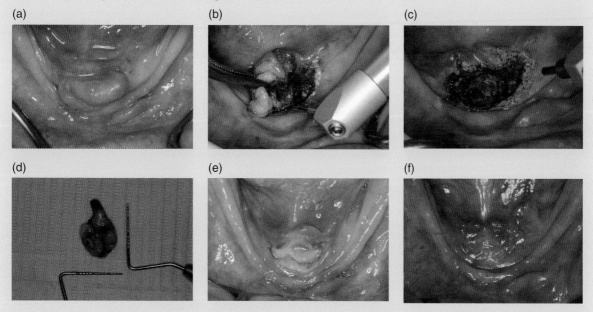

Figure 3.12 Lingual fibroma (a) excised with a focused non-contact CO_2 laser and 6 W average power (b). The wound was coagulated (defocused beam) to reduce the postoperative pain (c). The specimen (d) was examined histologically. Three weeks postoperatively a fibrin layer covered the wound (e). Uneventful healing was observed six weeks after surgery (f). *Source:* Dr. Georgios E Romanos.

The follow-up in three weeks presented fibrin formation covering the entire wound area (Figure 3.12e). The healing was uneventful six weeks after therapy (Figure 3.12f).

Removal of a Fibroma of the Buccal Mucosa

This clinical case presents a 55-year-old patient who was transferred with a small fibroma at the buccal mucosa (Figure 3.13a). The tumor was excised under topical anesthesia (xylocaine spray 2%) with the pulsed Nd:YAG laser (Figure 3.13b). The specified parameters were: power 2.0 W and frequency 30 pps (pulses per second). The coagulation was, in spite of the low energy settings, very good. One week later, a fibrin layer was present

covering the entire wound surface. Four weeks after surgery, excellent wound healing without scarring could be observed (Figure 3.13c).

Removal of a Fibroma of the Tongue with an Er:YAG Laser

An excision of a fibroma in the tongue (Figure 3.14a) was performed after local anesthesia using an Er:YAG laser (Figure 3.14b). The glass fiber was used in contact (focused beam) with an average power 2.5 W (250 mJ and 10 Hz). The bleeding was not easy to control (Figure 3.14c) using these parameters, and a suture was performed with absorbable suture material (Figure 3.14d). One week postoperatively the healing was uneventful (Figure 3.14e).

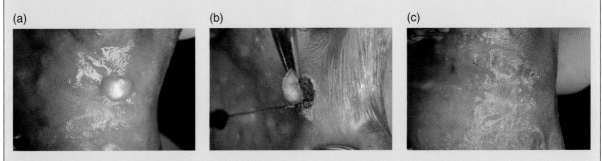

Figure 3.13 Fibroma at the buccal mucosa (a) removed with contact pulsed Nd:YAG laser (b). The wound healing completed after four weeks without complications and scar tissue formation (c). *Source:* Dr. Georgios E Romanos.

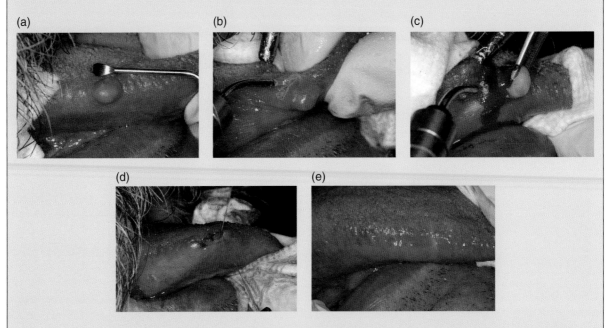

Figure 3.14 Excision of a fibroma in the tongue (a) using an Er:YAG laser (b) in a focused beam with an average power 2.5 W (c). The hemostasis was not adequate due to the strong tissue vascularization and therefore a suture was required (d); one week postoperatively the healing was uneventful without scar tissue formation (e). *Source:* Dr. Georgios E Romanos.

Removal of a Fibroma in the Maxillary Alveolar Ridge

A 63-year-old female patient presented with a large soft tissue tumor at the alveolar ridge (Figure 3.15a). The tumor was excised with a CO_2 laser (continuous beam; power of 6 W), after local anesthesia (Figure 3.15b). The whole area was finally sufficiently coagulated (Figure 3.15c). Wound healing succeeded with no complications, and a fibrin layer covered the wound one week after surgery (Figure 3.15d).

Removal of a Palatal Adenoma

A 43-year-old, hepatitis C–positive patient exhibited a round, approximately 8×10 mm wide soft tissue tumor (Figure 3.16a). The tumor had a normal consistency, was not painful at palpation, and showed, according to the patient, a relatively slow growth. The surgical excision occurred with the CO_2 laser to control bleeding because of the high risk of infection. After local anesthesia, the tumor was removed with the noncontact handpiece of the CO_2 laser and a continuous beam (power: 5 W) (Figure 3.16b). A

strong coagulation took place during the entire surgical procedure (Figure 3.16c). The surface was finally smoothed with the defocused beam, and the specimen was sent for histopathological examination (Figure 3.16d). Based on the pathology report the diagnosis was an adenoma of the small palatal salivary glands. Oral rinses with 0.12% chlorhexidine di-gluconate (three to four times daily) were recommended. Wound healing succeeded without any complications.

Removal of Fibroepithelial Palatal Hyperplasia

A 57-year-old patient was referred for surgical treatment of a wide lesion at his palate (Figure 3.17a) before fabrication of a new complete denture. After local anesthesia, a biopsy was taken with the CO_2 laser (focused beam) and the lesion was removed in layers with the defocused, continuous handpiece and power of 6 W (ablative mode). Finally, the entire wound area was coagulated (Figure 3.17b). The existing complete denture was soft-lined immediately after

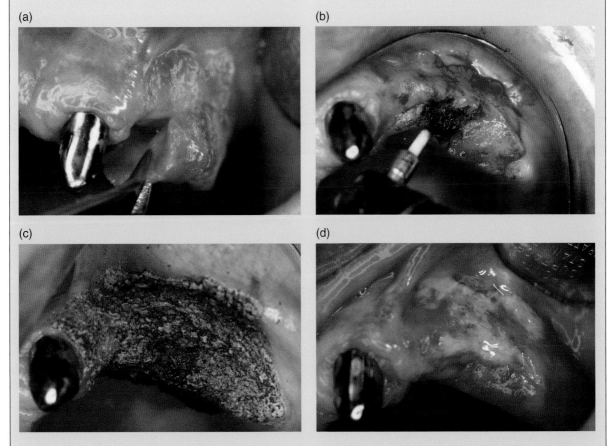

Figure 3.15 Soft tissue tumor of the alveolar ridge (a); excision with the CO_2 laser (b) and coagulation of the wound (c); fibrin coverage one week after surgery (d). *Source:* Dr. Georgios E Romanos.

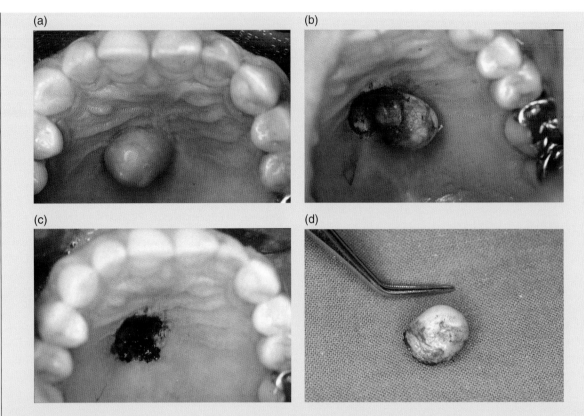

Figure 3.16 Soft tissue tumor in the palate (a). The surgical excision occurred with excellent bleeding control using the CO_2 laser (b, c). The specimen was examined histologically (d). *Source:* Dr. Georgios E Romanos.

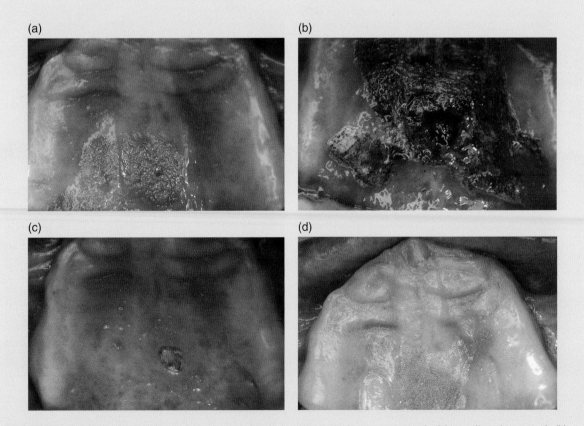

Figure 3.17 Palatal soft tissue lesion (a); using an ablative mode, the lesion was removed with excellent hemostasis (b); a thin fibrin layer was formed and covered the wound surface after one week (c), and after three weeks the tissue presented a completely healthy condition (d). *Source:* Dr. Georgios E Romanos.

surgery. Further postoperative measures were not necessary. The histopathological examination confirmed the clinical diagnosis. Wound healing succeeded without postoperative pain or bleeding. After one week, a thin fibrin layer was formed and covered the wound (Figure 3.17c), and after three weeks, wound healing was uneventful (Figure 3.17d).

Removal of Large Palatal Fibromas

A 52-year-old patient was referred by her dentist because of a large fibromatous tissue growth (approx. 4 × 2 cm) in the palatal aspect, respectively to teeth #1–4 (Figure 3.18a). The tumor was excised under local anesthesia with a scalpel due to the large size of the tumor, the bleeding (from the branches of the palatal artery) was controlled by the CO_2 laser (Figure 3.18b, c), and finally a eugenol-free periodontal pack (Coe-Pak®) was placed. The tumor was examined histologically to confirm the clinical diagnosis (Figure 3.18d). The diagnosis was a fibroma. Wound healing succeeded without complications.

Removal of Large Palatal Fibromas

A 67-year-old male patient presented for fabrication of a new complete denture in the maxilla. During the clinical examination, asymptomatic, bilateral soft tissue tumors with the clinical diagnosis of symmetric fibromas (Figure 3.19a) were observed. The surgical procedure was performed using the superpulsed CO_2 laser (Figure 3.19b). The patient denied use of any local anesthesia (he was afraid of needles) and confirmed that the surgery was acceptable only with topical anesthesia. The CO_2 laser was applied with 4W continuous wave (CW) mode for both sites, excising the two fibromas and coagulating at the same time the underlying tissues. An extensive coagulation was achieved after surgery with the defocused ablative handpiece (Figure 3.19c). The two specimens were examined by an oral pathologist, who confirmed the clinical diagnosis. The tissue healed without any complications, and in the first two weeks a fibrin layer covered the entire wound. Six weeks after treatment the tissue was completely healthy (Figure 3.19d), and the next steps were done in order to deliver the final prosthesis.

(a) (b) (c) (d)

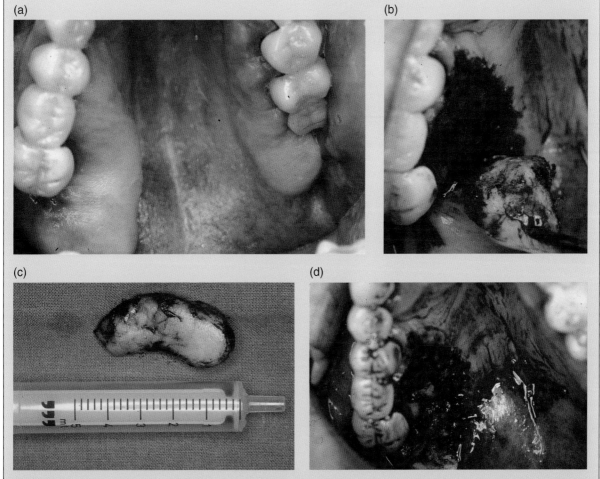

Figure 3.18 Excision of soft tissue tumor (a) with a scalpel and a CO_2 laser to control bleeding (b, c) followed by a SRP of the periodontally involved teeth. *Source:* Dr. Georgios E Romanos.

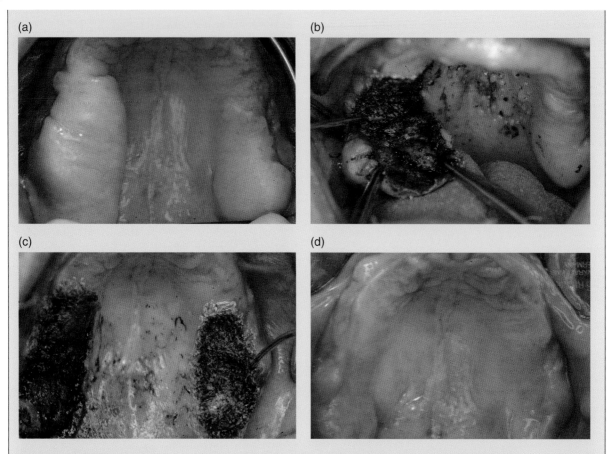

Figure 3.19 Clinical diagnosis of symmetric fibromas (a). The surgical procedure was performed using the superpulsed 4 W continuous wave CO_2 laser (b). An extensive coagulation was achieved after surgery (c). Six weeks after treatment the tissue was completely healthy (d). *Source:* Dr. Georgios E Romanos.

Removal of a Pyogenic Granuloma

A 37-year-old patient was referred for diagnosis and treatment of a mucous alteration or rather a tumor of the right side of her lower lip (Figure 3.20a). She reported slight pain, recurring bleeding, and a continuous growth of the tumor during the last two to three weeks. The clinical diagnosis was pyogenic granuloma. The tumor was excised under local anesthesia with the pulsed Nd:YAG laser and power of 6 W, and a histopathological examination took also place (Figure 3.20b, c). The surgical removal occurred mostly without pain and without any postoperative bleeding. Wound healing occurred without complications. The clinical situation after one month revealed a slight scar tissue formation (possibly due to the used relatively high-power settings), but without any other complications (Figure 3.20d).

Removal of a Fibroma at the Buccal Mucosa Using a Diode Laser

An excision of a fibroma in the buccal mucosa (Figure 3.21a) was performed under topical anesthesia using a diode laser (810 nm) with a 200 µm glass fiber in contact with the soft tissue. The fiber was initiated before surgery using an articulating paper. The tissue was excised completely (average power 2.5 W) for histological examination (Figure 3.21b). The coagulation was sufficient with the same fiber in noncontact, defocused beam (Figure 3.21c). No suture was necessary. Two weeks postoperatively, the healing was uneventful (Figure 3.21d).

Removal of a Fibroma at the Buccal Mucosa Using a CO_2 Laser

An excision of a fibroma in the buccal mucosa (Figure 3.22a) was performed under topical anesthesia using a CO_2 laser with a noncontact focused beam and a ceramic tip at a distance of 3–4 mm from the lesion. The tissue was excised completely (average power 4 W), and the excision line was within the healthy mucosa in order to preserve the complete size of the lesion for a better histological examination (Figure 3.22b). The coagulation was sufficient with the

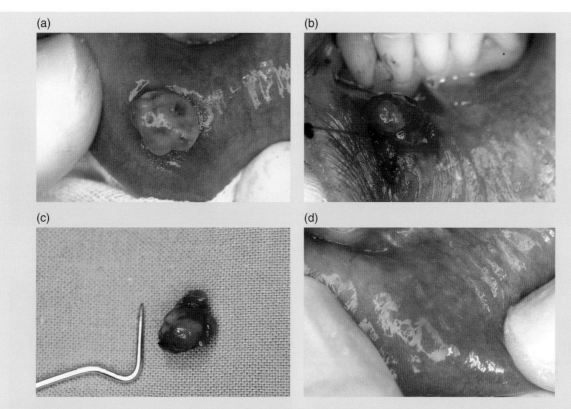

Figure 3.20 Pyogenic granuloma of the lower lip (a). The tumor was excised with the pulsed Nd:YAG laser and power of 6 W (b). The specimen was examined histologically (c). Due to tissue overheating, one month postoperatively, a slight scar tissue formation was demonstrated but without any other complications (d). *Source:* Dr. Georgios E Romanos.

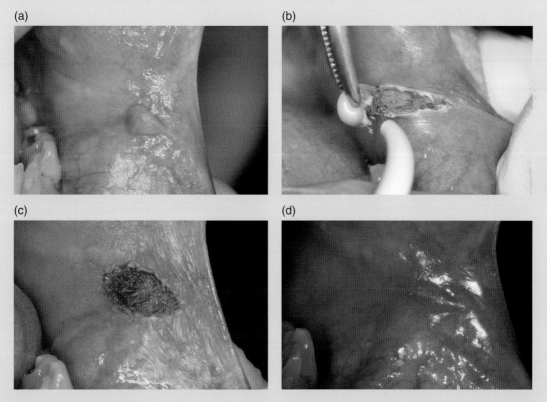

Figure 3.21 Fibroma in the buccal mucosa (a). The excision was performed using a diode laser (810 nm) with a 200 μm glass fiber and initiated tip in contact with the soft tissue (b). The coagulation was sufficient with the same fiber in noncontact, defocused beam (c). Two weeks postoperatively the healing was uneventful. Slight scar tissue was observed (d). *Source:* Dr. Georgios E Romanos.

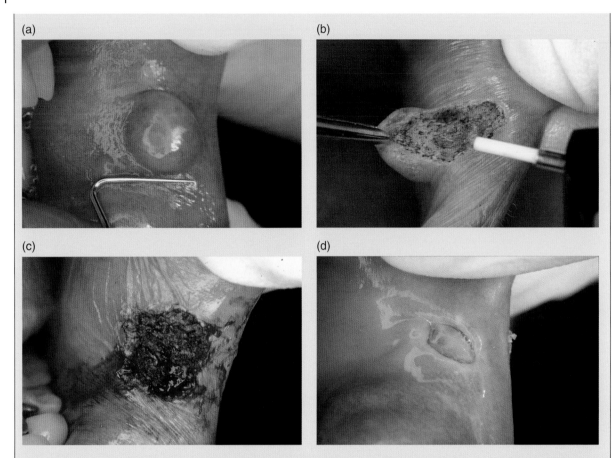

Figure 3.22 Fibroma of the buccal mucosa (a) excised with a CO_2 laser with a noncontact focused beam at a distance of 3–4 mm from the lesion (b). The coagulation was sufficient with the same handpiece in a defocused beam (c). No suture was mandatory. Three days postoperatively, a thick layer of fibrin covered the entire wound surface (d). *Source:* Dr. Georgios E Romanos.

same handpiece in a defocused beam (Figure 3.22c). No suture was mandatory. Three days postoperatively the healing was uneventful, and a layer of thick fibrin covered the wound surface (Figure 3.22d).

Removal of Hyperplastic Gingiva Underneath Bar Restoration

A 78-year-old patient was referred with the request to remove a hyperplastic gingiva underneath the bar restoration in the #22–27 teeth (Figure 3.23a). Because of the presence of the gingival hyperplasia, the oral hygiene of the patient was clearly affected, in such a way that the long-term prognosis of the abutment teeth #22 and #27 was questionable (very deep periodontal pockets, so-called pseudo-pockets were present). The hyperplastic tissues were excised under local anesthesia with the continuous noncontact beam of the CO_2 laser with an average power of 6 W (focused) (Figure 3.23b). After that the margins were smoothed in a defocusing beam. The hemostasis was

sufficient, and wound healing was completed without any complications (Figure 3.23c). The surgical site was healed three weeks later, and the plaque control was optimized (Figure 3.23d).

Removal of Hyperplastic Peri-implant Mucosa Underneath Bar Restoration

The case presented hyperplastic and inflamed mucosa with bleeding on probing around implants underneath a bar implant-retained restoration (Figure 3.24a). The excision was performed using a CO_2 laser and defocused beam in a continuous mode and 4–5 W average power setting. In addition, a partial vestibuloplasty was performed to improve the vestibule depth for better plaque control (Figure 3.24b). An excellent coagulation was achieved using this laser wavelength. Painkillers (Tylenol®) and antibiotics (Penicillin V®) were prescribed postoperatively (3x/die). After one week of healing (Figure 3.24c), a fibrin layer covered the entire wound surface. No swelling or other complications

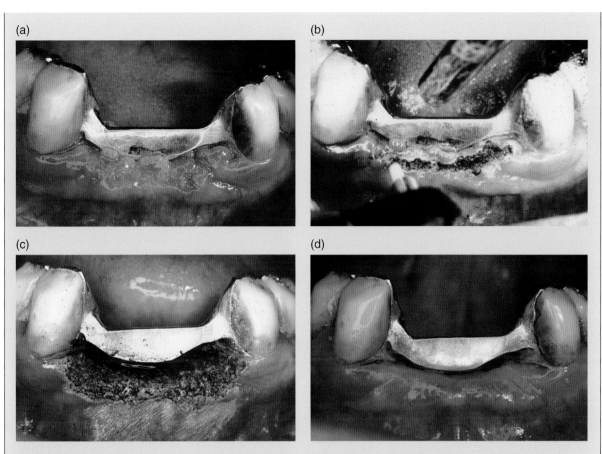

Figure 3.23 Surgical excision of the hyperplastic gingiva underneath the bar restoration (a) using a CO_2 laser with an average power of 6 W and focused beam (b); a good hemostasis (c) and an excellent wound healing was observed after three weeks (d). *Source:* Dr. Georgios E Romanos.

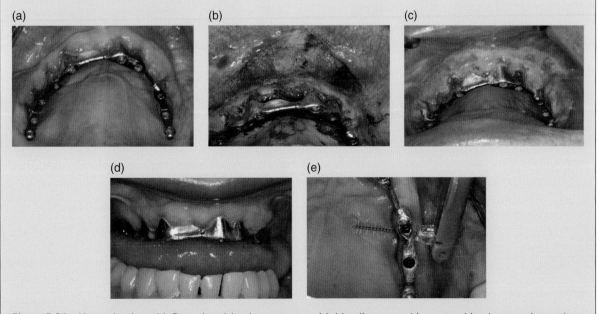

Figure 3.24 Hyperplastic and inflamed peri-implant mucosa with bleeding on probing around implants underneath a bar implant-supported restoration (a). The excision was performed using a CO_2 laser and defocused beam (CW) and 4–5 W average power (b). A partial vestibuloplasty was performed to improve the depth of the vestibule for better plaque control. An excellent coagulation was achieved using this laser wavelength. After one week of healing (c), a fibrin layer covered the entire wound. The tissue condition was evaluated after 1.5 months, and the prosthesis was relined permanently (d). Plaque control was optimized using interdental brushes (e) *(Surgery: Drs. G. Romanos and B. Katz, Stony Brook, NY). Source: Dr. Georgios E Romanos.*

were observed. The tissue condition was evaluated after 1.5 months, and the prosthesis was relined permanently in order to improve the soft tissue quality (Figure 3.24d). The patient's oral hygiene was optimized after the procedure using interdental brushes underneath the bar restoration (Figure 3.24e).

Removal of an Ossifying Fibroma Using a CO_2 Laser

A soft tissue tumor was present for almost two years according to the dental history of the patient (Figure 3.25a, b). The size of the lesion was 21 × 23 mm and was expanded in the palatal aspect as well (Figure 3.25c). Radiographical evaluation demonstrated a periodontal crestal bone loss as well as mineralized, calcified areas within the soft tissue tumor (Figure 3.25d). The excision was performed using the CO_2 laser under local anesthesia and an average power setting of 6 W in a continuous, noncontact handpiece and a focused mode (Figure 3.25e). During the entire surgical procedure, a hemostat was holding the tumor in order to visualize the underlying tissues during laser irradiation (Figure 3.25f). After excision a sufficient hemostasis was accomplished with the CO_2 laser in a defocused beam. In addition, irregularities of the tissue morphology, such as extensive frenulum and thick mucosa, were excised with the CO_2 laser in an ablative mode (Figure 3.25g). Sufficient coagulation was achieved in order to avoid postoperative bleeding (Figure 3.25h). The specimen (Figure 3.25i) was examined by an oral pathologist, who confirmed the diagnosis of the lesion. It was an ossifying fibroma. A follow-up of the case was not possible since the patient moved elsewhere.

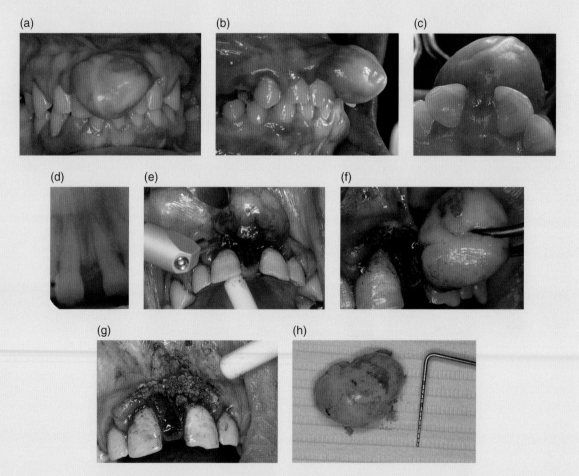

Figure 3.25 Clinical and radiographical examination of a patient with an ossifying fibroma of the gingiva (a–d). The excision was performed using the CO_2 laser under local anesthesia and an average power setting of 6 W in a continuous, noncontact handpiece and a focused mode (e, f). Sufficient bleeding control was accomplished with the CO_2 laser in a defocused beam. Irregularities of the tissue morphology, such as extensive frenum and thick mucosa, were excised with the CO_2 laser. Sufficient hemostasis was achieved in order to avoid postoperative bleeding (g). The specimen was examined by a maxillofacial pathologist, who confirmed the diagnosis of the lesion as an ossifying fibroma (h). *Source:* Dr. Georgios E Romanos.

Removal of an Ossifying Fibroma Using a Diode Laser

The soft tissue tumor of a female 25-year-old patient was present for almost three years in the same area (#8) and was associated with some bleeding (Figure 3.26a). The tumor was excised under local anesthesia and the use of a 980 nm diode laser (Figure 3.26b) with the glass fiber in contact with the lesion. The average power was 4 W (CW) with initiated handpiece. The surgical site was coagulated, and the margins of the defect were smoothed using the non-contact defocused beam and the same power. A conventional scaling and meticulous root planing were also performed (Figure 3.26c). The final result after six weeks presented excellent healing without recurrence (Figure 3.26d).

Removal of a Papilloma of the Lip

A soft tissue tumor of the lip (Figure 3.27a) was removed using an 810 nm diode laser (initiated tip) with contact handpiece and average power of 2 W (Figure 3.27b). The excision and coagulation were performed without complications (Figure 3.27c), and a suture was not necessary. The histopathological examination confirmed the diagnosis of a papilloma.

Removal of a Papilloma of the Lip

A 23-year-old female patient came with the request of the removal of a small tumor of her upper lip (Figure 3.28a). According to the medical history, the lesion was asymptomatic and existed for approximately three months. The clinical examination revealed a round lens-size and relatively hard superficial tumor with a wide base. It was excised, after local anesthesia, with the Nd:YAG laser. A contact fiber with a diameter of 300 μm, a power of 3 W, and a frequency of 30 pps was used for the excision (Figure 3.28b). Wound healing proceeded without complications (Figure 3.28c). The clinical result

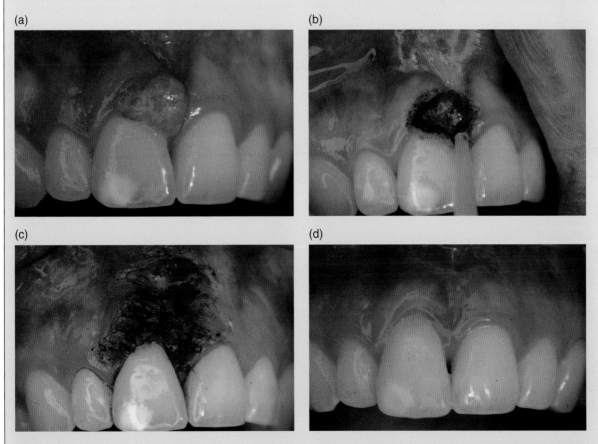

(a) (b) (c) (d)

Figure 3.26 Soft tissue tumor of the gingiva associated with some bleeding (a). The tumor was excised under local anesthesia using a 980 nm diode laser (b) and glass fiber in contact with the lesion (average power: 4 W/CW/initiated tip). The surgical site was coagulated, and the margins of the defect were smoothed using the noncontact defocused beam and the same power (c). The final result after six weeks presented excellent healing without recurrence (d). *Source:* Dr. Georgios E Romanos.

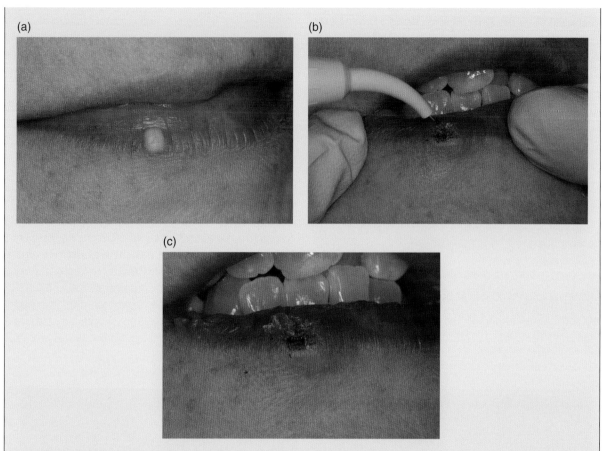

Figure 3.27 Soft tissue tumor of the lip (a) removed using an 810 nm diode laser with contact handpiece and average power of 2 W and initiated tip (b). Excision and coagulation performed without complications (c). *Source:* Dr. Georgios E Romanos.

remained stable and showed six months later no esthetic complications (Figure 3.28d).

Removal of a Lipoma in the Buccal Mucosa

The buccal mucosa of a male patient demonstrated a soft tissue tumor without symptoms but with hard consistency and slight yellow color (Figure 3.29a). The excision was performed with the CO_2 laser under local anesthesia (Figure 3.29b) and a power of 4 W in a CW mode. The coagulation was excellent. The specimen (Figure 3.29c) was examined by an oral pathologist to confirm the diagnosis. This was a lipoma of the buccal mucosa. The healing was performed by secondary intension, and fibrin covered the entire surgical area for the first two weeks (Figure 3.29d). No complications were found after three months of healing. A small scar was present but without any other clinical findings (Figure 3.29e).

Removal of a Lipoma of the Tongue

A 63-year old male patient presented with unusual swelling of his tongue (Figure 3.30a). The lesion had been there for many years according to the medical history, completely asymptomatic except sometimes in the last few weeks slight hypesthesia at the left tongue side. The motoric condition of the tongue was completely normal. Clinical examination showed a relatively round and hard lesion directly underneath the mucosa of the tongue. The patient was informed about the possible postoperative complications. Under local anesthesia, the CO_2 laser with a continuous wave mode and 6 W power setting was used in order to prepare and remove the lesion (Figure 3.30b). During the procedure, a round tumor was removed without bleeding but with an excellent dissection using the noncontact handpiece and a ceramic tip (Figure 3.30c). The tumor size was approximately 30×28 mm and was sent for histopathological

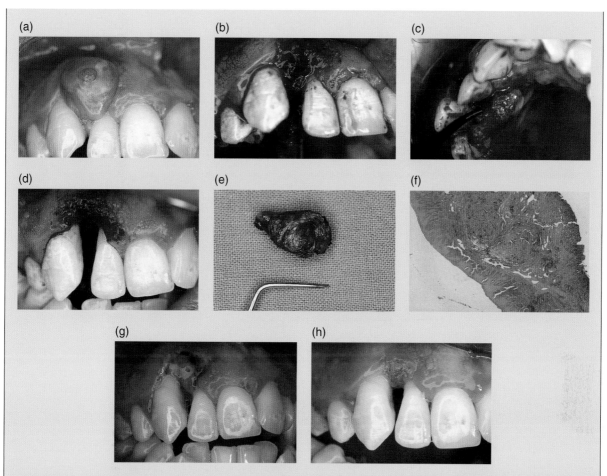

Figure 3.31 Soft tissue tumor of the gingiva (a); excision of the tumor using an Nd:YAG laser and power of 4 W, in a pulsed mode of 100 Hz frequency in order to provide sufficient hemostasis during surgery (b). The tumor was excised completely buccally and palatal and a meticulous scaling and root planing was performed (c). The interdental defect at #6–7 was sufficiently coagulated (d). The specimen (e) was examined by an oral pathologist who confirmed the diagnosis of a giant cell granuloma (f). Delayed wound healing was presented in the first two weeks (g). Three months after surgery the tissue presented no further signs of inflammation (h). *Source:* Dr. Georgios E Romanos.

the absence of marginal bone due to the tumor infiltration. Further follow-ups were not possible since the patient relocated, but the patient was informed about possible recurrence risks.

Removal of an Adenoma of the Sublingual Salivary Gland

A 73-year-old male patient presented a soft tissue tumor in the mouth floor causing a disturbance in the secretory function of the right sublingual salivary gland. A sialolith was not demonstrated radiographically. According to the clinical findings, the clinical diagnosis was adenoma of the sublingual salivary gland (Figure 3.32a). Demonstration of the

duct was performed initially with a dull needle (Figure 3.32b), and later on during the tumor preparation a plastic tube was inserted into the duct to demonstrate the duct orientation. The tumor was excised with the contact mode handpiece and at a power setting of 8–10 W (continuous wave) of a 980 nm diode laser because of the large tumor size (approximately 3 × 2 cm); finally the salivary gland was removed (Figure 3.32c). The hemostasis as well as the incision quality was excellent using this power (Figure 3.32d). The margins of the wound were sutured with Vicryl® suturing material. Postoperative medication with a wide spectrum of antibiotics (penicillin 3x/day) and painkillers was recommended. Postoperatively, no bleeding was

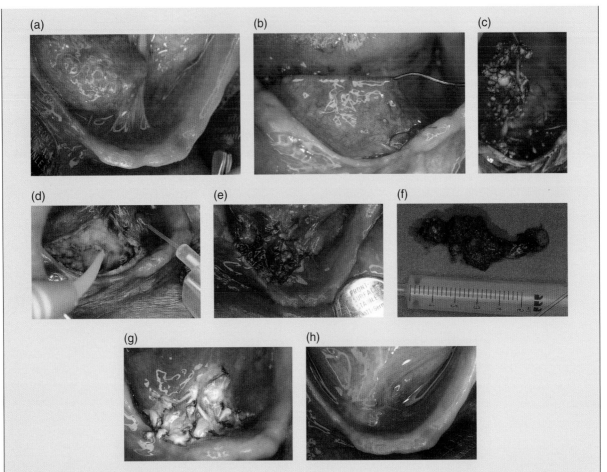

Figure 3.32 Soft tissue tumor in the mouth floor (a); a sialolith was not demonstrated radiographically. Demonstration of the duct with a dull needle (b); the tumor was excised in toto with the contact mode handpiece and at a power setting of 8–10 W (continuous wave) of a 980 nm diode laser (c, d); suturing of the wound margins with Vicryl absorbable material (e); the specimen (f) was examined histologically; Fibrin layer covers the wound (g); six weeks after surgery complete healing without scar tissue formation or sensory/functional disturbances was observed (h). *Source:* Dr. Georgios E Romanos.

observed. Only minor swelling was observed in the first three days (Figure 3.32e, f). The specimen (Figure 3.32g) was examined by an oral pathologist, who confirmed the diagnosis of an adenoma. The tissue was covered by fibrin during the first 10 days of healing. Six weeks after surgery there was complete healing without scar tissue formation or sensory/functional disturbances (Figure 3.32h).

3.5 Removal of Drug-Induced Gingival Hyperplasias and Epulides

3.5.1 Removal of Drug-Induced Gingival Hyperplasias

A gingival hyperplasia can be caused by systemic treatment with diphenylhydantoin-containing drugs (e.g. for epilepsy), cyclosporine-A (for immunosuppression after organ transplantations), calcium antagonists (for control of hypertension), and in particular nifedipine, but also diltiazem and amlodipine. A possible cause is the

dysfunctional collagen degradation as a result of a limited functional ability of the fibroblasts (Scully et al. 1996).

The gingival hyperplasia has, as a result, difficulties in plaque control and, if combined with insufficient oral hygiene, can lead to inflammatory reactions and further bone loss. The therapy of choice is the removal of the hyperplastic tissues. This is possible, according to the size of the hyperplasias, either with the CO_2 laser (Pick et al. 1985) alone, or in combination with Kirkland and Orban gingivectomy knives.

Initially, a measurement of the probing pocket depth with the Kaplan marking forceps allows determining the incision line. Two to three millimeters submarginal of this line, the incision will be initiated with the laser (see Figure 5.12 in chapter 5) in the focused mode. Because of the strong carbonization and the resulting hemostasis, the incision line is usually visible. For small-sized hyperplasias, the power of 4–6 W (CO_2 laser beam, CW) is sufficient for excellent cutting and coagulation. At the same time, the antimicrobial effect of the laser beam leads to a distinctive bacteria reduction in the entire surgical field (Pick et al. 1985; Pick 1993). For more extensive gingival hyperplasias, the excision is carried out in combination with conventional gingivectomy knives, in order to shorten the surgical procedure.

To protect the tooth surfaces, it is recommended (Neiburger and Miserendino 1988; Sievers et al. 1993) that metal matrix or special flat instruments (e.g. spatula, gingivectomy knives) be used, which can be placed within the periodontal pockets during excision. In order to control the potential risk of overheating due to the reflection of the laser beam from the metallic surfaces, other options have been recommended. Since the CO_2 laser beam is highly absorbed by wet surfaces, the use of a glycerin solution (or Vaseline®) over the tooth surface for further protection of the surrounding structures is strongly recommended.

After gingivectomy, the patients can be followed up in a strict recall program only when gingivoplasties can be successfully carried out with the help of a defocused laser beam, especially for medically compromised patients. The final hemostasis of the entire surgical area controls the bleeding and postoperative discomfort. The use of a periodontal pack (e.g. Coe-Pak, Peripak®) is not actually required. After approximately one week, new capillaries and blood vessels are formed. Two weeks after surgery wound healing is usually completed. If the medication can be substituted by another drug, no recurrences are expected. If a substitution is not possible, the regular application of the laser is of importance especially during whole periodontal maintenance appointments. From the clinical experience, three- to four-month intervals are recommended, where only topical anesthesia small, localized gingivectomies or gingivoplasties can be carried out.

The indication of the Nd:YAG, Er:YAG, or the diode lasers is in most cases restricted, since surgical procedures like that are time consuming and need also sufficient hemostasis. Therefore, the use of the CO_2 laser is in such cases strongly indicated.

3.5.2 Removal of Epulides

A frequent application of laser is performed for surgical removal of gingival epulides. As with the external gingivectomy, these lesions of the oral cavity can also be excised with the focused laser beam of CO_2, Nd:YAG, diode, or the Er:YAG laser. At the moment, there are no longitudinal studies to determine the long-term results after the removal of such tumors with different laser systems. The frequent recurrence after the removal of an epulis, without radical osteotomy of the adjacent bone and the extraction of the affected tooth, is given in the literature as between 5 and 70.6% (Giansanti and Waldron 1969; Eversole and Rovin 1972; Anderson et al. 1973; Benkert et al. 1982; Lee et al. 1986; Macleod and Soames 1987; Katsikeris et al. 1988; Mighell et al. 1995). A study of Gaspar and Szabo (1991) reported a recurrence rate of about only 7.9% after five years, if after the tumor excision with the CO_2-laser, an additional bone curettage and osseous decortication is carried out (Gaspar and Szabo 1991).

Clinical Cases

Removal of an Epulis Fibromatosa

A /6-year-old patient reported spontaneous bleeding from the interdental area #2–3 and a proliferation of the tissue especially in the last months (Figure 3.33a). A gingivectomy was carried out under local anesthesia with the pulsed Nd:YAG laser (power: 5 W, frequency: 50 Hz), and a curettage of the periodontal pocket was also accomplished (Figure 3.33b, c). Wound healing developed without any complications. Due to the better oral hygiene in this area, the clinical condition was improved and remained stable after six months (Figure 3.33d).

Removal of an Epulis Granulomatosa (Pregnancy Epulis)

A 58-year-old, nine-months pregnant patient complained about intense bleeding at the left site of the mandible, which was provoked during chewing. During the comprehensive clinical examination of the oral cavity, a gingival tumor (Figure 3.34a) was found. It had a size of 25 × 12 × 9 mm and was strongly inflamed, because of the excessive vascularization (Figure 3.34b). Directly next to that were two hopeless, asymptomatic teeth, which did not cause any problem to the patient. The patient was afraid of any

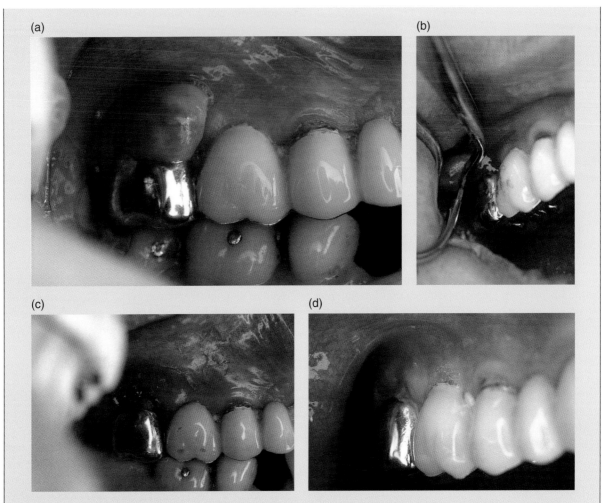

Figure 3.33 Epulis in the interdental area #2–3 (a). A gingivectomy was carried out under local anesthesia with the pulsed Nd:YAG laser (power: 5 W, frequency: 50 Hz), and a curettage of the periodontal pocket was also accomplished (b, c). Due to the better plaque control in this area, clinical improvement after six months was observed (d).

kind of treatment. The tumor was excised using only topical anesthesia with an Nd:YAG laser and average power of 4 W. The used glass fiber had a diameter of 300 μm. The tumor was removed completely and sent for histopathological examination. The surgical field was clearly visible during surgery, due to the good hemostasis. Two weeks postoperatively, a complete healing of the tissue could be observed (Figure 3.34c).

The remaining roots were extracted after the baby's delivery. The clinical diagnosis was confirmed histologically as an epulis granulomatosa. The strong vascularization of the connective tissue and the coagulation of the numerous vessels, due to the Nd:YAG laser's deep penetration, could be seen in the histopathological specimen (Figure 3.34d; see also Chapter 1, "Laser Tissue Interactions"; Figure 1.38).

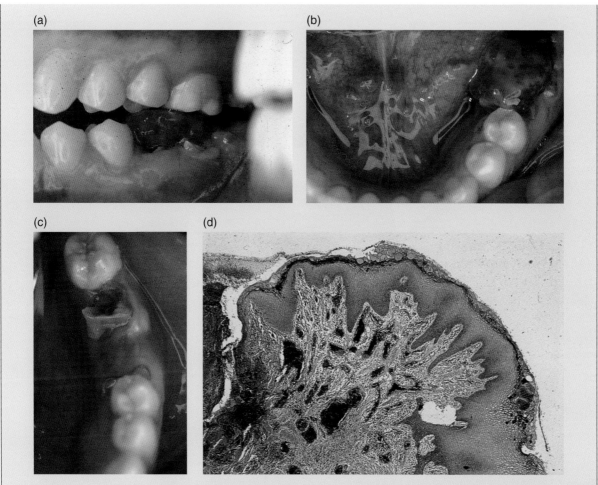

Figure 3.34 A gingival tumor in a buccal aspect and occlusal view (a, b). Directly next to that were two asymptomatic hopeless teeth. The tumor was excised under topical anesthesia with an Nd:YAG laser and average power of 4 W and a glass fiber with diameter of 300 µm. Two weeks postoperatively, a complete healing of the tissue could be observed (c). The histopathological evaluation of the specimen presented a strong vascularization of the connective tissue and coagulation of the numerous vessels, due to the Nd:YAG laser's deep penetration (d) and high absorption of hemoglobin.

3.6 Removal of Soft Tissue Cysts

Soft tissue cysts of the salivary glands (mucous retention cysts and extravasation cysts) are relatively common in the practice of the oral surgeons, particularly in relatively young patients. The cause is either trauma or obstruction of drainage ("retention" cysts) of the glandular excretory duct (Figure 3.35a), with a further retention or accumulation of saliva, or a cystic change of the duct position, thereby causing secretion accumulation into the gland ("extravasation" cysts). The surgical excision is under topical or local anesthesia if possible. A half-moon-shaped incision is usually performed on the roof of the cyst (Figure 3.35b). A blood-free continuous incision in the depth follows (Figure 3.35c). For this intervention the CO_2 as well as the Nd:YAG lasers are suitable.

With an average power of 4–6 W and continuous (for the CO_2 laser) or pulsed beam (for the Nd:YAG laser), a relatively quick incision is possible with good precision and quality. The blood-free surgical field allows clear differentiation between pathological and healthy tissues and enables a complete excision of the cyst, without any complications. After the complete removal of the cyst, an ablation of the excision borders (defocused beam) and the entire surgical field is recommended, so that postoperative pain, swelling, and other complications can be decreased (Figure 3.35d). The specimen is examined by an oral pathologist, who confirms the diagnosis (Figure 3.35e and f). In most cases healing by secondary intention will be performed with fibrin layer formation within the first 10 days (Figure 3.35g), and wound healing is uneventful after a couple of weeks (Figure 3.35h).

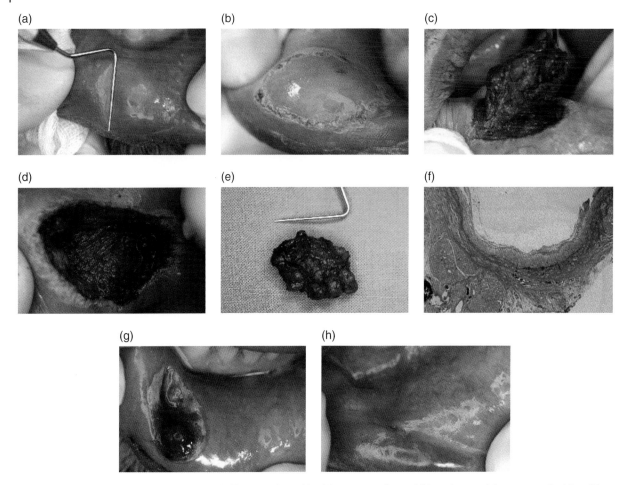

Figure 3.35 Mucocele of the low lip (a); a half-moon-shaped incision was performed (b) and an excision occurred with a CO_2 laser (c); a surgical field was presented with excellent hemostasis (d); the specimen (e) was examined by an oral pathologist who confirmed the diagnosis of a mucocele (f); the healing was done by secondary intention after 10 days (g) and after a couple of weeks with slight scar tissue formation (h). *Source:* Dr. Georgios E Romanos.

Clinical Cases

Removal of a Mucous Retention Cyst in the Lower Lip

A 25-year-old patient presented with a soft tissue lesion at her lower lip (Figure 3.36a). She reported a persistent swelling for approximately five weeks with slight pain on palpation. The clinical diagnosis was a mucus retention (salivary gland) cyst. After topical anesthesia the cyst was extirpated with a CO_2 laser.

As an alternative to the classical incision, before surgery an injection of an impression material can be applied into the cystic cavity, which changes the tissue color and differentiates normal from pathologic tissues. In addition, the removal of the mucoid saliva from the cyst is necessary by means of a trocar. After the setting time of the material, the incision is relatively easy, so that the cyst can be removed without complications (Figure 3.36b).

The average power of the CO_2 laser was 4 W (continuous wave) in a focused noncontact beam (Figure 3.36c). After the complete excision of the lesion, the entire surgical field was smoothed with a defocused laser beam (Figure 3.36c). Suturing was not required, and wound healing was uneventful. One week after surgery, a fibrin layer covered the surgical field. One month later, excellent wound closure without any complications and slight scar was observed (Figure 3.36d).

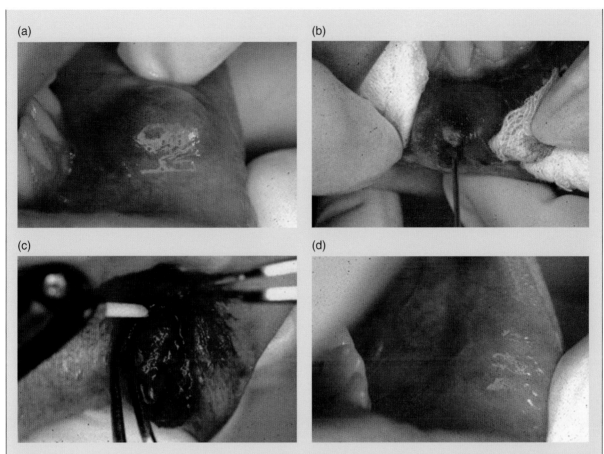

Figure 3.36 Mucus retention cyst of the lower lip (a). After topical anesthesia, an injection of an impression material was applied into the cystic cavity, changing tissue color in order to differentiate normal from pathologic tissues. The cyst was extirpated with a CO_2 laser and average power of 4 W (CW) in a focused noncontact beam (c). After the complete excision of the lesion, the entire surgical field was smoothed with a defocused handpiece (c). One month postoperatively, an excellent wound closure was observed (d). *Source:* Dr. Georgios E Romanos.

Removal of a Ranula

A 29-year-old female patient was referred by her dentist because of a swelling in the mouth floor on the left side (Figure 3.37a). She reported alternating pain for approximately one year. The clinical diagnosis was an extravasation cyst of the sublingual gland (ranula). Under local anesthesia, the excretory gland was demonstrated, and a plastic catheter was inserted and fixated with 4-0 silk. The excision of the ranula was performed with a CO_2 laser (average power: 6 W, CW) with special care to avoid injury of the gland duct. The surgical procedure was completed without bleeding (Figure 3.37b). Wound healing was performed without surgical complications. The catheter was removed after almost 10 days. Three weeks later, the incision area had no pathological findings or scar tissue formation (Figure 3.37c).

Intraoral Removal of an Epidermoid Cyst

A 56-year-old female patient came to the Department of Oral Surgery and Implant Dentistry at the University of Frankfurt, Germany, with swelling in her right cheek (Figure 3.38a) and sensitivity to palpation. The swelling was there for at least six months according to patient statement. Clinical evaluation showed a swelling (without liquid drainage) in the buccal oral mucosa with well-defined margins of the lesion. The examination showed also that the lesion was relatively subcutaneous, and the patient was referred to a dermatologist. She refused

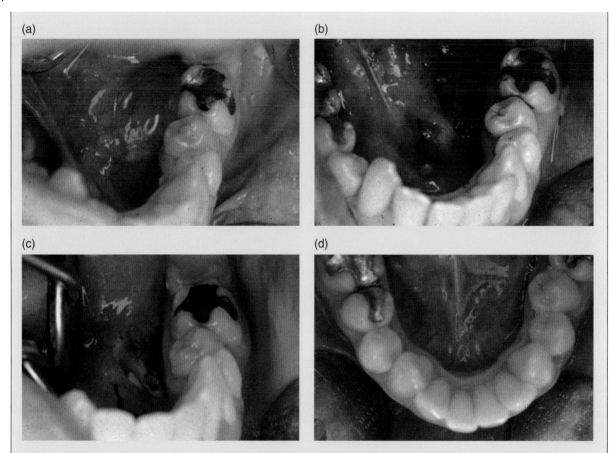

Figure 3.37 Extravasation cyst of the sublingual gland (a). A plastic catheter was inserted and fixated with 4-0 silk sutures (b). The excision of the ranula was performed with a CO_2 laser (average power: 6 W, CW) with special care to avoid injury of the gland duct (c). The surgical procedure was completed without bleeding. Three weeks later, the incision area had no pathological findings or scar tissue formation (d). *Source:* Dr. Georgios E Romanos.

the referral due to previous experience in a dermatology clinic, and she was not interested in having an extraoral incision. After an extensive informed consent about possible surgical complications, such as bleeding, swelling, infection, numbness, and motoric problems due to injury of the facial nerve, the patient accepted the treatment with removal of the lesion using intraoral incision. After local anesthesia, the excision was performed with the focused beam of the CO_2 laser and continuous wave mode (Figure 3.38b). The average power was 6 W in order to create an excellent hemostasis for a better dissection of the lesion. Careful dissection was performed under compression from the extraoral area of the cheek and a relative, large white lesion was completely removed (Figure 3.38c). After irrigation of the wound with saline, the wound margins were closed with conventional sutures (Figure 3.38d). The specimen (Figure 3.38e) was examined histologically. After four weeks of healing the oral mucosa showed an excellent condition without scar (Figure 3.38f). Postoperatively, the patient did not experience any complications, such as numbness or motoric damage of the facial nerve and was very happy with the final clinical outcome (Figure 3.38g). After histological examination, the lesion was diagnosed as an epidermoid cyst. Clinical photographic documentation in various movements of the lips and cheek were able to prove after three months an excellent result of the surgical procedure (Figure 3.38h–i) without motoric or sensation complications.

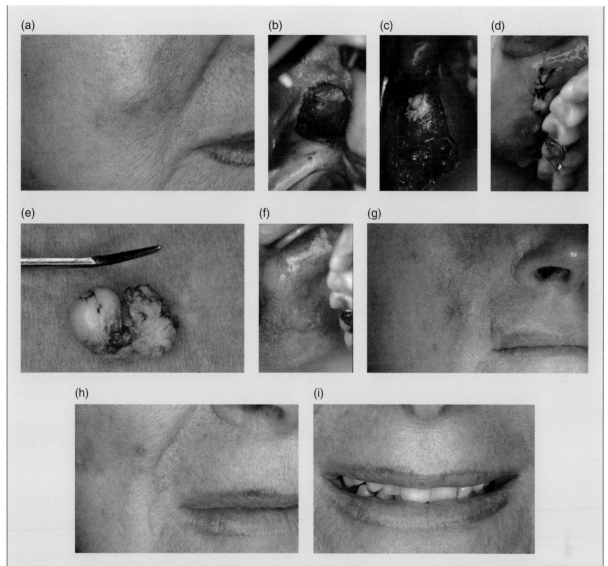

Figure 3.38 Swelling of the cheek (a) and sensitivity to palpation for at least six months. The excision was performed intraorally with the focused beam of the CO_2 laser and continuous wave mode (b). The average power of 6 W provided excellent hemostasis visibility during surgery without bleeding (c). The wound margins were closed with conventional sutures (d). Specimen for histological examination (e). After four weeks of healing the oral mucosa showed lack of scar tissue (f), no numbness or motoric complications from the facial nerve (g). Clinical photographic documentation after three months was able to prove the excellent clinical outcome (h, i). *Source:* Dr. Georgios E Romanos.

3.7 Frenectomies and Vestibuloplasties

There are indications for surgical removal of lip or tongue frenum especially for orthodontic, pre-prosthetic, and phonetic reasons. Vestibuloplasties serve as pre-prosthetic surgical procedures for improvement of denture retention. Denture stability and wearing comfort are improved by the relative increase of the height of the alveolar ridge. In comparison to conventional methods, surgical interventions with the CO_2, Nd:YAG, or diode lasers are associated with low intra- and postoperative complications and good wound healing.

3.7.1 Frenectomies

Labial or lateral frenum is indicated very often for surgical excision, when muscular attachments can negatively affect the periodontal condition of the adjacent teeth, speech, and also esthetics, especially in patients with a high smile line.

There are controversial aspects about the indication of the labial frenectomy when a median diastema is involved, and different authors suggest a frenectomy before orthodontic therapy (Edwards 1977; Zachrisson 2003).

However, there is common agreement between clinicians that frenectomy should be performed after complete eruption of the permanent canines, which determine the final position of the six anterior teeth and therefore may close the median diastema. According to the literature, this diastema may close in 96% of cases (AAP 1996). However, the frenum tension should be evaluated from the periodontal standpoint, and there is our recommendation for frenectomy if there is mobility of the attached gingiva of the teeth during function or if a speech therapist makes this suggestion.

The laser frenectomy can be performed with almost all different laser wavelengths. The clinician is advised to read carefully the laser-tissue interactions (Chapter 1) since tissue color and used laser wavelength determine power settings and certainly penetration within the tissue. This is significant in order to provide a clinical outcome without complications (Table 3.3).

An average power between 4–6 W is sufficient for frenectomies of the lip or lingual frenum with the CO_2 laser. Using the Nd:YAG laser, a power of 4 W should not

Table 3.3 Tissue color and relationship to laser wavelengths and power settings.

Tissue Color	Laser Wavelength	Power Settings
Whitish (under tension)	CO_2 laser	2–4 W (CW) or 4–6 W (pulsed)
Yellow	Diode lasers	3–5 W (CW) or 5–6 W (pulsed)
	Er:YAG laser	1.2–3 W, 20–30 Hz frequency
	Nd:YAG laser	1.5–3 W, 50–100 Hz frequency
Pink	CO_2 laser	3–5 W (CW) or 5–6 W (pulsed)
	Diode lasers	2–4 W (CW) or 3–5 W (pulsed)
	Er:YAG laser	1.5–5 W, 30–50 Hz frequency
	Nd:YAG laser	1.5–2.0 W, 50–100 Hz frequency

be exceeded in order to avoid pain and postoperative scar tissue formation. The incision design in a V-shape allows removing the muscular attachment over the periosteum creating a new established vestibule. Suturing is usually not necessary. The final tissue ablation in the entire surgical field allows a wound dressing, protecting the tissue from infections, as well as relief of postsurgical pain.

Clinical Cases

Removal of a Lingual Frenum

A 63-year-old male patient was referred for the removal of a pronounced lingual frenulum (Figure 3.39a), which led to a limited mobility of his tongue and slight speaking problems. With the CO_2 laser and a power of 4 W in a continuous mode, the lingual frenum was excised using only topical anesthesia. The excision was carried out using a V-shape incision (Figure 3.39b). Suturing was not necessary. After excision, the wound was coagulated with the defocused beam (Figure 3.39c). Bleeding and pain were absent. After two weeks only, a slight scar tissue was observed due to tongue mobility, but nevertheless did not affect the tongue movements (Figure 3.39d).

Removal of Frenum in the Maxilla and Mandible

The excision of the two frenula (Figure 3.40a, b) was performed, in order to have better soft tissue stability of a new fabricated full denture, in the maxilla and

mandible. The surgical procedure with the CO_2 laser (4 W, CW) under local anesthesia presented an excellent hemostasis (Figure 3.40c, d) and the follow-up after three weeks was uneventful (Figure 3.40e, f).

Frenectomy with CO_2 Laser

The excision was performed due to referral by a speech therapist, treating a young patient for two years (Figure 3.41a). The CO_2 laser with 2 W continuous wave focused beam was used to excise the frenulum in the mucogingival junction and to dissect the muscle attachment over the periosteum (Figure 3.41b). The surgical procedure was done using only topical anesthesia. The hemostasis was sufficient, and no additional sutures were required. After three days the tissue was healed without complications (Figure 3.41c). The patient came back after eight months for reevaluation (Figure 3.41d), and the speech therapist reported significant

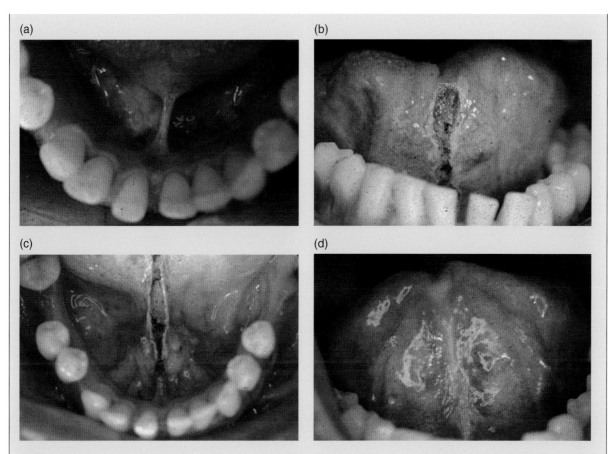

Figure 3.39 Excision of the lingual frenum (a) with a CO_2 laser (4 W; continuous mode) using a V-shape incision (b, c) and complication-free wound healing two weeks after surgery (d). *Source:* Dr. Georgios E Romanos.

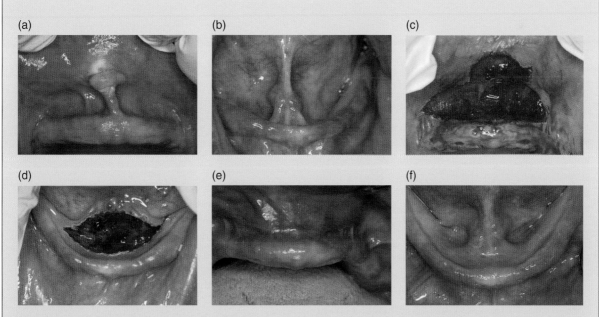

Figure 3.40 The excisions of the two frenula (a, b) in the maxilla and the mandible were performed with the CO_2 laser (4 W, CW) with an excellent coagulation (c, d); follow-up after three weeks was uneventful without scar tissue formation (e, f). *Source:* Dr. Georgios E Romanos.

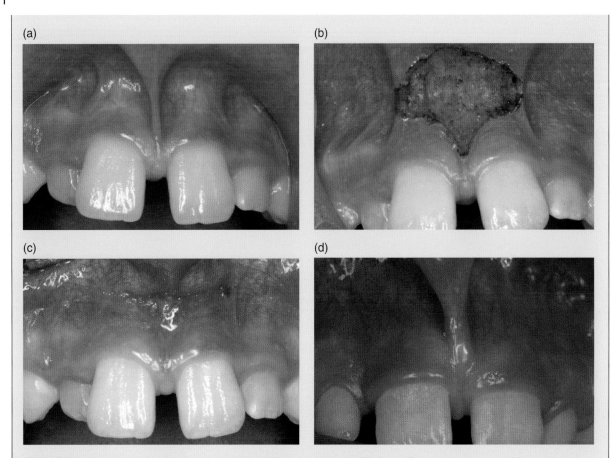

Figure 3.41 Tight frenum in the anterior maxilla (a). Excision with the CO_2 laser (2 W, continuous wave, focused beam) with dissection of the muscle attachment (b). After three days, the tissue was healed without complications (c). Follow up after eight months without complications (d). *Source:* Dr. Georgios E Romanos.

improvement in the speaking ability of the patient after laser surgery.

Frenectomy of Labial Frenum with a Diode-Pumped Nd:YAG Laser

The chief complaint of the patient was an esthetic problem in the anterior teeth due to a high smile line and papilla overgrowth at #8–9 (Figure 3.42a). The clinical examination showed excessive labial frenum and close relationship to the labial papilla in this area. The excision of the labial frenum was performed using a focused diode-pumped Nd:YAG laser (1064 nm; Diodium®, Weil Dental, Rosbach, Germany) with a glass fiber and in contact with the tissue during excision (Figure 3.42b). The average power was 4 W, in a pulsed mode with a frequency of 400 Hz under local anesthesia. The laser was able to sufficiently coagulate the surgical field (Figure 3.42c). After four days the healing was uneventful, and no complications were associated with the procedure (Figure 3.42d).

Frenectomy in the Mandible with a Diode (810 nm) Laser

An excision of the labial frenulum (Figure 3.43a) was performed in order to prepare the bed for further implant placement. A focused 810 nm diode laser was used with initiated fiber, in contact with the tissue during excision. The average power was 3 W (CW) under local anesthesia. The laser was able to sufficiently coagulate the surgical site (Figure 3.43b). The muscle fibers were transferred apically using a wet gauze especially close to the mental nerve for better visualization of the anatomical structures before final coagulation (Figure 3.43c). After seven days the healing was uneventful, and no complications were observed.

Frenectomy in the Anterior Maxilla with a Diode (810 nm) Laser

The excision of the labial frenum (Figure 3.44a) was performed in order to improve plaque control and to reduce the gingival recession of the adjacent

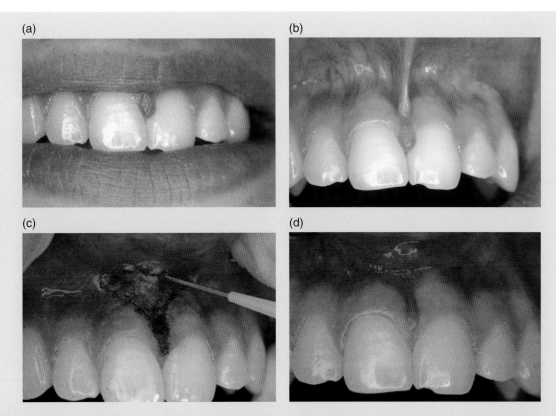

Figure 3.42 Hypertrophic papilla creating esthetic problems for the patient (a). The labial frenum was excised (c) using a focused diode-pumped Nd:YAG laser with a glass fiber and in contact with the tissue (average power: 4 W, pulsed mode; frequency: 400 Hz). The laser was able to coagulate sufficiently the surgical site. After four days, the healing was uneventful (d). *Source:* Dr. Georgios E Romanos.

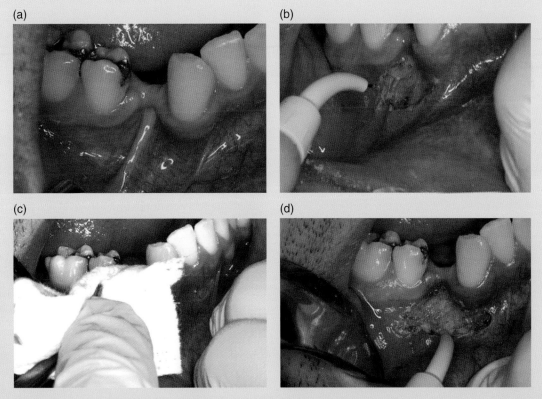

Figure 3.43 Excision of the labial frenulum (a) with a focused 810 nm diode laser and initiated fiber (average power: 3 W, CW). The muscle fibers were transferred apically using a wet gauze (c), close to the mental nerve for better visualization of the anatomical structures before final coagulation (d). *Source:* Dr. Georgios E Romanos.

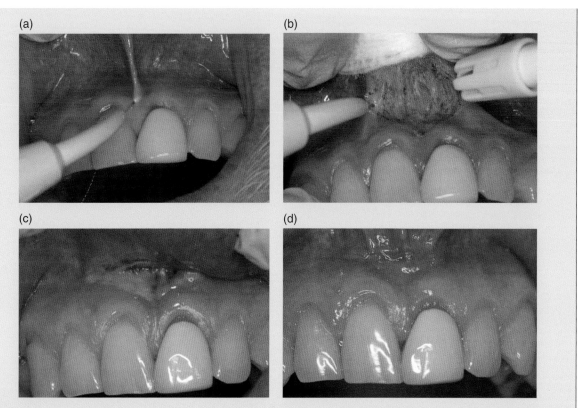

Figure 3.44 Excision of the labial frenum (a) using a focused 810 nm diode laser with initiated fiber, in contact with the tissue during excision. The average power was 2 W (CW) providing sufficient bleeding control (b). A fibrin layer covered the wound four days after surgery (c) and showed a complete healing two weeks after surgery (d). *Source:* Dr. Georgios E Romanos.

teeth due to the tension of the marginal attached gingiva (#8, 9). A focused 810 nm diode laser was used with initiated fiber, in contact with the tissue during excision. The average power was 2 W (CW) under local anesthesia. The laser was able to sufficiently coagulate the surgical site (Figure 3.44b). After four days the healing was uneventful with a fibrin layer covering the wound (Figure 3.44c). Complete healing was observed two weeks after surgery (Figure 3.44d).

3.7.2 Vestibuloplasties

Vestibuloplasties are surgical procedures indicated to improve the depth of the vestibule in the maxilla and/or mandible (pre-prosthetic surgical interventions). These procedures are performed to increase the retention of partial or full dentures allowing better adaptation of the denture flange to the alveolar ridge after dissection of the muscular attachment. Since the height of the alveolar ridge is increased, such procedures can be considered as "relative augmentations."

The problem of the relapse of the vestibule depth is the main complication after this kind of procedure and was studied many years ago (Szaba 1916).

Considering that the primary goal in the vestibuloplasty is the increase of the vestibule depth, the incision can be performed in the deepest part of the vestibule.

However, the simultaneous increase of the width of keratinized mucosa should be considered since this can be a benefit in case of a later implant placement. From the periodontal standpoint, the recommendation is to make the incision at the mucogingival margin as a partial thickness flap.

The wound will be left either to heal by secondary intention or will be covered by a soft tissue graft (autogenous free gingival, skin graft or also allograft). Numerous studies show that the recurrence (relapse) is frequent especially after vestibuloplasty with secondary intension in the mandible (almost 100% rebound) (Baumann 1976; Hillerup 1980) but only 50% in the maxilla (Neidhardt 1963; Lambrecht and Härle 2003).

Specifically, early clinical observations especially from Europe showed that the vestibuloplasty in the mandible without the use of a skin graft is not indicated due to complete recurrence and scar tissue formation (Obwegeser 1965; Baumann 1976; Lambrecht and Härle 2003).

The healing of the wound after vestibuloplasty, with secondary epithelialization (intention) was studied in dogs. The focus of this study was the nature of the relapse. The attachment of new mucosa (gained from secondary epithelialization of the periosteum) to the bone eventually becomes loose in the muscle-bearing region of the jaw. Based on this study, the detached muscles reinsert into scar tissue near their preoperative attachment. Thus, the relapse seems to be the result of muscle reattachment, loosening of new mucosa, and an interaction of wound contraction. Other surgical techniques were recommended, such as the use of grafting of skin or mucosa to the periosteal wound as a logical approach to the prevention of this relapse (Hillerup 1980, 1987).

Further clinical studies compared two vestibuloplasty methods and a muscle-formed method for improving the retention and stability of complete mandibular dentures in 19 edentulous patients with advanced mandibular bone resorption. The resorptive changes in the alveolar ridge and any potential relapse in the extended vestibule depth after surgery were monitored for two years. Simultaneous production of the first new complete dentures, to which the labial plate is delivered after the surgical procedure, and fixated with circumferential wiring around the mandible during primary healing showed the best surgical and prosthetic results. A muscle-formed method for extending the base of a complete mandibular denture was found to be a useful alternative for patients with highly advanced mandibular bone resorption (Kotiranta et al. 1986).

The CO_2 laser is particularly suitable for these surgical procedures because of its good incision quality and the relative short surgical time. The muscular attachment will be excised over the periosteum in order to create an optimal extension of the vestibule depth. This improves the mechanical retention of the prosthesis. The maximum power of dental CO_2 lasers is usually 10W in the continuous mode even though there is no need for high power settings for this procedure. The incision is carried out with the noncontact handpiece. The charring (with a defocused beam) of the entire surgical area allows good hemostasis and visualization during the procedure as well as a wound dressing.

In a previous study with 27 patients requiring soft tissue pre-prosthetic surgery, the surgical carbon dioxide laser was used to vaporize soft tissues on an ambulatory basis causing little bleeding, pain, swelling, or wound contraction. The laser was evaluated on vestibuloplasties and demonstrated no postoperative bleeding or infections. Swelling was minimal and pain, as measured

on a linear pain scale, was moderate. One third of the patients required no analgesics. Wound contraction did occur but was less than is historically quoted for scalpel wounds (Pogrel 1989).

In comparison to the CO_2 laser, the diode lasers provide better hemostasis. Although the Nd:YAG laser allows excellent coagulation, it has the risk of scar tissue formation and is associated with a longer operation period.

After surgery, with an intact periosteum, the mobile mucosa will be immobilized with sutures in the deepest point of the vestibular fold. The flanges of the existing denture will be extended to provide compression of the underlying tissues and relined to use as a surgical stent for 7 to 10 days. Special postsurgical measures are in general not necessary. Routine oral hygiene is adequate thereafter. Four weeks later, there are normally no pathological conditions observed. Postsurgical bleeding or swelling do not usually appear. The pain is significantly reduced in comparison to conventional (or electrosurgical) procedures and can be successfully controlled, if necessary, using pain killers.

- In cases, where an increase of the width of keratinized mucosa is indicated, the incision line will be performed at the border between keratinized and not keratinized mucosa.
- If there is no keratinized mucosa, the incision is initiated in the middle of the alveolar crest. After the separation of the existing muscle fibers from the underlying periosteum, a partial thickness flap lingually as well as in the buccal extension provides an excellent recipient site for a graft harvested from the palate. The graft fixation succeeds by sutures or topical tissue adhesive (Histoacryl®, Braun Medical Inc., Bethlehem, PA, USA). In this case the carbonization of the recipient site should be avoided in order to allow sufficient blood supply and nutrition of the graft. For this purpose, a careful removal of the superficial tissue layer should be performed with wet (soaked in saline) gauze or cotton swabs. The carbonization (charring) of the donor site is recommended to establish good hemostasis and control postoperative complications.

During the preparation of a partial thickness flap and dissection of the attached muscle fibers, a safety zone from the underlying alveolar bone is absolutely necessary in order to avoid bone exposure and dehiscence. Therefore, regular bone sounding with a dull probe is recommended during surgery. If it comes to a bone exposure and carbonization of the bone, the superficial layer of the bone should be curetted carefully, and the wound will heal by secondary intention. In case of larger dehiscence, an additional dressing with local antibiotics is indicated.

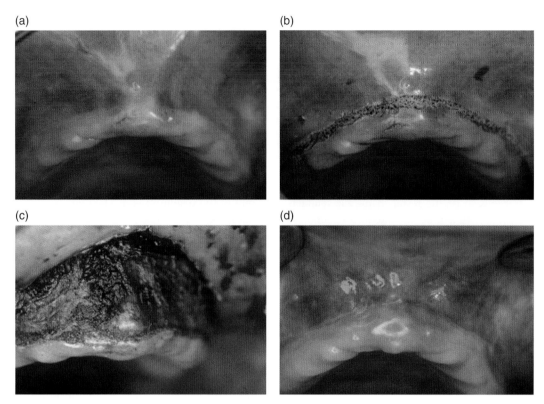

Figure 3.45 Insufficient vestibule in the maxilla (a) associated with lack of retention for the upper full denture. Incision was performed at the mucogingival junction with a CO_2 laser (b). Superficial coagulation to create a type of wound dressing and control postoperative bleeding and discomfort (c). The clinical situation after approximately six weeks after surgery was not associated with pathological findings or recurrence (d). *Source:* Dr. Georgios E Romanos.

Clinical Cases

Vestibuloplasty in the Maxilla

A 75-year-old female patient with maxillary full denture and insufficient retention was referred by her general dentist requesting increase in the height of the alveolar ridge in order to provide better retention of the prosthesis (Figure 3.45a). Several attempts to improve the denture stability were not successful. The incision was performed with a CO_2 laser under local anesthesia between the keratinized and non-keratinized mucosa (Figure 3.45b). The preparation and separation of the muscle fibers in a width of at least 10 mm were carried out in the continuous mode (CW) and with an average power of 8–10 W. The entire surgical field was finally coagulated to create a wound dressing in order to avoid postoperative bleeding and discomfort (Figure 3.45c). The flanges of the existing denture were extended immediately after surgery, and the base was soft relined. Pain medication was prescribed after surgery, and cooling of the extraoral region was advised for the first three to four days. No antibiotics were prescribed. The wound healing

developed without complications. A fibrin layer covered the entire surgical area one day after the procedure and was present for the first 7 to 10 postoperative days. The clinical condition was without pathological findings after approximately four weeks and after six weeks remained without recurrence (Figure 3.45d). The new prosthesis was fabricated by the general dentist with high retention.

Vestibuloplasty in the Maxilla

This case presents a 62-year-old patient with insufficient stability of his full denture due to insufficient vestibule depth (Figure 3.46a). After incision (under local anesthesia) with the noncontact handpiece of a CO_2 laser and an average power between 6–10 W (CW), the tissue was separated from the underlying attached muscle fibers with simultaneous coagulation of the blood vessels and capillaries. The mucosa was then fixated in a new, more apical position, using absorbable polyglactin pins (Figure 3.46b). The new denture was fabricated within the next two weeks.

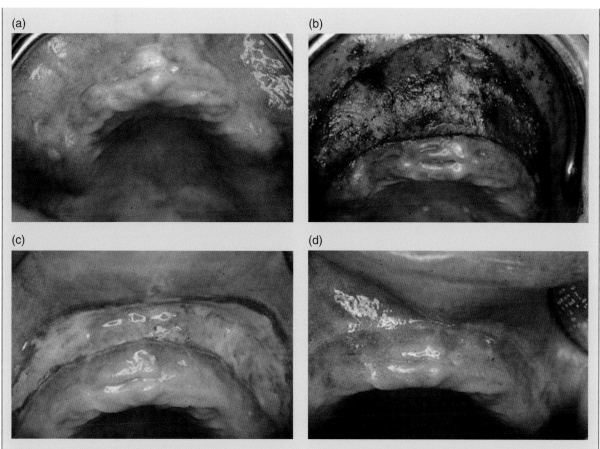

Figure 3.46 Lack of vestibule depth before surgery (a); the incision was performed with a noncontact handpiece of a CO_2 laser (average power: 6-10 W, CW), separating the underlying attached muscle fibers from the periosteum with simultaneous coagulation of the blood vessels (b); fibrin layer covered the wound surface seven days after surgery (c). At the three month-follow up, the tissue was free of scar or muscular reattachment (recurrence), and an increased vestibule depth allowed the retention of the full denture (d). *Source:* Dr. Georgios E Romanos.

Bleeding, swelling, and intense pain were absent. In the first days after surgery, fibrin covered the entire wound surface (Figure 3.46c). After approximately three months, the tissue was free of scar or muscular attachment (recurrence), and no pathological findings were observed (Figure 3.46d).

Vestibuloplasty with a Diode (980 nm) Laser as a Complication of Wrong Power Settings

The 49-year-old patient was referred with the request of vestibuloplasty in the mandible (Figure 3.47a). The mucosa was dissected at the height of the mucogingival junction (Figure 3.47b) with the diode laser (980 nm) and a maximum power of 12 W and frequency of 10 pps (pulse duration: 0.3 seconds). After separation of the muscle fibers, the entire wound was coagulated. A fibrin layer was formed after one week (Figure 3.47c). After three months, no pathological findings were found except an extensive scar tissue

without significant improvement of the vestibule depth (Figure 3.47d). This can be considered as a complication due to the use of high-power diode laser.

Vestibuloplasty to Increase Keratinized Tissue Width with a Nd:YAG Laser

A frenectomy (Figure 3.48a) was performed without local (only topical) anesthesia in a male patient (60 years old) in area #20–21 in combination with routine periodontal treatment of the teeth #20–23. The Nd:YAG laser was used with 30 pps frequency and 2.0 W power in contact fiber (focused beam) to remove the frenum, which was the reason for the reduced amount of the attached, keratinized gingiva of the teeth #20, 21 (Figure 3.48b). There was no bleeding during the entire postoperative period. The clinical situation after one month was very good with no tension in the attached mucosa, and the keratinized gingiva in the healed area was continuously increased

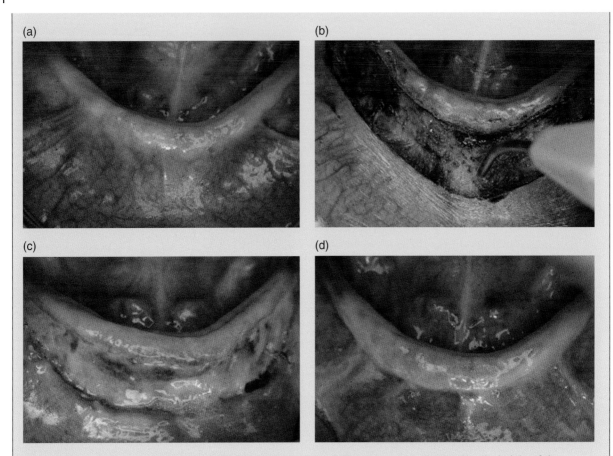

Figure 3.47 Insufficient depth of the vestibule in the mandible (a). The mucosa was dissected at the height of the mucogingival junction (b) with the diode laser (980 nm) and a maximum power of 12 W and 10 pps (pulse duration: 0.3 seconds). After separation of the muscle fibers, the entire wound was coagulated. A fibrin layer was formed after one week (c). After three months, an extensive scar was observed without improvement of the vestibule depth (d). *Source:* Dr. Georgios E Romanos.

(Figure 3.48c). After periodontal treatment of the remaining teeth and crown preparation (including post and core) of the premolars, the clinical situation presented an excellent soft tissue healing.

Vestibuloplasty with an Er:YAG Laser

The vestibuloplasty using an Er:YAG laser may be performed under local anesthesia using pulsed mode and power settings, such as 250 mJ and 10 Hz. The tissue could be excised easily, but the hemostasis is usually not adequate compared to other laser wavelengths, such as the CO_2, diode, or Nd:YAG lasers (Figure 3.49).

Vestibuloplasties in Conjunction with Soft Tissue Tumors

A 94-year-old patient presented with insufficient vestibule depth in the maxilla and mandible including presence of a large soft tissue tumor covering the entire alveolar ridges (Figure 3.50a). The patient was referred by his dentist for tumor removal and pre-prosthetic therapy in order to be able to get new full dentures. The excision occurred under antibiotic therapy (2 g Amoxicillin one hour before surgery) in two different sessions. For the surgical procedure in the maxilla, under local anesthesia, a noncontact handpiece of the CO_2 laser (6 W, CW)

(a)
(b)

(c)

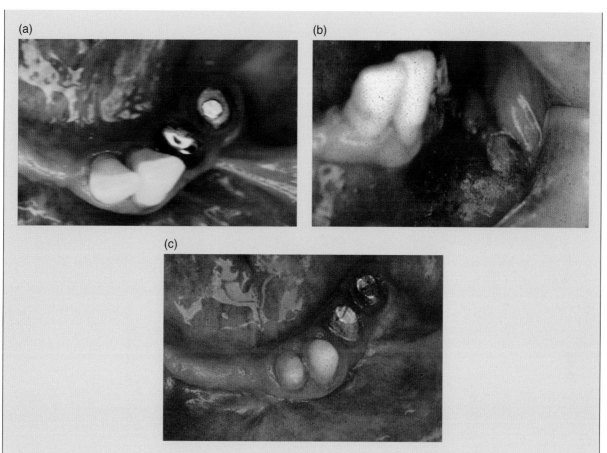

Figure 3.48 A frenectomy (a) was performed using a pulsed Nd:YAG laser (2.0 W power, 30 pps frequency) in contact with the tissue. No bleeding was observed during surgery (b); the clinical situation after one month presented no tension of the attached mucosa and the keratinized gingiva width was improved (c). *Source:* Dr. Georgios E Romanos.

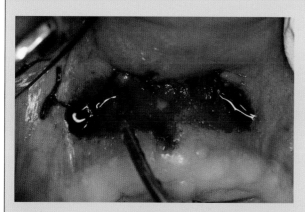

Figure 3.49 Vestibuloplasty with an Er:YAG laser. Observe the insufficient bleeding control. *Source:* Dr. Georgios E Romanos.

marked the incision line (at the mucogingival junction) (Figure 3.50b), and the tumor was separated from the periosteum (Figure 3.50c). The hemostasis was adequate using these power settings. The apical margin of the partial flap was fixed in place with 4-0 silk suture material (Figure 3.50d). The specimen (Figure 3.50e) was sent to an oral, maxillofacial pathologist to confirm the clinical diagnosis. One week after surgery, no postoperative complications were reported, and a thick fibrin layer covered the entire wound surface (Figure 3.50f). The patient was followed up after two weeks to remove the sutures (Figure 3.50g), and two months later (Figure 3.50h) wound healing was completed and the patient was referred to his general dentist for fabrication of new full dentures.

Similarly, the protocol in the mandible was performed using a 980 nm diode laser (Spectra laser) providing excellent bleeding control and healing without complications (Figure 3.51).

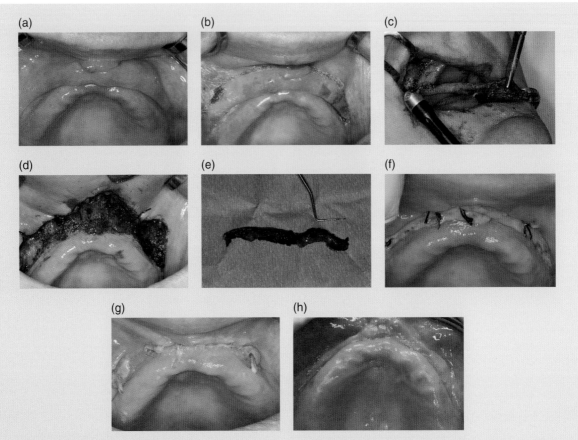

Figure 3.50 Insufficient vestibule depth in the maxilla including soft tissue tumor covering the entire alveolar ridge (a); for this surgical procedure, a noncontact CO_2 laser (6 W, CW) beam marked the incision at the mucogingival junction (b); the tumor was separated from the underlying periosteum using the focused beam (c); the apical margin of the partial flap was fixed in place with 4-0 silk suture material (d); the specimen was sent to an oral, maxillofacial pathologist (e); one week after surgery (f) fibrin covered the entire wound. The patient was followed up after two weeks for suture removal (g) and two months later wound healing was completed (h). *Source:* Dr. Georgios E Romanos.

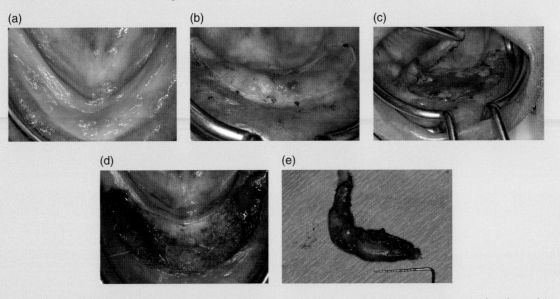

Figure 3.51 Insufficient vestibule depth in the mandible due to the presence of a soft tissue tumor covering the entire alveolar ridge (a); for the surgical procedure a contact diode laser (980 nm; 4 W, CW) beam with initiated tip, marked the incision at the mucogingival junction (b); the tumor was separated from the underlying periosteum (c); the entire wound bed was coagulated using the defocused beam (d); the specimen was sent to an oral, maxillofacial pathologist (e). *Source:* Dr. Georgios E Romanos.

Vestibuloplasty in Conjunction with Soft Tissue Tumor Using a CO₂ Laser

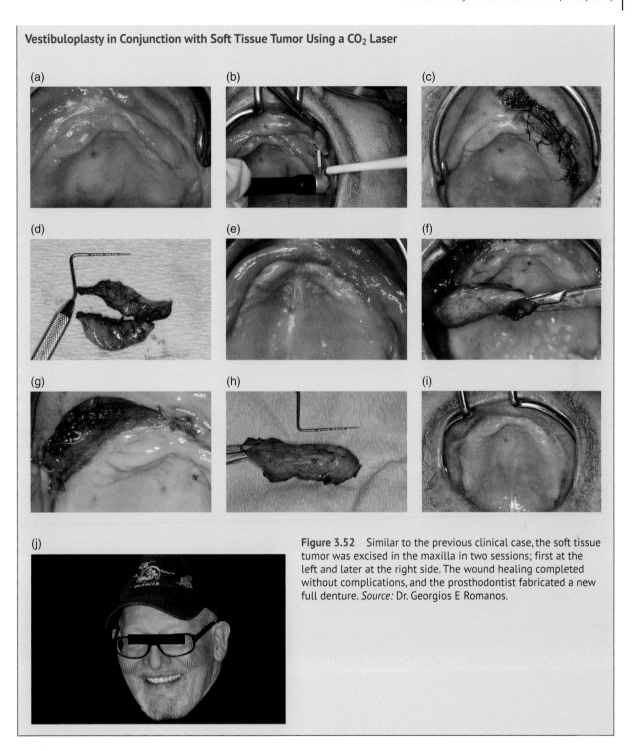

(a)

(b)

(c)

(d)

(e)

(f)

(g)

(h)

(i)

(j)

Figure 3.52 Similar to the previous clinical case, the soft tissue tumor was excised in the maxilla in two sessions; first at the left and later at the right side. The wound healing completed without complications, and the prosthodontist fabricated a new full denture. *Source:* Dr. Georgios E Romanos.

3.8 Removal of Precancerous Lesions (Leukoplakia)

Leukoplakia of the oral mucosa is defined, according to the World Health Organization (WHO), as a white, non-wipeable alteration of the mucosa, which cannot be characterized clinically or pathologically as any other pathologies. Leukoplakia is considered to be a common oral premalignant lesion (Pindborg 1980; Silvermann et al. 1984).

They can be subdivided in:

- simple form (the so-called leukoplakia simplex)
- verrucous form and
- erosive form

Histologically, leukoplakia is subdivided according to the dysplasia grade in four different groups, namely slight, moderate, and extreme dysplasia of the epithelium. The fourth stage is the so-called carcinoma in situ, which is characterized by an extensive differentiation of the cells, but without perforation of the basement membrane. Malignant transformations were described in up to 43% of cases (Vesper 1996). The mouth floor and the margin of the tongue are especially high-risk regions because the most malignant transformations are discovered here (Dunsche et al. 1994).

A correct and early-as-possible diagnosis, the respective therapy measures, wound healing follow-up, and effective aftercare are essential for successful treatment.

As therapy measures, reported in the literature are conventional surgical measures, cryosurgery, and drug therapy with vitamin A compounds (Mincer et al. 1972; Sako et al. 1972; Hausamen 1973, 1974; Schettler and Koch 1976; Esser 1979). The CO_2 laser provides a therapeutic alternative, which allows a removal of the leukoplakia without complications, also in difficult-to-access regions (Horch et al. 1983; Roodenburg et al. 1983; Gerlach et al. 1993; Dunsche et al. 1994). Smaller leukoplakia lesions can be removed easily with various laser systems, whereas the excision of wider lesions is better with the CO_2 laser (see also case presentation "Removal of a leukoplakia of the gingiva"). Also, diode lasers (810 nm) have been used for the removal of homogenous oral leukoplakia and reticular oral lichen planus without any postoperative complications, and it was concluded that the laser may prevent the risk of malignant transformation (Arora et al. 2018).

Prior to the actual surgical procedure, a small biopsy should be taken from the clinically suspected regions to confirm clinical diagnosis. After confirmation of the clinical diagnosis, the actual surgical laser treatment may be performed.

The treatment occurs usually under local anesthesia. The ablation of the affected oral mucosa occurs with the defocused, noncontact laser beam and an average power of 4–6 W. The surfaces, which are superficially carbonized from the laser treatment, are removed in layers using a wet gauze, in order to visualize the laser effect on the underlying tissues (complete removal of the epithelium). Finally, the whole surgical field will be coagulated for hemostasis and to control postoperative pain.

For the first three postoperative days, soft/liquid food is recommended. The diet should be followed carefully, so that the charring remains as long as possible in place, in order to avoid wound healing complications and eventually scar tissue formation or wound contraction. Painkillers are usually sufficient for pain relief.

Depending on the size of the lesion, the formation of the new epithelium is concluded within two to four weeks.

The advantages of the CO_2 laser for the removal of leukoplakia in the oral cavity are reported in the international literature (Horch et al. 1983, 1986; Horch 1992; Dunsche et al. 1994). The CO_2 laser is superior in comparison to conventional methods because it results in greater pain reduction, good intra- and postsurgical hemostasis, and the lack of functional impairment. Follow-ups have also clinically confirmed complete lesion removal (Romanos and Nentwig 1997a). In comparison to scalpel excision, CO_2 laser surgery is associated with less scar tissue formation (Tambuwala et al. 2014).

After the removal of a wide leukoplakia, no dressing is necessary. This results in a clearly diminished surgical time and avoidance of a second intervention in the donor's site.

Although most authors recommend a high power of 15–20 W (Seifert and Burkhardt 1977; Horch et al. 1983; Roodenburg et al. 1983, 1991; Gerlach et al. 1993) for the treatment of leukoplakia. Dunsche et al. (1994) were able to successfully treat leukoplakia using a power of 3–5 W. From our clinical experience, good results can be achieved with a power of 4–6 W and therefore, there is no need of the use of CO_2 lasers in private practice with power higher than 10 W. Our success rate of 84% (Romanos and Nentwig 1997a) is comparable to the results of other multicenter studies such as Gerlach et al. (1993), although in this study the size of the lesion played no significant role. Vesper (1996) reported a success rate of 100% within six months from the removal of wide lesions with a power of 10 W.

In comparison to the conventional methods of treatment or systemic use of vitamin A, which are associated with a recurrence rate from up to 34% or respectively 55%, the laser use is clearly more effective (Mincer et al. 1972; Schettler and Koch 1976).

Delayed wound healing due to thermal effects from the laser application (Horch and Rehrmann 1978; Fisher et al. 1983; Horch et al. 1983; Fisher and Frame 1984; Grossenbacher 1985; Rossmann et al. 1987; Goultschin et al. 1988; Keller et al. 1990) is nevertheless better than the that resulting from cryosurgery (Table 3.4).

The low recurrence rate, the relatively easy use of the CO_2 laser, and the healing process without complications make this procedure the therapy of first choice. Dental CO_2 lasers (with relative low power) can be used successfully for leukoplakia removal in clinical settings.

Table 3.4 Studies on leukoplakia removal and recurrence rate.

Study	Method	Leukoplakia Size	Follow-up	Recurrence
Horch et al. (1983)	15–20W (CO_2)	small and big	9 months	21.9%
Roodenburg et al. (1983)	15–20W (CO_2)	small and big	36 months	6.9%
Frame (1985)	10W (CO_2)	small and big	29 months	2.6%
Gerlach et al. (1993)	15–20W (CO_2)	small and big	46.4 months	14.2%
Dunsche et al. (1994)	3–5W (CO_2)	small and big	21 months	0%
Vesper (1996)	10W (CO_2)	big	6 months	12%
Romanos and Nentwig (1997a)	4–7W (CO_2)	big	27 months	17.4%
Mincer et al. (1972)	scalpel	small and big	18 months	34%
Hausamen (1973)	cryosurgery	small and big	18 months	0%

Clinical Cases

Removal of a Verrucous Leukoplakia in the Alveolar Ridge

This case presents an 85-year-old patient with a total prostheses. She was referred by her general dentist with the request of diagnosis and treatment of a white, non-wipeable alteration of her hard palate and alveolar ridge at #1–4. The size of the lesion was approximately 1.8 × 4.0 cm. The diagnosis was, according to the clinical and histopathological examination (a biopsy was performed before complete removal), of a verrucous leukoplakia without dysplasia (Figure 3.53a). The lesion was removed layer by layer under local anesthesia with a defocused laser beam of the CO_2 laser and with a power of 5 W in the continuous mode (Figure 3.53b, c). The tissue was finally coagulated. Wound healing completed without severe pain, swelling, or bleeding within a period of three weeks (Figure 3.53d), and no recurrence was observed after 2.5 years (Figure 3.53e).

Removal of Multiple Leukoplakia Lesions

This case demonstrated a flat and verrucous leukoplakia of the tongue (Figure 3.54a), the mouth floor (Figure 3.54b), and the palate of a 55-year-old female patient. In the last approximately eight years, she had noticed such alterations of her oral mucosa, but a clear diagnosis was not confirmed. The patient was eventually referred to our clinic by her general dentist for diagnosis and further treatment. Small biopsies were taken to confirm the clinical diagnosis of verrucous leukoplakia at the tongue and the mouth floor. After that, the leukoplakia was removed with the defocused CO_2 laser and with a power between 4–6 W in the continuous mode (noncontact) (Figure 3.54c, d). After one week, a fibrin layer covered the wound (Figure 3.54e), and superficial necrotic tissue (thermal damage) could be observed at the areas where high power was used. After approximately three months, excellent healing without any pathological findings was observed (Figure 3.54f). The clinical result remained stable and recurrence-free for the entire observation period of five years when the patient was seen for the last time (Figure 3.54g, h).

Removal of a Leukoplakia in the Gingiva

A 62-year-old patient was referred for removal of a leukoplakia at the attached gingiva in the area #20–21. A previous sample biopsy confirmed the clinical diagnosis (Figure 3.55a). The lesion was ablated under topical anesthesia with the noncontact CO_2 laser and a power of 4 W in the continuous mode. During irradiation, the laser was used in a defocused beam (ablative mode) at a distance of approximately 4–5 mm from the tissue (Figure 3.55b). At the same time, the tissue was strongly coagulated to ensure the complete ablation of the pathologic epithelial surface. The charred field of the lesion was removed with wet gauze, and the underlying layer was superficially coagulated. Postoperative complications, such as postoperative bleeding and pain, were not observed. The use of a periodontal dressing was not required. The healing process occurred without complications. Three days after the surgery, a fibrin layer was formed and remained for another 10 days (Figure 3.55c). One month after surgery, the situation remained without recurrence (Figure 3.55d).

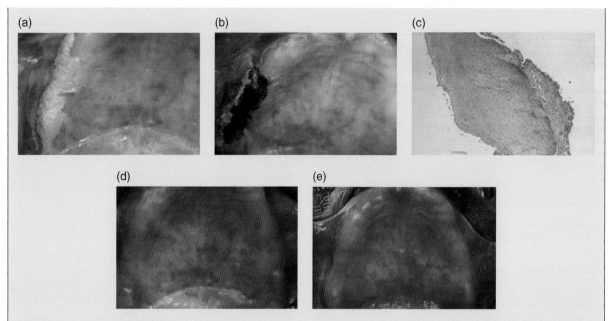

Figure 3.53 Oral leukoplakia in the alveolar ridge of the maxilla before excision (a), during excision presenting an excellent hemostasis (b), and the histological specimen under light microscope confirming the clinical diagnosis of simple leukoplakia (c). Wound healing without recurrence after three weeks (d) and after 2.5 years (e). *Source:* Dr. Georgios E Romanos.

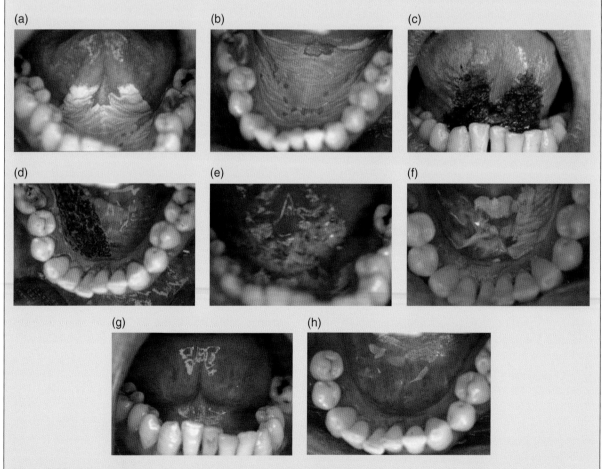

Figure 3.54 Oral leukoplakia of the tongue (a) and mouth floor (b); charring after removal with a CO_2 laser to ensure the complete removal of the epithelial cells (c, d); this carbonized layer was removed immediately after surgery to ensure bleeding of the underlying tissue (connective tissue exposure ensures that the complete epithelial cells have been removed; thermal effect with necrosis after one week (e, f) and after five years (g, h). *Source:* Dr. Georgios E Romanos.

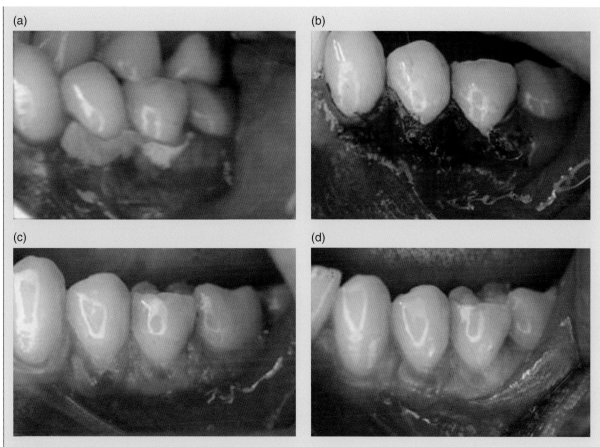

Figure 3.55 Leukoplakia of the gingiva (a); removal of the lesion using a CO_2 laser (b); complete healing of the surgical site after 10 days (c) and after four weeks (d). *Source:* Dr. Georgios E Romanos.

Removal of Leukoplakia in the Periodontal Tissues with Recurrence

A 76-year-old female patient was referred for diagnosis and treatment of excessive leukoplakia of the keratinized gingiva in the anterior teeth of the mandible. The lesion was extended within the periodontal pockets of the teeth (Figure 3.56a) and was present for almost two years without any progression. Histological evaluation confirmed the presence of a simple leukoplakia, and under local anesthesia the gingiva was excised with a scalpel using a submarginal incision. The CO_2 laser was used in a defocused beam with a power of 4W to coagulate the wound after excision (Figure 3.56b). The tissue healed initially without complications, but three months later the patient visited another clinic, where an oral and maxillofacial surgeon decided to extract the teeth adjacent to the lesion. The lesion presented again a couple of weeks later (Figure 3.56c), but the teeth were missing. The patient visited again our clinic with an interest in complete treatment of the remaining lesion. After a new excision with a CO_2 laser in a

focused beam (4W power), the tissue healed without complications and recurrence (Figure 3.56d).

Removal of a Leukoplakia of the Gingiva with an Nd:YAG Laser

A 33-year-old patient came for diagnosis and treatment of a white lesion at her gingiva in the area #12–13. The patient had observed changes in her mouth for the last six months and reported a stable size of the lesion (Figure 3.57a). The clinical findings indicated a simple leukoplakia of the gingiva. The topography of the lesion (interdental papilla of the gingiva), as well as its small size, permitted the excision of the leukoplakia with the glass fiber of a Nd:YAG laser (3W power, pulsed mode, and 30 pps frequency). The fiber was in contact with the tissue and was held in a direction of approximately 30–45° to the axis of the tooth or interdental space (Figure 3.57b), so that strong penetration of the energy and further transmission in the narrow interdental space (narrow alveolar bone, narrow papilla) could remain under control. After the excision of the lesion, the tissue was examined histologically.

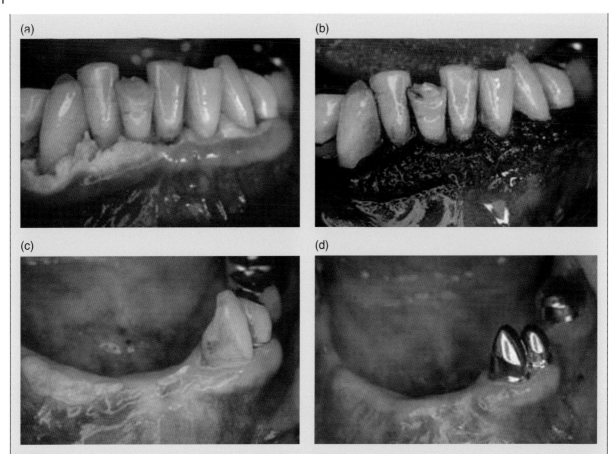

Figure 3.56 Leukoplakia of the gingiva (a); coagulation after laser excision (b); rebound of the lesion after extraction of the teeth (c); and complete healing after second surgery (d). *Source:* Dr. Georgios E Romanos.

Finally, the area of the excision was coagulated. For this purpose, the glass fiber was applied without contact with the tissue. The healing process developed without complications, and after two weeks there were no pathological findings (Figure 3.57c). Regular postoperative follow-up after nine months showed no recurrence (Figure 3.57d).

Removal of Leukoplakia in the Tongue

An excision was performed for complete removal of a large leukoplakia at the right side of the tongue (Figure 3.58a). The contralateral side did not present any pathological findings. The excision was performed using local anesthesia and the focused beam of the CO_2 laser (5 W power, in CW) within the normal surrounding healthy tissues (Figure 3.58b) in order to evaluate the lesion by an oral and maxillofacial pathologist. The separation of the lesion from the underlying healthy mucosa was not very easy, but with the advantage of a sufficient hemostasis, the tissue was excised (Figure 3.58c) and the defect was not covered with dressing (Figure 3.58d). The patient took postoperative pain medication and was advised to avoid spicy food, which may irritate the wound. Healing was without complications and three days postoperatively presented fibrin tissue (Figure 3.58e). Six weeks after surgery the tissue demonstrated a complete normal consistency and no signs of pathology (Figure 3.58f).

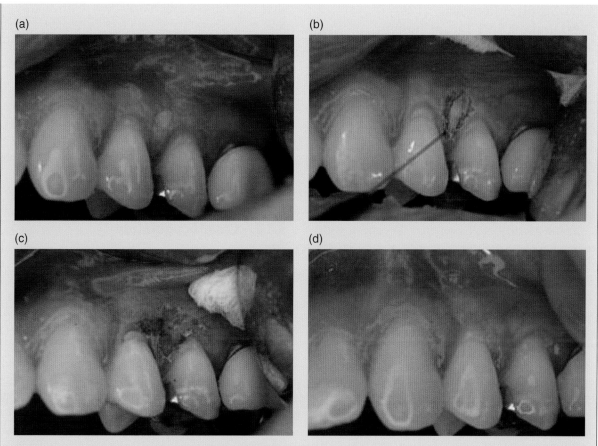

Figure 3.57 Oral leukoplakia in the interdental papilla (a); excision with an Nd:YAG laser using the glass fiber in contact (b); coagulation of the surgical field (c); and follow-up after nine months demonstrating complete healing (d). *Source:* Dr. Georgios E Romanos.

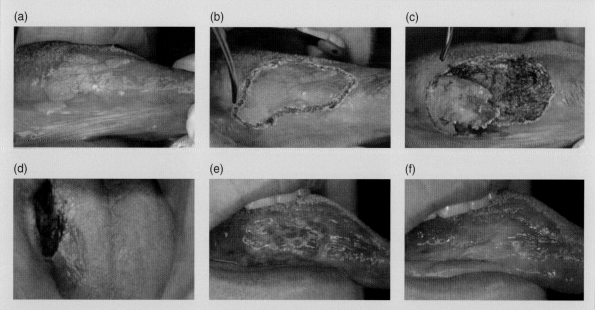

Figure 3.58 Oral leukoplakia at the right side of the tongue (a); excision using a focused beam of the CO_2 laser (b); separation of the lesion from the underlying normal, healthy mucosa (c, d); three days postoperative wound healing presenting fibrin (e); six weeks after surgery no signs of pathology were found (f). *Source:* Dr. Georgios E Romanos.

3.9 Surgical Removal of Malignant Soft Tissue Tumors

The surgical removal of malignant tumors in the oral cavity can be also carried out with the laser as different studies have shown (Carruth 1982; Pecaro and Garehume 1983; Horch 1985; Duncavage and Ossoff 1986). Only a short overview about the surgical removal of such tumors is described here, for interested, surgically oriented clinicians, since a referral is recommended to an experienced oral and maxillofacial surgeon, or head and neck surgeon, who will be responsible for the diagnosis and the treatment of the malignant tumor.

Clinical research has proven that, for patients with a compromised general condition and serious diseases, the CO_2 laser provides special advantages in tumor surgery. Advanced bleeding is prevented by complete sealing of the blood vessels (Horch 1995). Until recently, it was not confirmed whether the sealing of the vessels actually decreased the risk of metastases, due to the lack of clinical trials focused on this question. However, available studies indicate that the use of the CO_2 laser clearly reduces the local recurrence of tumors in comparison to conventional methods (Lanzafame et al. 1986a, b). The first resection of a tumor in the oral cavity with a CO_2 laser was performed by Strong et al. (1979a, b).

The noncontact CO_2 laser or the Nd:YAG laser are currently used for laser surgery of malignant tumors in the oral cavity. For this purpose large CO_2 laser devices with an output power of 20–30 W are required or Nd:YAG lasers with a power of 15–20 W and a fiber of 800 μm in diameter, so that bleeding during surgery can be under control. In addition, a reduced number of postoperative complications, such as infections with fistula formation and pain, were observed during the first five postoperative days (Horch 1985; Gaspar and Szabo 1990; Galucci et al. 1994). From 548 surgical interventions with the CO_2 laser, only 31.2% of the patients needed analgesics, in cases of advanced surgeries, and only in the first postoperative day (Gaspar and Szabo 1990).

3.10 Laser Coagulation

The coagulation of blood vessels, in order to achieve adequate hemostasis, is very important for every surgical intervention. This is of particular importance, especially for patients with coagulopathies or large vessel defects.

The CO_2 laser is indicated for the quick hemostasis of smaller, peripheral vessels, and due to the coagulation, an additional dressing of the wound is not necessary. In most clinical cases, a power of 4–10 W is used, depending on the vessel thickness and the bleeding tendency.

Certainly, in case of arterial bleeding, the traditional surgical techniques to achieve a hemostasis are required, namely the visualization and ligature of the injured blood vessel.

Clinical Case

Coagulation in Patients with Coagulopathies

The patient presented here was referred for the removal of hopeless tooth #19. The patient suffered from a mild von Willebrand disease. Around tooth #19, a soft tissue tumor was found (Figure 3.59a). The gingival tumor was excised under anesthesia with a pulsed Nd:YAG laser (power: 8 W, frequency: 100 pps).

The excision was carried out without bleeding tendency (Figure 3.59b). After the tumor excision, the hopeless tooth was extracted, the alveolar socket was curetted, and further coagulation with the Nd:YAG laser was performed (Figure 3.59c). The wound margins were adapted using conventional silk sutures (Figure 3.59d), and excellent wound healing was observed without complications.

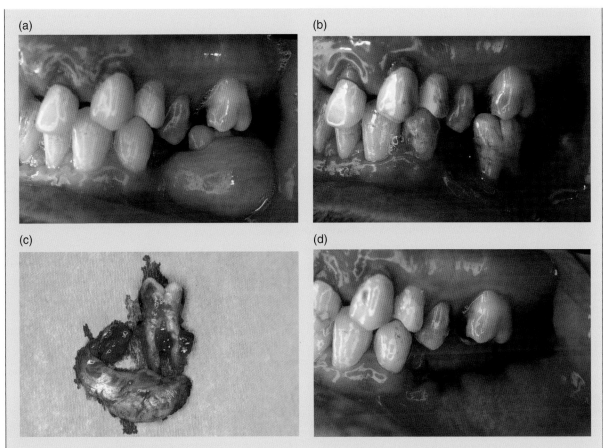

Figure 3.59 Soft tissue tumor in a patient with von Willebrand disease before laser excision (a); after laser excision, tooth extraction, and coagulation with an Nd:YAG laser (b); specimen in toto (c) and clinical condition after suture (d). *Source:* Dr. Georgios E Romanos.

3.11 Lasers in Vascular and Pigmented Lesions

The removal of vascular and lesions rich in pigments with a laser is possible intraorally, as well as extraorally, thanks to the selective absorption of the laser light from the hemoglobin and the specific chromophores. The color of the tissue changes because of the absorption, and at the same time a coagulation of the blood vessels takes place. Therefore, vascular lesions can be removed without excision or thermal damage of the surrounding tissues. The exact underlying mechanism is until today not identified.

Such skin lesions can be treated primarily with the argon, the Nd:YAG laser, the dye laser, as well as the Q-switched Nd:YAG laser.

3.11.1 Laser Types

The argon laser light has a wavelength in the electromagnetic spectrum between 488 and 514 nm and can be absorbed by hemoglobin and skin pigments (Olbricht and Arndt 1987). Its penetration depth is 1–1.5 mm within the epidermis and, so, clearly deeper than the wavelength of the CO_2 laser. By means of an optical fiber and the defocused mode, the vessels of the connective tissue can be well sealed.

This procedure can be performed under local anesthesia and, if possible, without the use of vasoconstrictors, which negatively affect the vascular dilatation during laser therapy.

The surgical intervention is blood-free, thanks to the superficial thermal damage of the tissue during the operation and, thus, a suturing is not required. Initially, a coagulation occurs, and afterwards a whitish discoloration of the treated surface is formed. This alteration is reversible after a few days and functions as a protective wound dressing (Sexton and O'Hare 1993).

A common complication with the use of an argon laser is the contraction of the wound and scarring, particularly when laser has high power (Noe 1988). In normal clinical practice a power of 0.5–1.5 W is applied.

Directly after the surgical intervention with the argon laser, the application of ice is recommended for the first two postoperative days. Hot and crunchy food, which can affect the wound healing and can irritate the irradiated area, should be avoided at least one week after surgery. In order to avoid dehydration of the extraoral area, the use of a hydrating cream is recommended.

The Nd:YAG laser is today the alternative to the argon laser for the removal of vascular lesions. With a wavelength of 1064 nm a selective coagulation effect is achieved on vessels with a diameter of 2–3 mm. Its penetration depth in the tissue is 2–3 mm and is definitely greater than that of the argon laser (Castro 1992). Specifically, using high power, the risk for tissue necrosis definitely increases. The handpiece is suitable for the contact as well as the noncontact use. This characteristic feature permits control of the penetration depth of the laser and therefore further tissue damage and scarring (Romanos and Nentwig 1997b).

The pulsed dye laser has a wavelength of 575–587 nm, which is an advantage in particular for the coagulation of vessels. The coagulation's effect causes no pain, and scarring is significantly reduced. With the dye laser not only small vessels, but also telangiectasias can be removed without causing any damage in the adjacent regions. This is why this laser type is applied at esthetically critical areas and used for the treatment of children and adolescents.

The Q-switched Nd:YAG laser is the most suitable laser type for the removal of pigmentations. A large number of patients present intraoral amalgam tattoos, whereas extraorally, various pigmented alterations are often seen. The laser light is selectively absorbed by the pigments and leaves an esthetically favorable result. The tattoos are treated with high power and usually need repeated treatment sessions. For this reason, a precise informed consent of the patient is necessary. In contrast, pigmented alterations of the skin are to be removed with low power. The application spectrum of this laser type is relatively limited in dentistry and its indication is primarily set in dermatology.

3.11.2 Removal of Vascular Alterations with the "Ice Cube" Method

This method was developed and described earlier (Romanos 1999) and is recommended for the removal of large vascular lesions, mainly in esthetically critical areas. For this purpose, an ice cube is placed on the vascular lesions. It has to be transparent, so that transmission and better focusing of the beam can occur. The glass fiber is directed through the ice cube onto the vascular tumor, and the tissue is irradiated without contact with the laser. Pain is rare, thanks to the simultaneous cooling effect. The entire size of the vascular lesion can be reduced very quickly. The tissue becomes grayish or whitish, and after healing, the results are impressive, particularly in esthetically critical areas.

This surgical procedure can be described with the help of the theoretical model illustrated in the Figure 3.60. Due to the cooling, a contraction of the tissue occurs. The erythrocytes of the blood vessels are thereby gathered in smaller areas within the vascular lesion, so that the hemoglobin content increases in selective fields, and thus the laser light is absorbed faster. A relatively quick reduction of the size of the vascular lesion is therefore reached with a comparably low power. For very large vascular lesions, this procedure is repeated in several therapeutic sessions in weekly intervals.

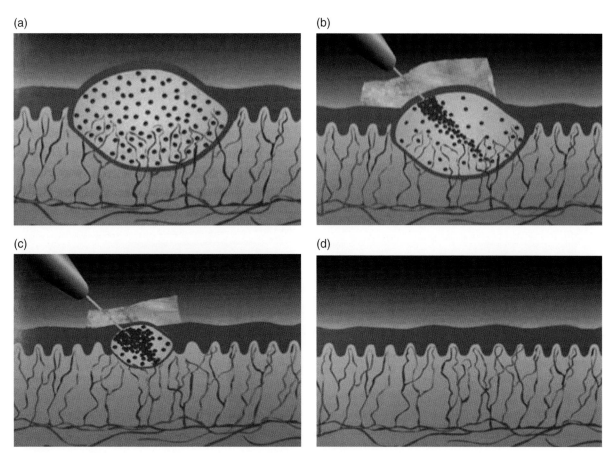

Figure 3.60 Schematic illustration of the ice cube technique in conjunction with treatment of a vascular lesion (a); the ice cube is placed on the surface of the lesion (b) simultaneously with the irradiation of the lesion accumulating hemoglobin content close to the irradiation field. Reduction of the lesion size (c) will be followed by subsequent irradiations until the lesion is completely healed (d). *Source:* Dr. Georgios E Romanos.

Clinical Cases

Removal of Hemangioma of the Buccal Mucosa

This clinical case demonstrates a 49-year-old patient with a vascular lesion at the mucous mucosa of the left cheek. A large hemangioma was found (Figure 3.61a). With the help of the 980 nm diode laser (Ceralas D15®, CeramOptec, Bonn, Germany) and with an output average power of 8.0 W, the glass fiber was focused under the ice cube and the rich-in-vessels tumor was coagulated from the surface into its depth (Figure 3.61b). The healing, one week after surgery, was good, and fibrin deposition was found (Figure 3.61c). The tumor was removed completely, and thus a further laser treatment was not necessary. After four weeks there was no recurrence or any functional complication in the area of the excision (Figure 3.61d).

Removal of a Hemangioma of the Lower Lip

A 45-year-old patient was referred by her general dentist with the request of removal of two vascular lesions at the lower lip (Figure 3.62a). The lesions were filled by blood and had a size between 0.6 × 0.7 cm and 0.3 × 0.4 cm. The clinical diagnosis was hemangioma of the lower lip. Both hemangiomas were coagulated with an Nd:YAG laser under topical anesthesia. The laser used was a pulsed noncontact Nd:YAG-Laser with an average power of 6 W. It was focused under an ice cube (Figure 3.62b), and a selective, specific coagulation of the blood vessels of the hemangioma was performed. This led to an obvious contraction of the entire tumor. After laser treatment, a considerable discoloration was seen, which was caused by the strong vascular contraction (Figure 3.62c). A frequent application of

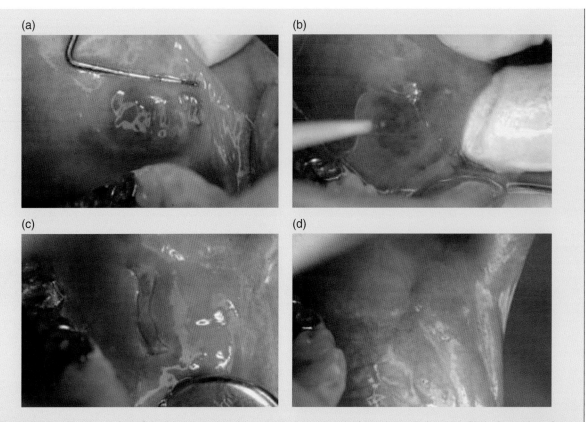

Figure 3.61 Vascular lesion of the buccal mucosa (a); coagulation using the ice cube technique (b); fibrin formation after one week of healing (c); complete wound healing four weeks after surgery without recurrence or any other complications (d). *Source:* Dr. Georgios E Romanos.

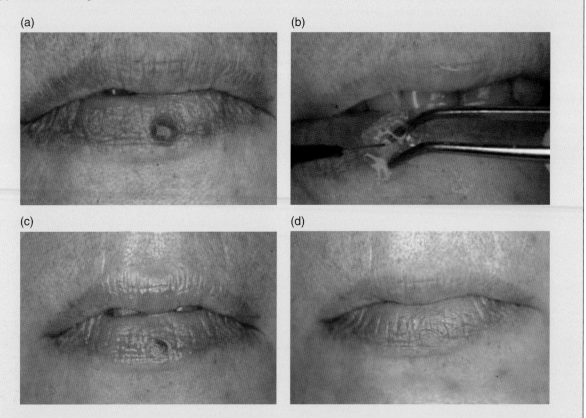

Figure 3.62 Hemangiomas of the lower lip (a); the lesions were coagulated using the ice cube technique (b) following to significant size reduction after one week (c) and without rebound four years later (d). *Source:* Dr. Georgios E Romanos.

Vaseline on the entire treated area was recommended. Four weeks later there was no color differentiation from the neighboring tissue to be seen. The result was without any changes for many years (Figure 3.62d).

Removal of Telangiectasias in Morbus Osler's Disease

The 62-year-old patient with Osler's disease was presented for the removal of multiple telangiectasias on the skin of his cheek (Figure 3.63a, b) and the treatment of intraoral lesions with frequent spontaneous bleeding. After an extensive informed consent, the telangiectasias were treated under topical anesthesia with a pulsed Nd:YAG laser and with the use of the ice cube technique. The power used was 6–10 W and the tissue was treated without contact. The application of a sunscreen was recommended. The healing developed without complications, and a successful esthetic result in the skin was finally achieved (Figure 3.63c, d).

In addition, lesions at the lip (Figure 3.63e) and intraoral telangiectasias of the tongue (Figure 3.63f) were coagulated with the noncontact pulsed Nd:YAG laser (power: 4–6 W, frequency: 30–50 Hz) under topical anesthesia. The result was excellent after four weeks of healing (Figure 3.63g, h) and stable after two years (Figure 3.63i).

Removal of a Large Hemangioma of the Lower Lip

The patient's lower lip hemangioma (Figure 3.64a) was coagulated in five different visits with two-week intervals. The size was larger than 1×1 cm (Figure 3.64b). The coagulation was performed with an Nd:YAG laser (pulsed, defocused beam; 6 W power and 200 Hz frequency) using the ice cube technique (Figure 3.64c). The size of the lesion was continuously reduced, and the tumor disappeared within five months (Figure 3.64d).

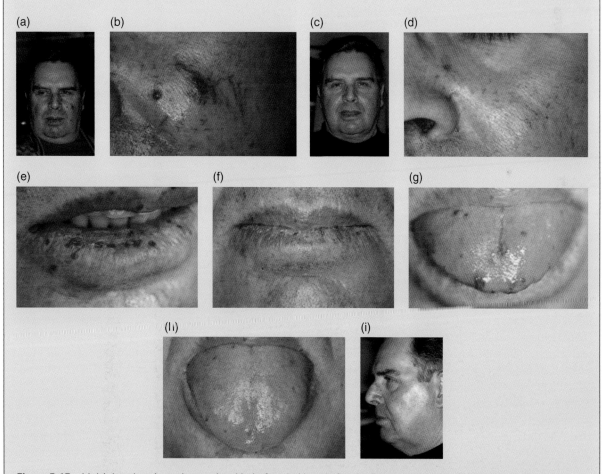

Figure 3.63 Multiple telangiectasias on the skin before (a, b) and after (c, d) treatment using the ice cube technique as well as the lower lip (e, f) and intraoral vascular lesions (g, h) after six months. The esthetic result after two years was very successful without any type of scar tissue (i). *Source:* Dr. Georgios E Romanos.

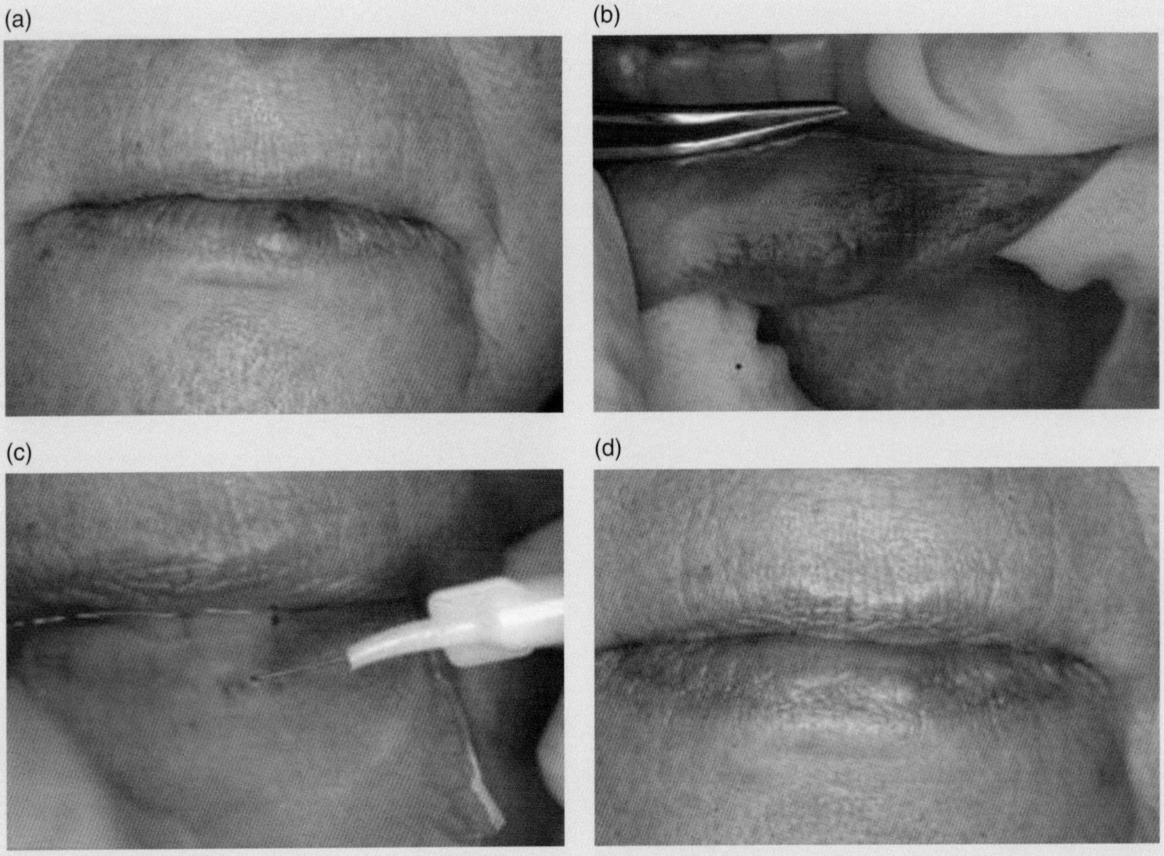

(a)

(b)

(c)

(d)

Figure 3.64 Hemangioma of the lip (a) in a size larger than the width of a tooth (b); during the coagulation with the ice cube technique (c); presenting complete healing without rebound and scar after five months (d). *Source:* Dr. Georgios E Romanos.

Removal of a Large Hemangioma of the Tongue

A 67-year-old patient presented for the removal of a cherry-size tumor on her tongue (Figure 3.65a). The tumor was coagulated under local anesthesia in several visits, after each of which it was reduced in size. For this purpose, the pulsed Nd:YAG laser beam was defocused by means of a cold glass plate and with a high power of 10 W. During the entire intervention, the fiber had no contact with the tissue. Directly after the coagulation, an obvious tissue necrosis was observed with postoperative pain (Figure 3.65b). Later on, contraction of the entire tumor and a whitish alteration of its surface were found. The postoperative pain could be controlled only with mild analgesics, such as paracetamol (Tylenol®) pain medication. Five weeks after the intervention (Figure 3.65c), there was a slight scar. After approximately two years of follow-up, no recurrence of the tumor appeared (Figure 3.65d).

Removal of a Large Hemangioma of the Tongue

The 58-year-old patient exhibited a large hemangioma on the tongue (Figure 3.66a). The vascular tumor was coagulated under local anesthesia with the glass fiber of a Nd:YAG laser and with the use of an ice cube on its surface (Figure 3.66b). The tissue was subsequently penetrated by the fiber (intraluminal method) and, with circulating movements of the fiber, coagulated from the deepest point toward the surface (Figure 3.66c). For the determination of the exact expansion of the tumor, an aspiration of blood was necessary before the laser use. The coagulation of the vessels and the final size reduction of the tumor were performed at two different therapy sessions. The output power of the Nd:YAG laser was 8 W and a frequency 100 pps (Hz). Wound healing developed without complications or functional problems (Figure 3.66d).

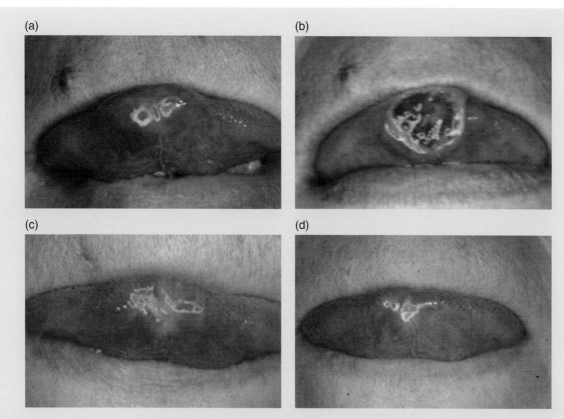

Figure 3.65 Conventional method of coagulation of the hemangioma of the tongue (a) using the Nd:YAG laser leading to necrosis (b), scar tissue after five weeks (c), and stable condition after two years (d). *Source:* Dr. Georgios E Romanos.

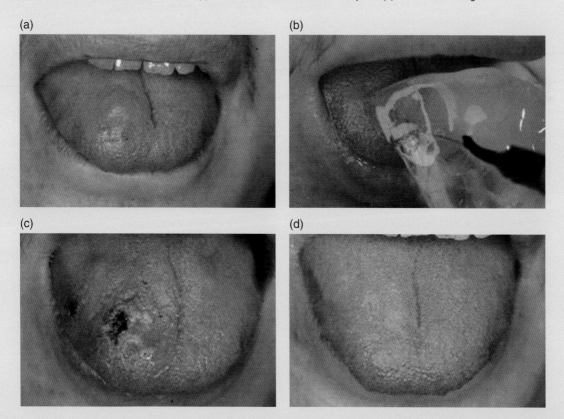

Figure 3.66 Large hemangioma on the tongue (a) coagulated with the intraluminal method and ice cube technique (b) leading to contraction of the tumor and complete healing after five irradiations in a period of five months (d). *Source:* Dr. Georgios E Romanos.

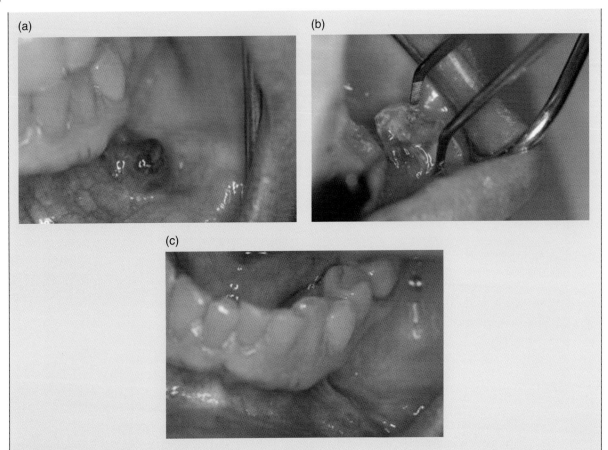

Figure 3.67 Hemangioma of the oral mucosa (a) irradiated with the ice cube technique and an noninitiated tip of the glass fiber of a 980 nm diode laser and a noncontact mode (b); the result was excellent after three months (c). *Source:* Dr. Georgios E Romanos.

Removal of a Hemangioma in the Oral Mucosa with a Diode Laser

A hemangioma in the oral mucosa (Figure 3.67a) was removed after topical anesthesia and a noninitiated tip of the glass fiber of a 980 nm diode laser (Gentleray®, KaVo Dental, Charlotte, NC) in a noncontact mode, 4 W power setting, and continuous wave using the ice cube technique (Figure 3.67b). The result was excellent after three irradiation visits (Figure 3.67c) within three months.

Removal of a Hemangioma in the Lower Lip with a Diode Laser

A hemangioma of the lower lip (Figure 3.68a, b) was removed after topical anesthesia and a noninitiated tip of the glass fiber of a 980 nm diode laser in noncontact mode, 4–6 W average power setting and continuous wave beam using the ice cube technique (Figure 3.68c). The hemangioma was continuously reduced in size after one month (Figure 3.68d), and the final result was excellent after three irradiation visits (Figure 3.68e, f) and one year follow-up (Figure 3.68g, h).

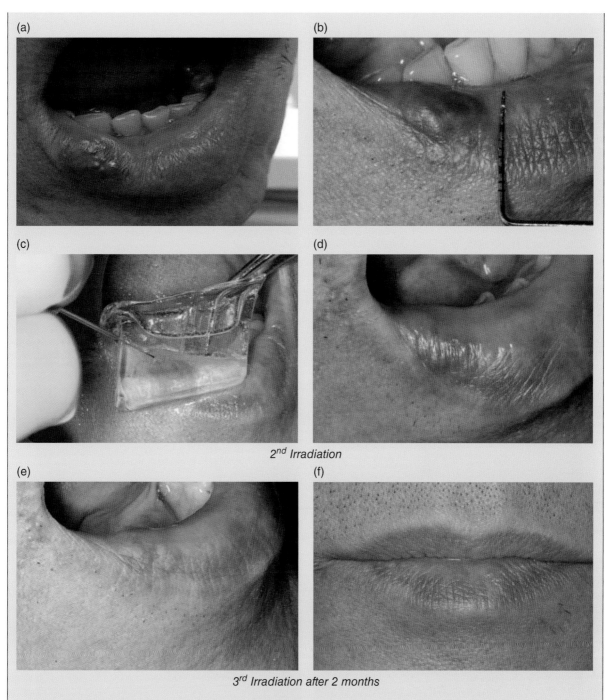

Figure 3.68 Hemangioma of the lower lip (a, b) removed with a diode laser and noninitiated tip without contact through the ice cube (c); a reduction in size after one month (d), two months (e, f), and complete healing after one year (g, h).
Source: Dr. Georgios E Romanos.

(g)   (h)

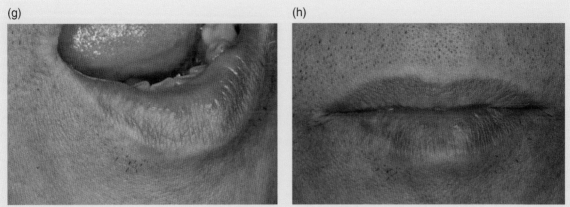

Final Outcome (1-year post op)

Figure 3.68 (Continued)

Other Clinical Examples of Hemangioma Removal Using the Ice Cube Technique

Case 1

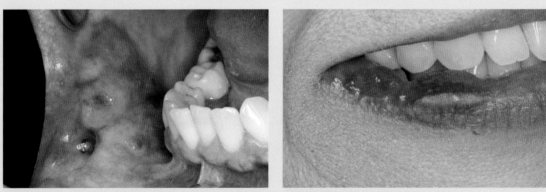

Initial Clinical Demonstration of the Large Hemangioma of the Oral Cavity

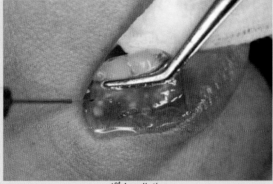

1st Irradiation

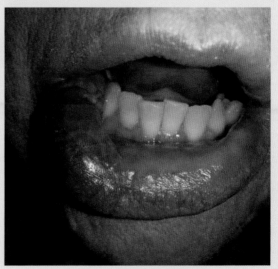

Postoperative clinical condition 3 days
after the first irradiation

Figure 3.69 Initial clinical demonstration of a large hemangioma of the oral cavity. First irradiation (a); postoperative clinical condition three days after the first irradiation (b); second radiation (c); third irradiation (d); sonography of the lower lip verifying the complete coagulation of the vascular tumor from the surface of the oral mucosa in order to control bleeding two years after therapy. *Source:* Dr. Georgios E Romanos.

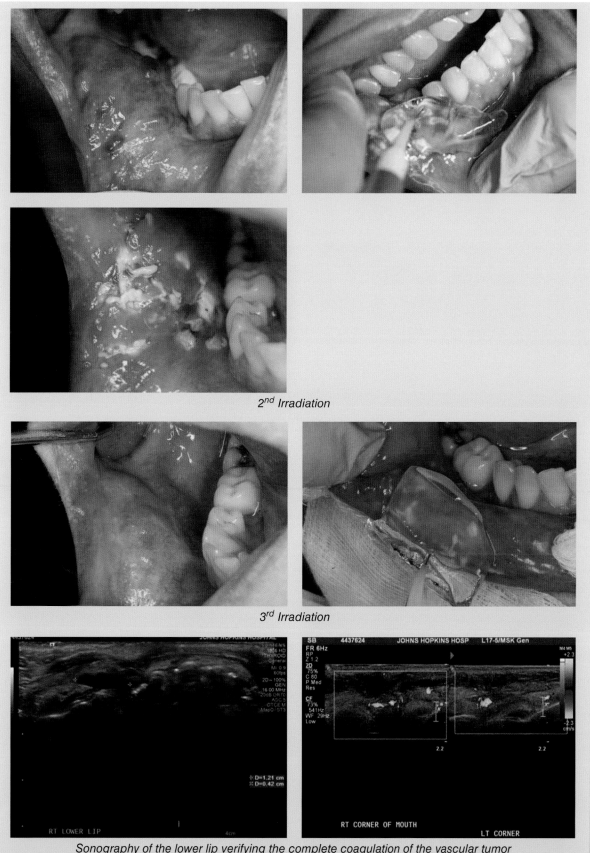

2*nd* Irradiation

3*rd* Irradiation

Sonography of the lower lip verifying the complete coagulation of the vascular tumor from the surface of the oral mucosa in order to control bleeding two years after therapy.

Figure 3.69 (Continued)

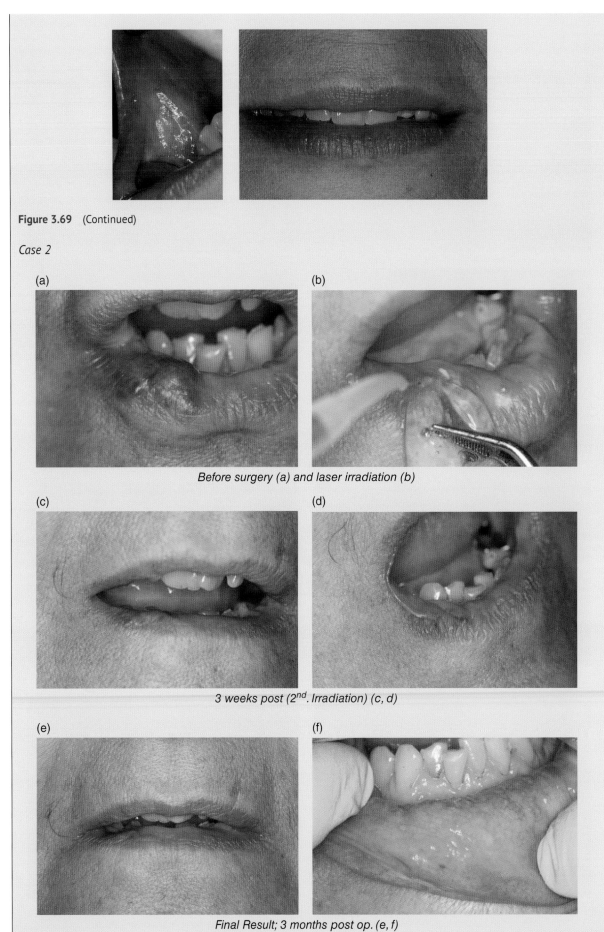

Figure 3.69 (Continued)

Case 2

Before surgery (a) and laser irradiation (b)

3 weeks post (2nd. Irradiation) (c, d)

Final Result; 3 months post op. (e, f)

Figure 3.70 Before surgery (a) and laser irradiation (b); three weeks post (second irradiation) (c, d); final result (e); three months post-op. (f). *Source:* Dr. Georgios E Romanos.

Case 3

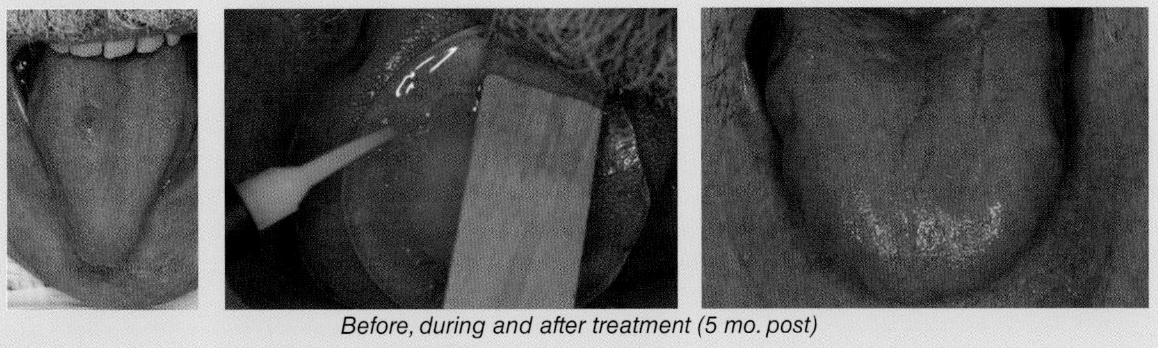

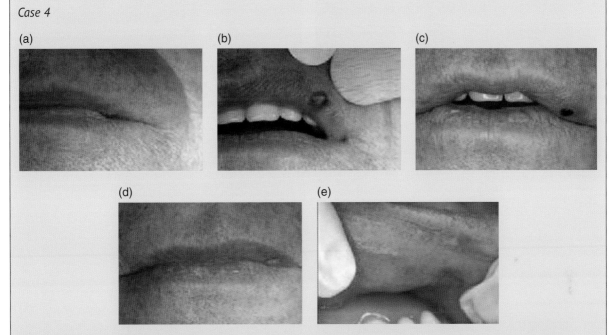

Before, during and after treatment (5 mo. post)

Figure 3.71 Before, during, and after treatment (five months post-op). *Source:* Dr. Georgios E Romanos.

Case 4

(a) (b) (c)

(d) (e)

Figure 3.72 Hemangioma of the upper lip associated with esthetic concerns (a, b); immediately after irradiation the vascular lesion was contracted (c) and covered with fibrin after one week (d); complete healing was observed after one month (e). *Source:* Dr. Georgios E Romanos.

Removal of an Amalgam Tattoo with an Nd:YAG Laser

A 76-year-old female patient was referred by a general dentist for diagnosis and treatment of a lesion in the area #1–3. The clinical diagnosis was of an amalgam tattoo of the oral mucosa associated with the restored teeth #2–3 (Figure 3.73a). For the removal of the lesion, a pulsed Nd:YAlaser was applied at three different therapy sessions. The laser energy was applied in the noncontact mode (Figure 3.73b). The average power (at each irradiation visit) was between 6–8 W and frequency was 80–100pps. The lesion's size was reduced significantly within two weeks (Figure 3.73c). After two months, excellent healing was observed without scarring or color differences with the adjacent healthy mucosa (Figure 3.73d).

Removal of a Nevus of the Upper Lip

A 67-year-old patient was referred for the removal of a brown lesion of her upper lip. The clinical diagnosis was nevus in the upper lip (Figure 3.74a). The nevus was removed completely with an Nd:YAG laser (power: 1.75 W; frequency: 20 Hz) under topical anesthesia (Figure 3.74b) and examined histologically in order to get confirmation of the clinical diagnosis. Two weeks after the surgical intervention, a slight redness appeared at the excision area (Figure 3.74c). Five months postoperatively excellent healing without scar tissue was demonstrated. The patient was very happy with the final esthetic result (Figure 3.74d).

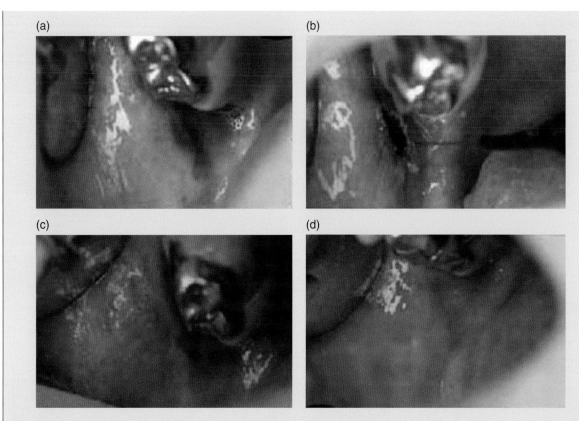

Figure 3.73 Amalgam tattoo removal (a) using a pulsed Nd:YAG laser (b); the lesion was reduced in size significantly within two weeks (c). After two months, excellent healing was observed, without scarring or discoloration (d). *Source:* Dr. Georgios E Romanos.

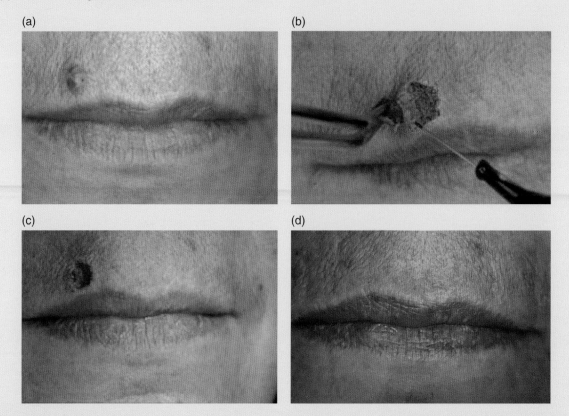

Figure 3.74 Removal of a nevus in the upper lip (a) using an Nd:YAG laser (b, c); five months postoperatively an excellent healing was demonstrated (d). *Source:* Dr. Georgios E Romanos.

3.12 Exposure of Impacted, Unerupted Teeth

The exposure of impacted teeth is a frequent indication in the area of the oral surgery (operculectomy). Considering the mucosa covering, partially impacted wisdom teeth, with available antagonists, an exposure is indicated in some cases, instead of an extraction or osteotomy. Another indication is the exposure of impacted teeth for orthodontic reasons. If the teeth are covered only by mucosa and not by bone, this intervention can be easily carried out with any type of laser. The CO_2 laser wavelength, as well as the diode and the Nd:YAG laser are applicable for this purpose since they provide an excellent coagulation. Certainly, lasers of the erbium family (Er:YAG, Er, Cr: YSGG lasers) can be used as well without to provide an excellent coagulation. The surgical procedure is performed usually without complications and if the exposure is sufficient, there are no recurrences are usually to be expected.

Clinical Cases

Exposure of a Semi-impacted Tooth During Pregnancy

A 28-year-old pregnant patient (in the ninth month of pregnancy) was referred by her general dentist because of severe pain and slight swelling in the region of tooth #17. The patient showed a pronounced sensibility to pain and the intraoral findings indicated a pericoronitis (Figure 3.75a). After detailed informed consent about the excision of the mucosa of the impacted tooth #17 with a pulsed Nd:YAG dental laser, the hyperplastic, inflamed tissue was removed under topical anesthesia.

The excision was performed using the glass fiber in contact with the soft tissues, and a relative low power (3.0 W and frequency of 50 Hz) due to deep penetration of the laser light to the inflamed tissues. The coagulation during the excision was sufficient (Figure 3.75b). Cooling of the submandibular region with cold water was recommended as the only postoperative instruction. Oral hygiene and sufficient plaque control was recommended after one week to 10 days. A follow-up evaluation three weeks after surgery revealed good and healthy conditions around tooth #17 (Figure 3.75c).

(a) (b) (c)

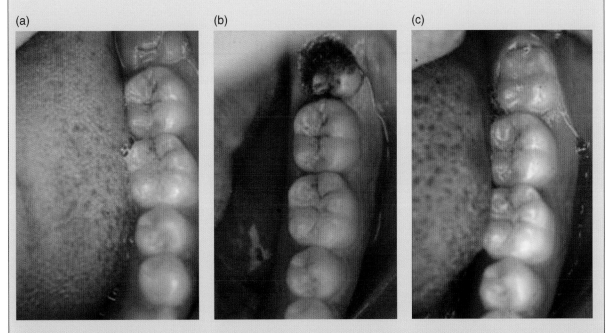

Figure 3.75 Pericoronitis around tooth#17 (a); excision of the mucosa with a pulsed Nd:YAG dental laser and subsequent hemostasis (b); the follow-up after three weeks presents healthy and asymptomatic tissues around tooth #17 (c). *Source:* Dr. Georgios E Romanos.

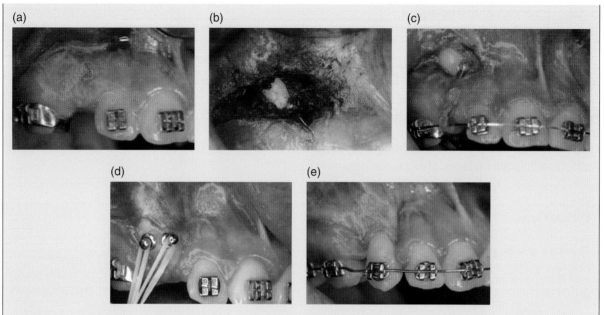

Figure 3.76 Unerupted tooth (a) exposed with a CO_2 laser (b) after placement of a bracket one week after laser surgery (c); orthodontically dynamic movement of the tooth two weeks later (d) and after one year of orthodontic treatment (e). *Source:* Dr. Georgios E Romanos.

Exposure of an Unerupted Canine for Orthodontic Reasons

A 17-year-old patient was referred by her orthodontist with the request of the exposure of unerupted tooth #6. An attempt to expose the tooth, which took place five months previously, failed because the exposed area was covered again, due to delayed orthodontic movement. In addition to that, the intervention left a large scar in the mucosa (Figure 3.76a). After careful radiographic evaluation (Figure 3.76b), a wrong position of the orthodontic bracket was diagnosed (contact with the alveolar bone), possibly the main reason for the unsuccessful long-term tooth movement. After an extensive informed consent about the alternative options, such as the conventional technique or use of another laser wavelength, the mucosa covering the tooth was excised, under topical anesthesia (with Xylocaine spray 2%) with the CO_2 laser in a continuous mode. The surgery was performed without complications. A strong hemostasis was attempted during the entire surgery with the defocused beam to control postoperative bleeding (Figure 3.76b). The patient was subsequently referred back to her orthodontist. After 10 days, a fibrin layer was observed at the surgical field (Figure 3.76c). Active tooth movement was initiated (Figure 3.76d). The tooth could be moved further orthodontically, and the treatment was completed within one year (Figure 3.76e). The initial large scar was clearly reduced by the laser surgical procedure.

3.12.1 Exposure of an Unerupted Teeth for Orthodontic Reasons

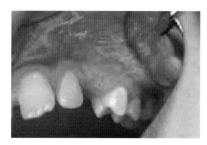
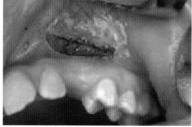
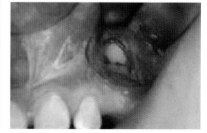

Figure 3.77 CO_2 laser-assisted surgical exposure of an impacted tooth for orthodontic reasons. *Source:* Dr. Georgios E Romanos.

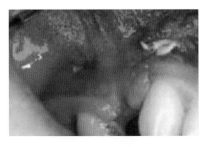
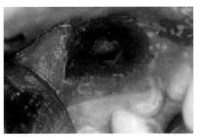
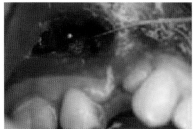

Figure 3.78 Surgical exposure of an impacted tooth for orthodontic reasons using a CO_2 laser and placement of the bracket due to the good coagulation immediately after surgery. *Source:* Dr. Georgios E Romanos.

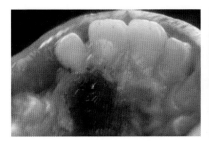
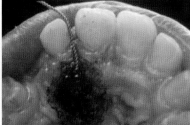
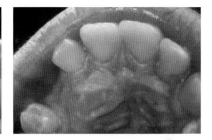

Figure 3.79 Surgical exposure of an impacted tooth for orthodontic reasons using the CO_2 laser. *Source:* Dr. Georgios E Romanos.

3.13 Removal of Sialoliths Using the Laser

Due to the presence of salivary duct stones (so called "sialoliths"), obstruction of the excretory ducts and, as a result, massive saliva deposits (with calcium) within the duct or the gland may occur. The conventional surgical procedures include the preparation of the excretory duct by introducing a narrow catheter for drainage and then incision to remove the salivary stone; from the deeper areas of the parenchyma of the gland requires a bigger surgical effort. The complete removal of the salivary gland is sometimes necessary. As an alternative to the scalpel, the removal of sialoliths (in different sizes) is also possible with the laser. Numerous case reports recommend the use of different lasers for intraoral lithotripsy and sialolithectomy (Azaz et al. 1996; Ito and Baba 1996). Recent studies showed the clinical benefits of the diode lasers for the surgical removal of sialoliths (Angiero et al. 2008; Luers et al. 2014).

Clinical Case

Removal of Deeply Localized Sialoliths of the Submandibular Gland

A 51-year-old patient exhibited pronounced pain at the right submandibular region during chewing and swallowing. During the clinical examination, a deeply localized salivary stone could be palpated (Figure 3.80a). A thin plastic catheter was inserted under local anesthesia in the excretory duct of the gland, in order to present the orientation of the duct. An incision was performed with the Nd:YAG laser (contact glass fiber and focused beam) close to the area of the palpated salivary stone. The output average power was 3 W and the frequency 60 pps (Figure 3.80b). Three sialoliths were removed, and the wound was left to heal for secondary intension (Figure 3.80c, d). The catheter was removed from the excretory duct after approximately 10 days. Wound healing took place without complications, and after approximately three weeks a complete wound closure was observed.

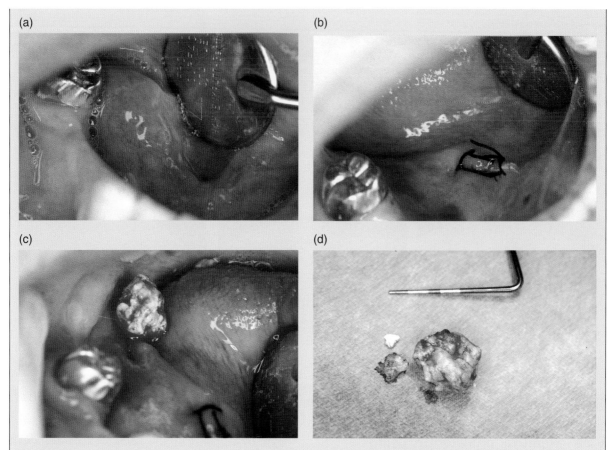

Figure 3.80 A deeply localized salivary stone was palpated in the submandibular area (a); a thin plastic catheter was inserted in the excretory duct of the gland, in order to present better orientation and location of the duct (b); the incision was performed with the Nd:YAG laser (c); three salivary stones were removed from the duct (d). *Source:* Dr. Georgios E Romanos.

References

Abt, E.H., Wigdor, R., Lobraico, B. et al. (1987). Removal of benign intraoral masses using the CO_2 laser. *JADA* 115: 729–731.

American Academy of Periodontology (1996). Proceedings of the 1996 World Workshop of Periodontics. Lansdowne, Virginia, July 13–17. Ann Periodontol 1:1–947.

Anderson, L., Fejerskov, O., and Philipsen, H.P. (1973). Oral giant cell granulomas: a clinical and histological study of 129 cases. *Acta. Pathol. Microbiol. Scand. Sect A: Pathol.* 81: 606–616.

Angiero, F., Benedicenti, S., Romanos, G.E., and Crippa, R. (2008). Sialolithiasis of the submandibular salivary gland treated with the 810- to 830-nm diode laser. *Photomed. Laser Surg.* 26 (6): 517–521.

Arora, K.S., Bansal, R., Mohapatra, S. et al. (2018). Prevention of malignant transformation of oral leukoplakia and oral lichen planus using laser: an observational study. *Asian Pac. J. Cancer Prev.* 19: 3635–3641.

Azaz, B., Regev, E., Casap, N., and Chicin, R. (1996). Sialolithectomy done with a CO_2 laser: clinical and scintigraphic results. *J. Oral Maxillofac. Surg.* 54 (6): 685–688.

Baumann, M. (1976). Partial vestibuloplasty with secondary epithelization. *SSO Schweiz. Monatsschr. Zahnheilkd.* 86 (1): 17–28. (German).

Benkert, P., Passler, L., and Seidl, R. (1982). Die Epuliden-klinische und histologische von 208 Faellen. *Stomatol DDR* 32: 426–431. (German).

Carruth, J.A.S. (1982). Resection of the tongue with the carbon dioxide laser. *J. Laryngol. Otol.* 96: 529–543.

Castro, D.J. (1992). The physical principles of lasers. In: *Atlas of Cutaneous Laser Surgery* (ed. D.B. Apfelberg), 235–256. New York: Raven Press.

Duncavage, J.A. and Ossoff, R.H. (1986). Use of the CO_2 laser for malignant disease of the oral cavity. *Lasers Surg. Med.* 6: 442–444.

Dunsche, A., Fleiner, B., and Hoffmeister, B. (1994). Die Exzision von Mundschleimhautveraenderungen mit dem CO_2- Laser. *Dtsch. Zahnarztl. Z.* 49: 148–150. (German).

Edwards, J.G. (1977). The diastema, the frenum, the frenectomy: a clinical study. *Am. J. Orthod.* 71: 489–508.

Esser, E. (1979). Therapie der intraoralen Leukoplakie. *Dtsch. Z Mund. Kiefer GesichtsChir.* 3: 201–208. (German).

Eversole, L.R. and Rovin, S. (1972). Reactive lesions of the gingiva. *J. Oral Pathol.* 1: 30–38.

Fisher, S.E. and Frame, J.W. (1984). The effect of the CO_2 surgical laser on oral tissues. *Br. J. Oral Maxillofac. Surg.* 22: 414–425.

Fisher, S.E., Frame, J.W., Browne, R.M., and Tranter, R.M. (1983). A comparative histological study of wound healing following CO_2 laser and conventional surgical excision of canine buccal mucosa. *Arch. Oral Biol.* 28: 287–291.

Frame, J.W. (1985). Removal of oral soft tissue pathology with the CO_2 laser. *J. Oral Maxillofac. Surg.* 43: 850–855.

Galucci, J.G., Zeltman, D., and Slotman, G. (1994). Nd:YAG laser scalpel compared with conventional techniques in head and neck surgery. *Lasers Surg. Med.* 14: 139–144.

Gaspar, L. and Szabo, G. (1989). Removal of benign oral tumors and tumor-like lesions by CO_2 laser application. *Laser Med. Surg.* 7: 27–31.

Gaspar, L. and Szabo, G. (1990). Manifestation of the advantages and disadvantages of using the CO_2 laser in oral surgery. *J. Clin. Laser Med. Surg.* 8: 39–43.

Gaspar, L. and Szabo, G. (1991). Removal of epulis by CO_2 laser. *J. Clin. Laser Med. Surg.* 9: 289–294.

Gerlach, K.L., Pape, H.D., de Lacroix, W.F. et al. (1993). Die Therapie oraler Praekanzerosen mit dem CO_2-Laser. Behandlungsergebnisse aus drei Kliniken. *Dtsch. Zahnaerztl. Z.* 48: 48. (German).

Giansanti, J.S. and Waldron, C.A. (1969). Peripheral giant cell granuloma: review of 720 cases. *J. Oral Surg.* 27: 787–791.

Goultschin, J., Gazit, D., Bichacho, N., and Bab, I. (1988). Changes in teeth and gingiva of dogs following laser surgery. *Lasers Surg. Med.* 8: 402–408.

Grossenbacher, R. (1985). Laserchirurgie in der Oto-Rhino Laryngologie. In: *Aktuelle Oto-Rhino-Laryngologie*, I-19. S. 1-69. (eds. W. Becker, H.G. Boenninghaus and H.H. Naumann). Stuttgart, New York: Thieme Publ (German).

Hausamen, J.E. (1973). Kryochirurgische Behandlung von Leukoplakien der Mundschleimhaut. *Dtsch. Zahnaerztl. Z.* 28: 1032–1036. (German).

Hausamen, J.E. (1974). *Klinische und experimentelle Untersuchungen zur Kryochirurgie im Kiefer-Gesichts-Bereich*. Berlin: Quintessenz.

Hillerup, S. (1980). Healing reactions of relapse in secondary epithelization vestibuloplasty on dog mandibles. *Int. J. Oral Surg.* 9 (2): 116–127.

Hillerup, S. (1987). Preprosthetic mandibular vestibuloplasty with split-skin graft. *Int. J. Oral Maxillofac. Surg.* 16: 270.

Horch, H.H. (1985). Die Laser-Chirurgie im Mund-, Kiefer-Gesichtsbereich. *Zahnaerztl. Mitt.* 75: 2554–2568. (German).

Horch, H.H. (1992). Laser in der Mund -Kiefer-Gesichtschirurgie. In: *Laser in der Zahnmedizin* (eds. J. Yahl and H. van Benthem), 43. Berlin: Quintessenz (German).

Horch, H.H. (1995). Laser in der Zahn-, Mund-, Kiefer- und Gesichtschirurgie. In: *Angewandte Laserzahnheilkunde* (eds. G. Mueller and T. Ertl). Landsberg: Ecomed (German).

Horch, H.H. and Rehrmann, A. (1978). Tierexperimentelle Studien zur oralen Laserchirurgie der Weichteile. *Dtsch. Z Mund. Kiefer GesichtsChir.* 2: 67–71. (German).

Horch, H.H., Gerlach, K.L., Schaefer, H.E., and Pape, H.D. (1983). Erfahrungen mit der Laserbehandlung oberflaechlicher Mundschleimhauterkrankungen. *Dtsch. Z Mund. Kiefer GesichtsChir.* 7: 31–35. (German).

Horch, H.H., Gerlach, K.L., and Schaefer, H.E. (1986). CO_2 laser surgery of oral premalignant lesions. *Int. J. Oral Maxillofac. Surg.* 15: 19–24.

Ito, H. and Baba, S. (1996). Pulsed dye laser lithotripsy of submandibular gland salivary calculus. *J. Laryngol. Otol.* 110 (10): 942–946.

Katsikeris, N., Kakarantza-Angelopoulou, E., and Angelopoulos, A.P. (1988). Peripheral giant cell granuloma. Clinicopathologic study of 224 new cases and review of 956 reported cases. *Int. J. Oral Maxillofac. Surg.* 17: 94–99.

Keller, U., Hibst, R., and Mohr, W. (1990). Tierexperimentelle Studien zur Laserablation von Mundschleimhauterkrankungen mit dem Er:YAG-Laser. *Oesterr. Z. Stomatol.* 87: 475–480. (German).

Kotiranta, J., Virtanen, K., and Pernu, H. (1986). Surgical and prosthetic treatment of the atrophic mandible. *Scand. J. Dent. Res.* 94 (2): 146–153.

Lambrecht, J. and Härle, F. (2003). Präprothetische Chirurgie. In: *Zahnärztliche Chirurgie*, 4e (ed. H.H. Horch), 255–272. Munich: Urban and Fischer Publ (German).

Lanzafame, R.J., Rogers, D.W., Naim, J.O. et al. (1986a). The effect of CO_2 laser excision on local tumor recurrence. *Lasers Surg. Med.* 6: 103–105.

Lanzafame, R.J., Rogers, D.W., Naim, J.O. et al. (1986b). Reduction of local tumor recurrence by excision with the CO_2 laser. *Lasers Surg. Med.* 6: 439–441.

Lee, K.W. (1986). The fibrous epulis and related lesions. *Periodontics* 6: 277–291.

Luers, J.C., Petry-Schmelzer, J.N., Hein, W.G. et al. (2014). Fragmentation of salivary stones with a 980nm diode laser. *Auris Nasus Larynx* 41 (1): 76–80.

Macleod, R.I. and Soames, J.V. (1987). Epulides: a clinicopathological study of a series of 200 consecutive lesions. *Br. Dent. J.* 163: 51–53.

Mighell, A.J., Robinson, P.A., and Hume, W.J. (1995). Peripheral giant cell granuloma: a clinical study of 77 cases from 62 patients, and literature review. *Oral Dis.* 1: 12–19.

Mincer, H.H., Coleman, S.A., and Hopkins, K.P. (1972). Observations on the clinical characteristics of oral lesions showing histological epithelial dysplasia. *Oral Surg.* 33: 389.

Neiburger, E.J. and Miserendino, L. (1988). Laser reflectance: hazard in the dental operatory. *Oral Surg. Oral Med. Oral Pathol.* 66: 659.

Neidhardt A. (1963) Die Mundvorhofplastik mit sekundaerer Epithelisation am Oberkiefer. University of Zurich, Med. Dissertation. (German).

Noe, J.M. (1988). Laser therapy of port-wine stains. In: *Vascular Birthmarks: Hemangiomas and Malformations* (eds. J.B. Milliken and A.E. Young), 91–102. Philadelphia: W.B. Saunders.

Obwegeser, H. (1965). Zur Indikation fuer die einzelnen Methoden der Vestiulumplastik und Mundbodenplastik. *Fortschr. Kiefer-GesichtsChir.* 10: 1. (German).

Olbricht, A. and Arndt, K. (1987). Lasers in cutaneous surgery. In: *Surgical Lasers: A Clinical Guide* (ed. T.A. Fuller), 113–145. New York: MacMillan.

Pecaro, B.C. and Garehume, W.J. (1983). The CO_2 laser in oral and maxillofacial surgery. *J. Oral Maxillofac. Surg.* 41: 725–728.

Pick, R.M. (1993). Using lasers in clinical dental practice. *JADA* 124: 37.

Pick, R.M. and Colvard, M.D. (1993). Current status of lasers in soft tissue dental surgery. *J. Periodontol.* 64: 589–602.

Pick, R.M. and Miserendino, L.J. (1989). Lasers in dentistry. *J. Clin. Laser Med. Surg.* 7: 33–42.

Pick, R.M., Pecaro, B.C., Pecaro, B.C., and Silverman, C.J. (1985). The laser gingivectomy. The use of CO_2 laser for the removal of phenytoin hyperplasia. *J. Periodontol.* 56: 492–496.

Pick, R.M. and Powell, G.L. (1993). Lasers in dentistry. Soft tissue procedures. *Dent. Clin. N. Am.* 37: 281–297.

Pindborg, J.J. (1980). *Oral Cancer and Precancer*, vol. 15. Bristol: Wright.

Pogrel, M.A. (1989). The carbon dioxide laser in soft tissue pre-prosthetic surgery. *J. Prosthet. Dent.* 61 (2): 203–208.

Romanos, G.E. (1994). Clinical applications of the Nd:YAG laser in oral soft tissue surgery and periodontology. *J. Clin. Laser Med. Surg.* 12: 103–108.

Romanos, G.E. (1999). *Atlas der chirurgischen Laserzahnheilkunde*, 218. Munich: Urban und Fischer Verlag (German).

Romanos, G.E. and Nentwig, G.H. (1996). Present and future of lasers in oral soft tissue surgery: clinical applications. *J. Clin. Laser Med. Surg.* 14: 179–184.

Romanos GE, Nentwig GH. (1997a) Erfahrungen bei der chirurgischen Behandlung von grossflaechigen Leukoplakien mit dem CO_2-Laser. Vortrag bei der Jahrestagung der Deutschen Gesellschaft fuer Laserzahnheilkunde am 31.1.-2. 2. Frankfurt.

Romanos, G.E. and Nentwig, G.H. (1997b). Der Einsatz des Nd:YAG Lasers bei der hereditaeren haemorrhagischen Teleangiektasie (Morbus Osler). *Quintessenz* 48: 1613–1618. (German).

Roodenburg, J.L.N., Panders, A.K., Yenney, A., and Verschueren, R.C.J. (1983). Treatment of superficial les ion s of the oral mucosa with the carbon dioxide laser: a report of 58 cases with 5 years follow up. *J. Exp. Clin. Cancer Res.* 3: 283–286.

Roodenburg, J.L.N., Panders, A.K., and Vermey, A. (1991). Carbon dioxide laser surgery of oral leukoplakia. *Oral Surg. Oral Med. Oral Pathol.* 71: 670–674.

Rossmann, J.A., Gottlieb, S., Koudelka, B.M., and McQuacle, M.J. (1987). Effects of CO_2 laser irradiation on gingiva. *J. Periodontol.* 58: 423–425.

Sachs, S.A. and Borden, G.E. (1981). The utilization of the carbon dioxide laser in the treatment of recurrent papillomatosis: report of a case. *J. Oral Surg.* 39: 299.

Sako, K., Marchetta, F.C., and Hayes, R.L. (1972). Cryotherapy of intraoral leucoplakia. *Am. J. Surg.* 124: 482–484.

Schettler, D. and Koch, H. (1976). Langzeitbeobachtungen nach Vitamin-A-Saeure-Therapie bei Leukoplakien der Mundschleimhaut. In: *Fortschritte der Kiefer-Gesichts-Chirurgie*, vol. 21 (eds. K. Schuchardt and G. Pfeifer), 179. Stuttgart: Thieme.

Scully, C., Flint, S.R., and Porter, S.R. (1996). *Oral Diseases: An Illustrated Guide to the Diagnosis and Management of Diseases of the Oral Mucosa, Gingivae, Teeth, Salivary Glands, Bones*, 2e. Duntz M. Publ.

Seifert, G. and Burkhardt, A. (1977). Neue morphologische Gesichtspunkte bei malignen Tumoren der Mundschleimhaut. *Dtsch. Med. Wschr.* 102: 1596.

Sexton, J. and O'Hare, D. (1993). Simplified treatment of vascular lesions using the argon laser. *J. Oral Maxillofac. Surg.* 51: 12–16.

Sievers, M., Frentzen, M., and Koort, H.J. (1993). Reflectance of a CO_2 laser beam on metallic dental materials. *J. Dent. Res.* 72: 131. Abstract 223.

Silvermann, S. Jr., Gorsky, M., and Lozada, F. (1984). Oral leukoplakia and malignant transformation: a follow up study of 257 patients. *Cancer* 53: 563–568.

Strong, M.S., Vaughan, C.W., Jako, G.J., and Polanyi, T. (1979a). Transoral management of localized carcinomas of the oral cavity using the CO_2 laser. *Otolaryngol. Clin. N. Am.* 12: 207–218.

Strong, M.S., Vaughan, C.W., Healy, G.B. et al. (1979b). Transoral resection of cancer of the oral cavity: the role of the CO_2 laser. *Laryngoscope* 89: 897–905.

Szaba, J. (1916). Methode zur Verhinderung des Verwachsens der Mundbodenschleimhaut. *Österr. Vjschr. Zahnheilkd.* 32: 244. (German).

Tambuwala, A., Sangle, A., Khan, A., and Sayed, A. (2014). Excision of oral leukoplakia by CO_2 lasers versus traditional scalpel: a comparative study. *J. Maxillofac. Oral Surg.* 13: 320–327.

Vesper M. (1996) Untersuchung zur CO_2-Lasertherapie grossflaeachiger Leukoplakien. Lecture in the German Society of Laser Dentistry. February 2–4, Frankfurt, Germany (in German).

White, J.M., Goodis, H.E., and Rose, C.L. (1991). Use of the pulsed Nd:YAG laser for intraoral soft tissue surgery. *Lasers Surg. Med.* 11: 455–461.

Zachrisson, B.U. (2003). Orthodontics and periodontics. In: *Clinical Periodontology and Implant Dentistry*, 4e (eds. J. Lindhe, T. Karring and N.P. Lang), 744–779. Blackwell.

4

Lasers and Bone Surgery

Georgios E. Romanos

Stony Brook University, School of Dental Medicine, Stony Brook, NY, USA

4.1 Introduction

Medical advances for bone surgical procedures are, among others, facilitated by suitable and practice-oriented drilling and bone-cutting techniques. A promising alternative to drills, microsaws, trephines, and piezosurgery for osteotomy procedures (Al Asseri and Swennen 2018) is bone osteotomy using lasers.

Particularly in the oral cavity, the use of lasers is expected to result in a better quality of osteotomies due to the accessibility of the relatively small size of handpieces and laser delivery systems in intraoral conditions. The requirements of lasers for applications in the bone are much higher than of those for the soft tissues since complete bone evaporation is possible only with very high temperatures, because of the high mineral content of the bone.

In vitro osteotomies using human bone initially used industrial lasers, such as a 250-watt (W) carbon dioxide (CO_2) CW laser (Engelhardt and Bimberg 1972). Later on, experimental medical CO_2 CW systems were introduced as well as pulsed (superpulsed) CO_2 lasers in the ms range. Some studies were focused on the differences in the healing process among different CO_2 lasers, as well as comparisons to conventional osteotomies (Moore 1973; Gertzbein et al. 1981; Walsh et al. 1989). It has been reported that an intense carbonized zone at the osteotomy margins using CO_2 CW lasers is associated with the delay of wound healing. Therefore, mathematical models have been developed to control temperature rise and keep the temperature in constant conditions under CO_2 laser application (Lévesque et al. 2015; Levesque and Robaczewski 2017). Here, we demonstrate advances of laser-assisted bone osteotomies using different wavelengths or using shorter pulse widths, particularly in the μs-range.

4.2 CO_2 Laser

Clayman et al. (1978) demonstrated the influence of the CW and pulsed (superpulsed) CO_2 laser on bone healing in rabbits. In both groups, bone formation could be detected after four weeks, which was completed after two months with simultaneous formation of lamellar bone. The only significant clinical difference between the two laser systems is the much higher average speed of the osteotomy with the superpulsed CO_2 laser, with a pulse energy of 5 J, at an average power of 7 W, a pulse width of 50–200 ms, and a repetition rate of 25–250 Hz, compared to a CO_2 CW laser with energy of 10 J. The results of this study were compared to the wound healing processes with the use of high-speed drills on rabbit bone. It was found that the average quality of the incision with laser application was much better, and effective hemostasis could be achieved; yet the healing of the bone was significantly affected (Clayman 1976).

Studies performed by Small et al. (1979) in the rabbit tibia compared CO_2 laser osteotomies (both in the continuous and in superpulsed mode) with conventional drilling methods and concluded that an intense carbonized zone was formed at the laser-osteotomy, which during the laser use should be removed in order to allow better quality of the cut. The superpulsed lasers (with a maximum average output power of 6 W) showed a delay in wound healing by two to four weeks, in comparison to the CW laser systems with a maximum output power of 10 W. Significantly less lamellar bone formation and lower carbonization zone were shown. Cutting of the bone with 10 W CO_2 CW lasers was not possible (Small et al. 1979).

The bone healing processes were found to be fastest after conventional osteotomy, due to the reduced necrosis and lack of carbonization. A possible reason for these delayed healing processes after laser application is the strong thermal damage of the bone with the use of CW systems or systems that are pulsed in milliseconds. Another disadvantage of CO_2 lasers (CW or pulsed) is the limited visibility during the osteotomy due to the carbonization zone.

In summary, it has been proven that neither industrial nor medical CW and superpulsed CO_2 lasers for processing of bone have brought the desired results. The much-cited CW or superpulsed CO_2 laser cannot be used clinically, due to the thermal stressing of bone. Therefore, different laser systems, in particular with shorter pulse lengths, should be evaluated that would cause lower thermal damage on the bone during the osteotomy process.

Recent studies by Augello et al. (2018) showed that in adult sheep, using micro-CT and histological analysis, more mineralized bone was formed in the laser group compared to the piezoelectric group.

Also, Kuttenberger et al. (2008) used a technically demanding procedure to perform laser osteotomies in sheep tibia. The osteotomy depth was possible at a depth of 20 mm without visible thermal damage to the bone. The computer-guided CO_2 laser osteotomy demonstrated clinical and radiological healing patterns comparable to those seen with osteotomy done by standard mechanical instruments. The authors concluded that through the use of computer guidance, extremely precise osteotomies and sophisticated cut geometries are possible using this technique. For practical applications, precise control of the depth of laser cutting and easier manipulation of the osteotome are required.

Studies using transversaly excited atmospheric (TEA) pressure CO_2 laser systems operating at 9300 nm with pulse durations of 10–20 μs suggested that high repetition rates are well suited for dental applications. Specifically, these systems were used for dentin and bone ablation in vitro (Fan et al. 2006).

In contrast, TEA 9600 nm CO_2 lasers operating at the peak absorption wavelength of bone and with pulse durations of 5–8 μs showed approximately the same thermal relaxation rate as in hard tissue, produced high ablation rates, and minimal peripheral thermal damage. There was no discernible thermal damage and no need for water irrigation during ablation. In comparison, using a free-running Er:YAG laser the peripheral thermal damage measured 25–40 μm (Fried and Fried 2001). However, none of these systems have wide applications in clinical practice.

4.3 Excimer Laser

Due to the effect that CO_2 lasers are not routinely efficient without carbonization and thermal damage, high expectations were placed on the group of the excimer lasers (UV light). These lasers emit short pulses with durations in the nanosecond range in the wavelength range of 193–351 nm.

Comparative studies between the excimer laser (wavelength: 308 nm), the CO_2 CW laser, and an oscillating saw on rabbit bones showed that the excimer laser caused only a small delay in healing compared to the saw (Nelson et al. 1989a, b; Yow et al. 1989). Also, the cutting quality on the bone and cartilage was significantly improved (Nelson et al. 1988, 1989a,b; Walsh and Deutsch 1989; Walsh et al. 1989; Gonzales et al. 1990; Meyer et al. 1990). The healing rate of an excimer laser cut was not slower than mechanical treatments, and the quality of the osteotomy was comparable to mechanical treatment (Dressel et al. 1991).

The ablation rates of excimer lasers in their present form are too low to meet clinical requirements. However, increasing the pulse repetition rate, there is risk of thermal damage stress of the bone (Doerschel 1995), but there are no clinical applications of these systems today.

4.4 Er:YAG and Ho:YAG Lasers

An *in vivo* animal model osteotomy with an Er:YAG laser (full width half maximum [FWHM] 180 μs, 5 Hz) showed after eight weeks complete bone fill of the osteotomy gap (Scholz 1992). It showed no crystallization products and a moderate brown color of the crater rim, although no spray-cooling was used. The osseous structure and healing process were similar to conventional osteotomy methods and the application of the Er:YAG laser. Even after four weeks, the percentage of osseous construction in the osteotomy was more than 90%.

In contrast, the use of Ho:YAG laser ($\lambda = 2.1$ μm, FWHM 250 μs, repetition rate 5–10 Hz, pulse energy 400 mJ) showed a very strong destruction zone. When using a short-pulsed CO_2 laser (9.6 μm, ca. 65 μs FWHM and pulse energy 450 mJ, repetition rate 5 Hz) without spray-cooling, an approximately 5 μm thick carbonization zone was produced, forming a healing barrier, which was not reduced even eight weeks after surgery (Table 4.1).

Since the absorption coefficient of bone at the wavelength of Ho:YAG lasers is low, high-energy densities are necessary, but even then, a cut through the bone with this laser is very difficult. Moreover, complete bone healing was described only after a period of more than eight weeks (Nuss et al. 1988; Charlton et al. 1990).

However, recent studies were performed to explain the dynamic process of bubble evolution induced by Ho:YAG lasers underwater without and with bone tissue and its effects on hard tissue ablation. The results showed that the Ho:YAG laser was capable of ablating

Table 4.1 Bone healing in the osteotomies using different laser systems compared to conventional osteotomy. Quality assessment based on new osteon formation.

Bone Formation	After 4 Weeks	After 8 Weeks
Saw	+++	+++
Excimer laser	++ (+)	+++
Er:YAG laser	++ (+)	+++
Short pulsed CO_2 laser	++	+++
CW CO_2 laser	+	+
Ho:YAG laser	+	++

Bone formation (optimal: +++) (according to Scholz 1992).

hard bone tissue effectively in under water irrigation conditions. The penetration of the Ho:YAG laser can be significantly increased up to about 4 mm with the assistance of the bubble. The hydrokinetic forces associated with the bubble not only contributed to reducing the thermal injury to peripheral tissues but also enhanced the ablation efficiency and improved the ablation crater morphology (Zhang et al. 2016).

Results from studies in which ridge split was performed in pig mandible with Er:YAG laser, piezosurgery, and conventional drills showed that the maximum bone temperature of 7.3 °C was noted for a specimen prepared using piezosurgery devices. Furthermore, the bone temperature after irradiation with an Er:YAG laser with energy of 400 mJ increased more quickly (but less than the critical threshold) in comparison with the cases of energy equal to 200 mJ (Matys et al. 2016).

Besides, decortication for orthodontic implant placement with an Er:YAG laser compared to conventional osteotomy and piezosurgery methods was recently evaluated. The small diameter decortication by the Er:YAG laser appeared to provide better implant primary stability as compared to drill and piezosurgery (Matys et al. 2018).

4.5 Laser Systems for Clinical Dentistry

The currently published data and clinical practice have shown that bone removal and bone osteotomy are only possible with the Er:YAG or the Er,Cr:YSGG lasers. With the currently available applicators, the interventions on the bone, and with the necessary for the practice laser parameters, it is possible to use these laser wavelengths in clinical settings.

The use of special lenses (Zahn et al. 1997) or scanner systems for flat or geometry-based ablation and the use of sapphire fibers and rods as applicator's tail end allow osseous ablation with the Er:YAG laser. The quality of the osteotomy is comparable to the osteotomy performed by the Er,Cr:YSGG laser. Comparison with the conventional osteotomies using a Lindemann bur and piezosurgery showed a better precision in the osteotomy margins at the Er,Cr:YSGG and Er:YAG laser cuts according to Mueller and Romanos (2007) (Figure 4.1).

Besides, electron microscopic evaluation of the margins after Er:YAG or Er,Cr:YSGG laser showed a better cut quality using the Er,Cr:YSGG laser (Figures 4.2 and 4.3).

Sufficient cooling with an aerosol (Figure 4.4), preferably consisting of air and water (Ertl 1995), is essential for a good ablation of bone, as well as also every kind of treatment on biological hard tissues

Water amounts between 1 and 30 ml/min and air amounts between 1 and 10 l/min lead to good results. In this way, the risk of thermal damage can be reduced significantly, especially in the irradiation. Figures 4.2 and 4.3 show the detail of an osteotomy without melting, produced by an Er:YAG and Er,Cr:YSGG laser under spray cooling, respectively. Water spray also prevents the filling of the bone cut with blood, which would change the ablation with the laser, as the penetration depth is a few 10 μm, and therefore the treated osseous surface would be shielded.

Another way to reduce thermal damage on tissues during processing is to reduce the pulse length. However, even at pulse lengths of 50–40 μs, a spray cooling is unavoidable. However, a disadvantage of reducing the pulse length is the increase in pulse peak power. Especially, when using an optical fiber or a sapphire tip in the applicator, it may then lead to increased fiber burning at high energy densities.

In summary, the potential possibilities of bone removal using lasers today may occur in a thickness up to 3 mm. Advantages are the absence of contact with the tissue, the possible precision, and the lack of smear layer during bone cutting with bonemeal.

Clinical applications of bone removal in the oral cavity are:

- Removal of exostoses and alveolar ridge recontouring after multiple tooth extractions (Figures 4.4 and 4.5)
- Bone removal for root tip resection
- Crown lengthening procedures (Figure 4.6)
- Window preparation in sinus augmentations (Figure 4.7)
- Primary drill for implant placement (Figure 4.8)
- Implant removal (Figures 4.9 and 4.10)
- Bone splitting (Figure 4.11)

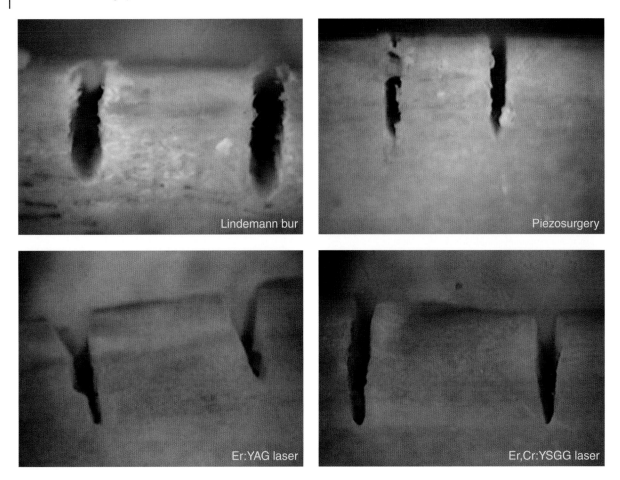

Figure 4.1 Comparison of the osteotomies performed by Lindemann bur, piezosurgery (Mectron), Er:YAG laser (KaVo) and Er,Cr:YSGG laser (Biolase, Inc.) illustrating an excellent quality of the osteotomies using the two laser systems. *Source:* Dr. Georgios E Romanos.

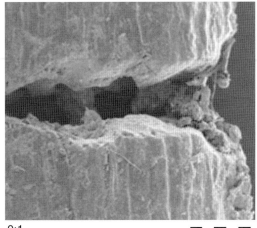

Er:YAG-Laser 300 mj and 15 Hz

0:1

1mm

Figure 4.2 Electron microscopic analysis of an osteotomy using Er:YAG laser (KaVo) and 300 mJ and 15 Hz. *Source:* Dr. Georgios E Romanos.

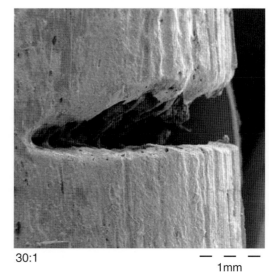

Er,Cr:YSGG-Laser
300 mj and 15 Hz

Figure 4.3 Electron microscopic analysis of an osteotomy using Er,Cr:YSGG laser (Biolase) and 300 mJ and 15 Hz presenting an excellent osteotomy margin. *Source:* Dr. Georgios E Romanos.

30:1

1mm

Case 1   Removal of Lingual Exostoses

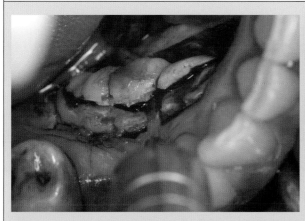

Figure 4.4a   Bone removal using an Er:YAG laser (Hoya, Japan). *Source:* Dr. Georgios E Romanos.

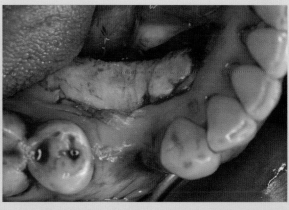

Figure 4.4b   Osteotomy site presenting a smooth surface after exostosis removal using an Er:YAG laser. *Source:* Dr. Georgios E Romanos.

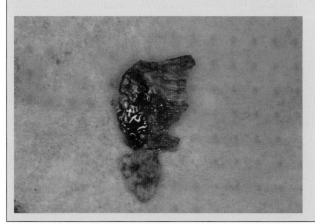

Figure 4.4c   Bone specimen removed with the Er:YAG laser presenting areas of carbonization due to possible overheating. This could lead to possible complications if this bone particle would be used for further grafting procedure. *Source:* Dr. Georgios E Romanos.

Case 2   Removal of Exostosis

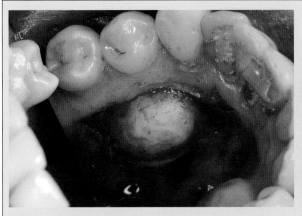 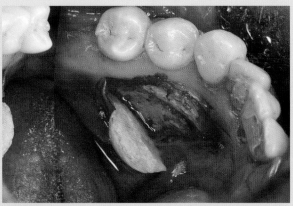

Figure 4.5a Preparation of an exostosis (tori mandibularis) after elevation of a mucoperiosteal flap with an Er:YAG laser. *Source:* Dr. Georgios E Romanos.

Figure 4.5b Osteotomy procedure for removal of a lingual exostosis using an Er:YAG laser. The smooth surface within the osteotomy area presents excellent margins and sufficient bleeding control. *Source:* Dr. Georgios E Romanos.

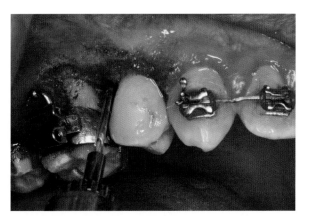 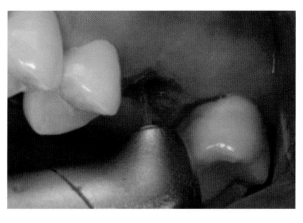

Figure 4.6 Crown lengthening using an Er:YAG laser for osseous reduction and soft tissue excision providing sufficient coagulation. *Source:* Dr. Georgios E Romanos.

Figure 4.8 Preparation of the cortical layer of the alveolar ridge using an Er,Cr:YSGG laser for implant placement. *Source:* Dr. D.S. Sohn, Daegu, Korea.

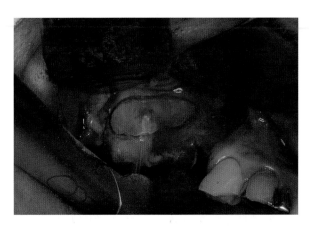 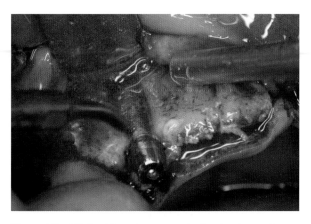

Figure 4.9 Minimal invasive removal of an implant using an Er:YAG laser (Hoya Conbio, Versawave, Tokyo, Japan) under water-cooling and air (parameters: 400 mJ pulse energy/ frequency: 20 Hz). *Source:* Dr. Georgios E Romanos.

Figure 4.7 Window preparation for sinus augmentation using an Er,Cr:YSGG laser. *Source:* Dr. D.S. Sohn, Daegu, Korea.

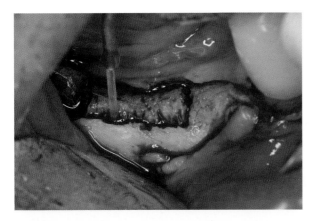

Figure 4.10 Block section using an Er:YAG laser (Hoya Conbio, Versawave, Tokyo, Japan) for removal of a fractured blade implant under water-cooling and air (parameters: 400 mJ pulse energy/frequency: 20 Hz). *Source:* Dr. Georgios E Romanos.

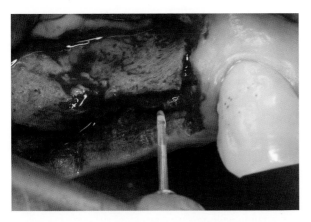

Figure 4.11 Bone splitting using the Er,Cr:YSGG laser (Waterlase® MD) with power of 6 W; hard tissue (H) mode, pulsed beam with duration of 140 µ, and repetition rate of 20 Hz in conjunction with the MG6 tip. *Source:* Dr. D.S. Sohn, Daegu, Korea.

Laser-assisted bone removal for crown lengthening procedures improves the quality of tissue around teeth leading to better aesthetics. This has been reported in various clinical case series (Lowe 2006; Sweeny and Romanos 2006).

However, implants can be placed in the bone after an Er:YAG laser osteotomy providing a significantly better rate of osseointegration (bone-to-implant percentages) in rabbits compared to the control group (Kesler et al. 2006). Recent information from the same specimens showed also that the expression of platelet-derived growth factor (PDGF) is greater in the Er:YAG laser-assisted osteotomy compared to the conventional osteotomy (Kesler et al. 2011).

The Er:YAG laser osteotomy can successfully be used in long bones with a depth of up to 22 mm without producing thermal damage (Stübinger et al. 2010).

Implants can be removed without complications from the surrounding bone. This technique seems to be minimally invasive and efficient (Smith and Rose 2010).

Bone ablation using the Er:YAG laser was studied recently in a pig model, where lateral maxillary windows were prepared for sinus lift procedures. It was shown that the Schneiderian membrane perforation rate during maxillary sinus floor elevation with the Er:YAG laser may significantly reduce the risk of iatrogenic perforation of the Schneiderian membrane and does not cause irreversible thermal damage in the bone. The lateral bony windows were created using an Er:YAG laser (200 mJ, 15 Hz, energy density, 25.48 J/cm^2) and a diamond bur (control). The average time necessary for the laser bony window osteotomy was 10 minutes and 37 seconds, whereas using the bur required middling 5 minutes and 50 seconds (Matys et al. 2017).

Osteotomies have been performed also with the Erbium,chromium:yttrium-scandium-gallium-garnet (Er,Cr:YSGG laser, 2780 nm), and it was found that the Er,Cr:YSGG laser allows for precise surgical bone cutting and ablation with minimal thermal damage to adjacent tissues. Irradiation in different methods may achieve different ablation rates and thermal damage (Wang et al. 2002). Osteotomies using the Er,Cr:YSGG laser utilizing water-air spray at 5 W and 8 Hz for 10 or 30 seconds were investigated, and the cutting effect on canine mandibular bone was evaluated in vitro. Temperature increases were measured in the irradiated areas by thermography. Based on the results of this study, the maximum temperature increase was an average 12.6 °C within 30 seconds irradiation period. The samples were then observed by stereoscopy and scanning electron microscopy to determine morphological changes and by energy-dispersive X-ray spectroscopy to evaluate atomic alterations.

Anatomic analytical examination revealed that the calcium phosphorus ratio was not significantly changed between the lased and unlased areas. No presence of burning, melting, or altering the calcium-phosphorus ratio of the irradiated bone was observed (Kimura et al. 2001).

Recent clinical studies showed the use of the Er,Cr:YSGG laser in sinus lift procedures without clinical complications. The perforation rate of the sinus membrane was relatively high (33.3%) but certainly can be reduced using the correct power settings and with an improvement of the surgical technique (Sohn et al. 2009).

Also, the bone preparation using laser technology (Er,Cr:YSGG laser) for dental implant placement does not compromise the primary stability of the implant compared to conventional techniques. The relationship between implant stability quotient (ISQ) values and implant insertion variables were comparable to those of conventional drilling (Lee et al. 2010).

The Er,Cr:YSGG laser was also used in removing implants in vitro providing superior results over the trephine bur in terms of bone preservation, thermal damage, and cutting efficiency (Hajji et al. 2016). The repair process after the Er,Cr:YSGG laser osteotomy was comparable clinically with the healing after conventional osteotomy (Esteves et al. 2016).

As a conclusion, the Er,Cr:YASGG laser seems to be today the only efficient laser wavelength for bone ablation and bone cutting, which can be used in oral surgery, periodontology, and implant dentistry with comparable results like the conventional osteotomy and therefore can be recommended for clinical use.

References

Al Asseri, N. and Swennen, G. (2018). Minimally invasive orthognathic surgery: a systematic review. *Int. J. Oral Maxillofac. Surg.* 47: 1299–1310.

Augello, M., Deibel, W., Nuss, K. et al. (2018). Comparative microstructural analysis of bone osteotomies after cutting by computer-assisted robot-guided laser osteotome and piezoelectric osteotome: an in vivo animal study. *Lasers Med. Sci.* 33 (7): 1471–1478.

Charlton, A., Dickinson, M.R., King, T.A., and Freemont, A.J. (1990). Er:YAG and Ho:YAG laser ablation of bones. *Lasers Med. Sci.* 5: 365–373.

Clayman, L. (1976). Bone response to carbon-dioxide, rapid-superpulse and continuous wave laser osteotomy in albino rats. *Bull. Sinai Hosp. Detroit.* 24: 189.

Clayman, L., Fuller, T., and Beckmann, H. (1978). Healing of continuous-wave and rapid superpulsed, carbon dioxide, laser-induced bone defects. *J. Oral Surg.* 36: 932–937.

Doerschel, K. (1995). Thermische und nicht-thermische Gewebewirkung. In: Angewandte Laserzahnheilkunde. II-4.3. ecomed. (eds. G. Mueller and T. Ertl). Landsberg/Lech. (German).

Dressel, M., Jahn, R., Neu, W., and Jungbluth, K.H. (1991). Studies in fiber guided excimer laser surgery for cutting and drilling bone and meniscus. *Lasers Surg. Med.* 11 (6): 569–579.

Engelhardt, A. and Bimberg, D. (1972). Osteotomie mit Lascr. *Laser und Elektrooptik* 3: 54. (German).

Ertl, T. (1995). Vermeidung thermischer Schaeden durch Kuehlung. In: Angewandte Laserzahnheilkunde. II-4.4. ecomed. (eds. G. Mueller and T. Ertl). Landsberg/Lech (German).

Esteves, J.C., de Souza Faloni, A.P., Macedo, P.D. et al. (2016). Effects on bone repair of osteotomy with drills or with erbium,chromium:yttrium-scandium-gallium-garnet laser: Histomorphometric and immunohistochemical study. *J. Periodontol.* 87 (4): 452–460.

Fan, K., Bell, P., and Fried, D. (2006). Rapid and conservative ablation and modification of enamel, dentin, and alveolar bone using a high repetition rate transverse excited atmospheric pressure CO_2 laser operating at lambda=9.3 micro. *J. Biomed. Opt.* 11 (6): 064008.

Fried, N.M. and Fried, D. (2001). Comparison of Er:YAG and 9.6-m TE CO_2 lasers for ablation of skull tissue. *Lasers Surg. Med.* 28 (4): 335–343.

Gertzbein, S.D., DeDemeter, D., Cruickshank, B., and Kapasouri, A. (1981). The effect of laser osteotomy on bone healing. *Lasers Surg. Med.* 1: 361.

Gonzales, C., van De Merwe, W.P., Smith, M., and Reinisch, L. (1990). Comparison of the erbium-yttrium Aluminium garnet and carbon dioxide lasers for in vitro bone and cartilage ablation. *Laryngoscope* 100: 14–17.

Hajji, M., Franzen, R., Grümer, S. et al. (2016). Removal of dental implants using the erbium, chromium:yttrium-scandium-gallium-garnet laser and the conventional trephine bur: an in vitro comparative study. *Photomed. Laser Surg.* 34 (2): 61–67.

Kesler, G., Romanos, G., and Koren, R. (2006). Use of Er:YAG laser to improve osseointegration of titanium alloy implants-a comparison of bone healing. *Int. J. Oral Maxillofac. Implants* 21 (3): 375–379.

Kesler, G., Shvero, D.K., Tov, Y.S., and Romanos, GE. (2011). Platelet derived growth factor secretion and bone healing after Er:YAG laser bone irradiation. *J. Oral Implantol.* 37 Spec No:195-204.

Kimura, Y., Yu, D.G., Fujita, A. et al. (2001). Effects of erbium,chromium:YSGG laser irradiation on canine mandibular bone. *J. Periodontol.* 72 (9): 1178–1182.

Kuttenberger, J.J., Stuebinger, S., Waibel, A. et al. (2008). Computer-guided CO_2 laser osteotomy of the sheep tibia: technical prerequisites and first results. *Photomed. Laser Surg.* 26 (2): 129–136.

Lee, S.Y., Piao, C., Heo, S.J. et al. (2010). A comparison of bone bed preparation with laser and conventional drill on the relationship between implant stability quotient (ISQ) values and implant insertion variables. *J. Adv. Prosthodont.* 2 (4): 148–153.

Levesque, L. and Robaczewski, A. (2017). Very accurate temperature control of bones by a CO_2 laser for medical applications. *Appl. Opt.* 56 (13): 3923–3928.

Lévesque, L., Noël, J.M., and Scott, C. (2015). Controlling the temperature of bones using pulsed CO_2 lasers: observations and mathematical modeling. *Biomed. Opt. Express* 6 (12): 4768–4780.

Lowe, R.A. (2006). Clinical use of the Er,Cr:YSGG laser for osseous crown lengthening: redefining the standard of care. *Pract. Proced. Aesthet. Dent.* 18 (4): S2–S9.

Matys, J., Flieger, R., and Dominiak, M. (2016). Assessment of temperature rise and time of alveolar ridge splitting by means of Er:YAG laser, piezosurgery, and surgical saw: An ex vivo study. *Biomed. Res. Int.* 2016: 9654975.

Matys, J., Hadzik, J., and Dominiak, M. (2017). Schneiderian membrane perforation rate and increase in bone temperature during maxillary sinus floor elevation by means of Er:YAG laser-an animal study in pigs. *Implant. Dent.* 26 (2): 238–244.

Matys, J., Flieger, R., Tenore, G. et al. (2018). Er:YAG laser, piezosurgery, and surgical drill for bone decortication during orthodontic mini-implant insertion: primary stability analysis-an animal study. *Lasers Med. Sci.* 33 (3): 489–495.

Meyer, D.R., Scholz, C., Klauke, J. et al. (1990). The short pulsed CO_2 laser 9.6µm wavelength in comparison to the Er:YAG laser at the laser osteotomy. *Laser Med. Surg.* 6: 150–155.

Moore, J.H. (1973). Laser Energy in Orthopedic Surgery, 1e. Amsterdam: Excerpta Medica.

Mueller C, Romanos GE. (2007) Microscopical examination of osteotomies with ultrasonic, laser- and classical procedures. European Association of Osseointegration. Barcelona, October 25–27.

Nelson, J.S., Yow, L., Liaw, L.H.L. et al. (1988). Ablation of bone and methacrylate by prototype and mid-infrared erbium:YAG laser. *Lasers Surg. Med.* 8: 494–500.

Nelson, J.S., Orenstein, A., Liaw, L.H.L., and Berns, M.W. (1989a). Mid-infrared Er:YAG laser ablation of bone: the effect of laser osteotomy on bone healing. *Lasers Surg. Med.* 9: 362–374.

Nelson, J.S., Orenstein, A., Liaw, L.H.L. et al. (1989b). Ultra-violet 308nm excimer laser ablation of bone: an acute and chronic study. *Appl. Opt.* 28: 2350–2357.

Nuss, R.C., Fabian, R.L., Sarkar, R., and Puliafito, C.A. (1988). Infrared laser bone ablation. *Lasers Surg. Med.* 8: 381–391.

Scholz, C. (1992). Neue Verfahren der Bearbeitung von Hartgewebe in der Medizin mit dem Laser. In: Advances in Laser Medicine (eds. G. Müller and H.-P. Berlien). Landberg/Lech: Ecomed Verlag. (German).

Small, I.A., Osborn, T.P., Fuller, T. et al. (1979). Observations of carbon dioxide laser and bone bur in the osteotomy of the rabbit tibia. *J. Oral Surg.* 37: 159–166.

Smith, L.P. and Rose, T. (2010). Laser explantation of a failing endosseous dental implant. *Aust. Dent. J.* 55 (2): 219–222.

Sohn, D.S., Lee, J.S., An, K.M., and Romanos, G.E. (2009). Erbium,chromium:yttrium-scandium-gallium-garnet laser-assisted sinus graft procedure. *Lasers Med. Sci.* 24 (4): 673–677.

Stübinger, S., Nuss, K., Pongratz, M. et al. (2010). Comparison of Er:YAG laser and piezoelectric osteotomy: An animal study in sheep. *Lasers Surg. Med.* 42 (8): 743–751.

Sweeny, S. and Romanos, G.E. (2006). Laser-assisted soft tissue management in esthetic dentistry. *J. Oral Laser Appl.* 6: 133–139.

Walsh, J.T. and Deutsch, T.F. (1989). Er:YAG laser ablation of tissue: measurement of ablation rates. *Lasers Surg. Med.* 9: 327–337.

Walsh, J.T., Flotte, T.J., and Deutsch, T.F. (1989). Er:YAG laser ablation of tissue: effect of pulse duration and tissue type on thermal damage. *Lasers Surg. Med.* 9: 314–326.

Wang, X., Ishizaki, N.T., Suzuki, N. et al. (2002). Morphological changes of bovine mandibular bone irradiated by Er,Cr:YSGG laser: an in vitro study. *J. Clin. Laser Med. Surg.* 20 (5): 245–250.

Yow, L., Nelson, J.S., and Berns, M.W. (1989). Ablation of bone and polymethylmethacrylate by an XeCl (308nm) excimer laser. *Lasers Surg. Med.* 9: 141–147.

Zahn, H., Jungnickcl, V., Eitl, T. et al. (1997). Knochenchirurgie mit dem Er:YAG Laser. *Lasermedizin* 13: 31–36. (German).

Zhang, X., Chen, C., Chen, F. et al. (2016). In vitro investigation on Ho:YAG laser-assisted bone ablation underwater. *Lasers Med. Sci.* 31 (5): 891–898.

5

Lasers in Periodontology

Georgios E. Romanos

Stony Brook University, School of Dental Medicine, Stony Brook, NY, USA

5.1 Introduction

The main goal in the treatment of periodontitis is the removal of subgingival biofilm, bacterial endotoxins, and calculus, which are localized in the hard tissues, such as cementum, enamel, and exposed dentin. The main aim of the treatment is entire removal of calculus (scaling) and planing of the root surface (root planing) without unnecessary removal of healthy tooth structures. In addition, the removal of periodonto-pathogenic bacteria, especially in areas not easily accessible to hand instruments, should be one of the main goals in the treatment of periodontal pockets. Biofilm penetrates the epithelium and the underlying connective tissue to a depth of 500 µm (Manor et al. 1984), releasing pro-inflammatory cytokines, collagenases, elastases, and others, destroying the foundation of the periodontal support and leading to a continuous loss of attachment.

Deep periodontal pockets cannot be cleaned sufficiently; periodonto-pathogenic bacteria support tissue destruction and, therefore, as a rationale of periodontal therapy a reduction of probing depth as well as gain of attachment should be considered. A sulcus with 1–3 mm probing depth controls the disease progression (Claffey and Egelberg 1995).

Nonsurgical and surgical periodontal therapy provide reconstruction of the periodontal sulcus (repair or regeneration), from the periodontal lesion having an inflamed pocket epithelium and connective tissue to a healthy periodontal support with a *reattachment* (reunion of the epithelium and connective tissue adherence with the root surface) and establishment of a long junctional epithelium or a *new attachment* (establishment of new stable connective tissue, which may include new

cementum). Different studies in Rhesus monkeys performed by Caton and Nyman (1980) and Caton et al. (1980) at Eastman Dental Center in Rochester, New York, showed that different periodontal treatment modalities, such as periodic root planing in conjunction with soft tissue curettage and Widman flap procedure with and without bone grafts, resulted in the reformation of an epithelial lining along the treated root surfaces (long junctional epithelium), with absence of new connective tissue attachment. In any case, the formation of a long junctional epithelium was achieved at the same level as before treatment. Further studies showed also that the Widman flap surgical procedure does not increase the bone fill in infrabony defects, and no connective tissue attachment has been proven after this procedure in monkeys (Caton and Nyman 1980). A long junctional epithelium was established after this procedure as well.

Further analysis of the literature shows evidence that healing without or minimal connective tissue attachment but migration of a long junctional epithelium is possible in humans today (Cobb 1996).

The ideal concept might be the retardation of the long junctional epithelium in the defect after scaling and root planing (SRP), providing a new connective tissue attachment with adaptation of dense collagen fibers (Caton and Zander 1979) for a better periodontal support without gingival recessions and improvement of esthetics.

From the biological standpoint the removal of inflamed tissues, such as pocket epithelium and connective tissue, allows the host to better eliminate bacterial toxins and regenerate lost tissues in the periodontal apparatus. Therefore, many studies have tried to prove the importance of removal of the inflamed epithelium in the pocket using excision with a hand instrument (curettage), a scalpel (excision new attachment procedure, ENAP), or flap elevation (Widman surgical procedure) (Yukna et al. 1976; Ramfjord et al. 1987). The main objective in all these approaches is the reduction of probing pocket depth and bleeding on probing, bacteria elimination, and the improvement of connective tissue attachment.

Other surgical approaches to improve connective tissue attachment have been developed with high sensitivity and costs using barriers (Guided Tissue Regeneration, GTR) with or without bone grafting materials. The exclusion of the migration of the epithelium and connective tissue fibers in the periodontal lesion will be attempted, promoting new cementum with inserting collagen (Sharpey's) fibers and also new bone formation. Even though GTR has a greater effect on probing reduction than open flap debridement, there is marked variability between studies, and the clinical relevance of these changes is unknown. Therefore, it is difficult to draw general conclusions about the clinical benefit of GTR and the factors affecting outcomes. There is a need to consider the predictability of this technique compared with other methods of treatment before making final decisions on use (Needleman et al. 2006).

However, a significant body of information has been produced in several clinical research centers evaluating the therapeutic responses of the periodontium to different treatment modalities. These studies provide evidence that periodontal therapy is effective in controlling periodontal inflammation, and that dentitions can be preserved for extended periods of time following treatments and proper maintenance. In general, there are no significant differences between the periodontal treatments evaluated. Therefore, the trend is from a resective to a more conservative, anti-infective therapeutic approach and evaluation of the patient (Caffesse and Quiñones 1993).

Dental lasers may contribute to the field of periodontology, where other types of therapy and protocols cannot achieve the best clinical outcome. Even though there is limited evidence supporting laser-mediated periodontal therapy over traditional treatment (Cobb 2006), there are reasons to include lasers in periodontal therapy as an adjunctive tool or as an alternative to conventional methods.

Due to the benefits of lasers, such as ablation or vaporization of the inflamed tissues, hemostasis and bactericidal effects may improve the periodontal condition and clinical outcomes. Less treatment time, less vibration and noise, as well as less operative pain, reduce the physical and mental stress of the patient and

dentist (Ishikawa and Sculean 2007). Certainly, disadvantages like the costs of the equipment and the thermal side effects in conjunction with high risk of tissue destruction have to be considered for clinical application in daily routine practice.

There are two terms important for laser-assisted periodontal therapy:

1) *Laser decontamination,* which defines bacteria reduction within the inflamed periodontium, implant surfaces, and the beneficial effects in the biofilm and
2) *Laser coagulation,* which means sealing of the blood vessels, capillaries, and lymphatic vessels in the inflamed tissues after laser decontamination.

Specifically, the following aims should be considered in the application of lasers during periodontal therapy:

- Bacteria reduction in the periodontal pockets
- Removal of dental calculus and subgingival hard deposits
- Root planing
- Removal of periodontal pocket epithelium and inflamed granulation tissue
- Retardation of the epithelial downgrowth in the defect

5.2 Laser-Assisted Bacteria Reduction in Periodontal Tissues

The current treatment concept for the therapy of periodontal disease focuses on the control of supragingival plaque and subgingival microflora. The standard therapy is to achieve supragingival plaque and calculus removal and reduction (and if possible elimination) of the attached plaque and "swimmers" in the biofilm with curettes, as well as special modified ultrasonic scalers. A complete removal of the pathogenic bacteria is currently not possible. For about 95% of patients, it is sufficient if plaque is reduced to under a certain value, which, in conjunction with the host response, corresponds with a clinically healthy periodontium. The host is, in general, able to maintain a good periodontal clinical condition independent of the bacteria presence. For most patients, the progress of the disease is under control only through local bacteria and endotoxin reduction.

Lasers, whose irradiation is transferred by glass fibers or other delivery systems, could be therefore used in order to support therapy by decontaminating root surfaces by means of their photoablation and thermal effects. In addition, laser irradiation (specifically the Er:YAG laser) in conjunction with scaling and root planing (SRP) may not only control the microorganisms in the periodontal pockets but also may be considered as a prophylactic method against transient bacteremia (Komatsu et al. 2012).

There is a plethora of in vitro studies demonstrating bacteria reduction using lasers, and these studies define the radiation parameters (Table 5.1) (Tseng et al. 1991b; White et al. 1991; Cobb et al. 1992; Ando et al. 1996; Coffelt et al. 1997; Gokhale et al. 2012; Komatsu et al. 2012).

The bactericidal effect is explained primarily by the photothermal effects of the laser irradiation on the tissues. For instance, the irradiation with the excimer laser is absorbed mainly from the bacterial DNA. In this case, substantially low energy density is necessary in comparison to other lasers to achieve a bactericidal effect (Purucker et al. 1994).

Encouraged by these positive in vitro results, single in vivo studies were carried out. According to studies performed by Liu et al. (1999) with a Nd:YAG laser as an adjunctive tool (mechanical + laser), a further bacteria reduction of 25–40% is possible. This effect becomes particularly obvious on black-pigmented microorganisms, because the laser irradiation is absorbed specifically by their melanin particles.

Working with high energies, which are necessary for the antibacterial effects, and without water-cooling produces an undesirable thermal effect of the laser radiation. In experiments with rabbits, it was proven that the critical temperature for the bone is only 10 °C above the body temperature within a period of 1 minute (Eriksson and Albrektsson 1983). Another in vivo study, in which gutta-percha was condensed in the root canal thermomechanically, showed that, in 28% of the cases cementum resorption was caused as a result of a temperature rise of about 18 °C (Saunders 1990). The study by Wilder-Smith et al. (1995) proved that this destruction of periodontal structures also happens in treatment with the Nd:YAG laser (5 W power, 1100 J/cm^2 energy density), in which a temperature rise was measured on the root surface of up to 22 °C after a treatment duration of 5 minutes with the Nd:YAG laser.

In vital teeth the applied thermal energy also affects the pulp tissue. According to Wilder-Smith et al. (1995), temperature rises up to 36 °C were measured in the pulp with Nd:YAG laser. These temperature rises are strongly dependent on the thickness of the dentin at the area of the laser application. Studies with Nd:YAG lasers have yielded temperature rises of 27 °C, with only 100 J/cm^2 (duration 30 seconds), if the dentin thickness is only 0.5 mm (White et al. 1994). A study with the Er:YAG laser revealed that an applied energy density of 2000 J/cm^2 (duration 20 seconds) caused a temperature rise of 18° C in the pulp (Aoki et al. 1994). This is due to the lower penetration depth of this laser radiation due to the tooth's hard substance (Table 5.2). The high

Table 5.1 Bactericidal effect of laser irradiation in vitro.

Study	Laser Wavelength	Bacteria	Power Density
Tseng et al. (1991b)	Nd:YAG	no defined	No defined
White et al. (1991)	Nd:YAG	B. subt., E. coli	No defined
Cobb et al. (1992)	Nd:YAG	A.a., P.g., P.i.	No defined
Purucker et al. (1994)	Excimer	A.a., P.g., P.i.	13 mJ/cm^2
Ando et al. (1996)	Er:YAG	A.a., P.g.	0.3 J/cm^2
Coffelt et al. (1997)	CO$_2$	E. coli	11 J/cm^2
Gokhale et al. (2012)	Er:YAG	Anaerobes	No defined
Komatsu et al. (2012)	Er:YAG	P.i., P.g., T.f., T.d.,F.n.	No defined

Table 5.2 Temperature increase during laser irradiation in vitro.

Study	Laser Wavelength	Power Density	Time	Pulp	Root
Aoki et al. (1994)	Er:YAG	2000 J/cm^2	20 sec	18 °C	39 °C
White et al. (1994)	Nd:YAG	100 J/cm^2	30 sec	6–43 °C	–
Wilder-Smith et al. (1995)	Nd:YAG	1100 J/cm^2	300 sec	36 °C	22 °C

temperatures resulting from the treatment with the laser are not acceptable. The corresponding water-cooling is therefore absolutely necessary, and similarly also in the use of ultrasonic scalers.

The bactericidal effects of the Nd:YAG laser (in vivo) on root surfaces and on the subgingival flora have been studied very early (Cobb et al. 1992; Ben Hatit et al. 1996). Other studies present contradictory results of the use of the Nd:YAG laser in periodontal therapy with no benefits to traditional SRP (Liu et al. 1999). However, a relatively recent review of the literature has been conducted to evaluate the evidence of the use of the Nd:YAG laser, supporting this treatment modality as mono-therapy or in conjunction with conventional non-surgical therapy (SRP). The review showed poor evidence of the benefits of the pulsed Nd:YAG laser in the treatment of periodontal disease (Thomas and Shafer 2011).

In contrast to the pulsed Nd:YAG laser, the bactericidal effects of the 980 nm diode laser (2.5 W, continuous wave in contact with the pocket epithelium in the pocket for subgingival curettage) as an adjunct to mechanical debridement were compared to conventional debridement and periodontal flap procedure and showed a greater reduction of the anaerobic bacteria in comparison to the control group (Gokhale et al. 2012).

Besides this thermal effect, changes on the root surfaces are also caused when using the Nd:YAG and CO_2 laser. When using the CO_2 laser for bacteria reduction in the periodontal tissues, damages, such as craters and microcracking, but also melting of the surface with increased porosity, can also occur with energy density levels of 41 J/cm^2 (Coffelt et al. 1997). Other studies have revealed that these damages lead to a bioincompatibility of the root surface for fibroblasts (Table 5.3) (Morlock et al. 1992; Trylovich et al. 1992; Thomas et al. 1994; Radvar et al. 1995; Wilder-Smith et al. 1995; Coffelt et al. 1997). In contrast to these studies Crespi et al. (2002) showed an increased fibroblast attachment

when root surfaces were irradiated with a defocused CO_2 laser, in pulsed mode with a low power of 2 W combined with mechanical instrumentation (ultrasonics) and was suggested as a useful tool for root conditioning.

With the evidence yielded by these studies, there is doubt whether treatment of the root surface with the currently available laser technologies in comparison to conventional therapy facilitates an improvement of the clinical outcome or leads to a more intense bacteria reduction.

5.3 Removal of Subgingival Calculus

The removal of calculus with hand instruments is a difficult technique, which requires advanced training and can be performed correctly only by well-trained, experienced clinicians. In addition to that, it is a procedure which cannot be tolerated by high number of patients due to discomfort. In contrast to that, the use of lasers to remove calculus seems to be a relatively simple technique with many advantages.

Tseng et al. (1991a) carried out the first studies with an Nd:YAG laser on freshly extracted molars. Although no better dental calculus removal was proven, there was a significant reduction of the processing steps which are necessary for its removal.

Selective dental calculus removal is in vitro possible with a Q-switched Nd:YAG laser using a certain energy density. Nevertheless, this laser is not yet available for dental applications. Furthermore, the removal rates, with the necessary settings for selective work, are very low. The excimer laser with wavelength of 193 nm also may be used for selective calculus removal without causing damage in the root structure (Frentzen et al. 1992).

Additional studies also showed the positive effects in the removal of calculus using the frequency-doubled

Table 5.3 Root surface changes due to laser irradiation *in vitro*.

Study	Laser Wavelength	Power Density	Changes
Morlock et al. (1992)	Nd:YAG	No defined	Craters, melting
Trylovich et al. (1992)	Nd:YAG	No defined	Craters, melting, Lack of biocompatibility
Thomas et al. (1994)	Nd:YAG	No defined	Lack of biocompatibility
Radvar et al. (1995)	Nd:YAG	No defined	Melting, porosity
Wilder-Wilder-Smith et al. (1995)	Q-switched Nd:YAG	922 J/cm^2	Craters, melting, substrate destruction
Coffelt et al. (1997)	CO_2	41 J/cm^2	Craters, melting, porosity

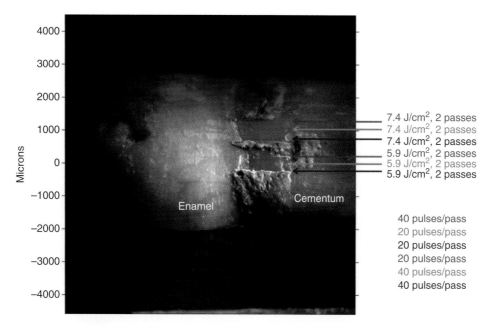

Figure 5.1 Removal of calculus in vitro using a new laser with wavelength of 400 nm. *Source:* (IPG Photonics, Oxford, MA.), J. Schoenly, PhD (IPG Photonics, Oxford, MA).

alexandrite laser (Rechmann and Henning 1995). The solid-state laser with a wavelength 337 nm, pulse duration 100 ns, removes dental calculus without damage to the cementum. However, recent experimental studies provide further information that a specific laser wavelength of 400 nm may be more efficient for calculus removal (Schoenly et al. 2010). Based on these studies with a scanning electron microscope (SEM), the 400 nm laser appears to be efficient for calculus removal resulting in a root surface more suitable for repair (Figure 5.1) in comparison to the conventional methods, such as use of ultrasonics and hand instruments (Schoenly et al. 2013).

All above laser wavelengths have no clinical applications, since they do not exist in the dental market today.

The only clinically used lasers for calculus removal are the Er:YAG laser (2940 nm) or the Er,Cr:YSGG laser (2790 nm) and the more recent CO_2 laser SOLEA (9300 nm). In vitro studies of Aoki et al. (1994) in Japan have shown the effective removal of calculus with an Er:YAG laser (Figure 5.2). The pulsed Er:YAG laser used with water irrigation was able to remove subgingival calculus from the tooth root effectively at an energy level of about 30 mJ/pulse (energy density: 10.6J/cm^2/pulse) and 10 pps, under in vitro conditions. Ablation of the tooth substance on laser-assisted scaling was generally observed within the cementum. However, the angle of the working tip of the Er:YAG laser seems to influence the amount of root substance removal and determines the clinical outcome. Angles of the working tip

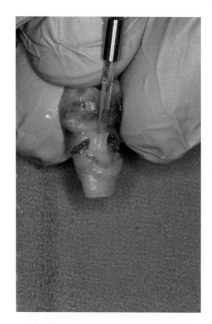

Figure 5.2 Calculus removal using the Er:YAG laser on an extracted tooth. *Source:* Dr. Georgios E Romanos.

less than 30° are beneficial without damage to the root surface (Folwaczny et al. 2001).

On the other hand, root surfaces temperatures rise to 39 °C, without cooling. On the pulp wall, there is a temperature rise of 18.4 °C. In order to avoid damage to the surrounding periodontal tissues and the pulp, water-cooling is of importance. Also problematic is the control of the substance removal, because not only hard deposits, but also dental hard tissue (cementum, dentin) is removed. Depending on the pulse energy (30–120 mJ/pulse, 10 pps frequency), the ablation depth of the dentin can be 74–136 μm (Aoki et al. 1994). This was found in studies of teeth of Asian patients. Because a potential complete removal of the cementum in the root surface cannot be avoided, an electronic control of lasers would be a possible solution for future clinical practice.

Other studies on calculus removal were performed by German groups of scientists and demonstrated the advantages of the Er:YAG laser for removal of subgingival calculus (Keller and Hibst 1995). Studies also showed increased loss of cementum and dentin, demonstrating roughened surfaces, which should be taken into account in clinical conditions (Frentzen et al. 2002). The used parameters were set at 160 mJ/pulse and frequency of 10 Hz. It has to be noted that there is a possible genetic difference in the cementum thickness between Caucasian and Asian teeth.

In an in vivo application of the laser, a sapphire tip (for the erbium family lasers) was used to remove calculus, which is in contact with the root surface or on an angle less than 30° in nonsurgical or surgical therapy to avoid deep crater formation (Folwaczny et al. 2001). Nevertheless, on the interproximal surfaces, there is no possibility of direct irradiation, in spite of the sufficient access, because the "side-firing fibers," which occur at the tip of the beam applicator with a deflection mirror, are not yet available.

Initial clinical studies presented an increase in attachment after nonsurgical periodontal therapy with an Er:YAG laser and maintenance of the clinical parameters for up to two years and is comparable to conventional scaling (Schwarz et al. 2003).

However, clinical studies by Sculean et al. (2004a) with nonsurgical periodontal therapy showed that sites treated with an Er:YAG laser demonstrated a mean gain of clinical attachment similar to a group where ultrasonics were used at three and six months. No statistically significant differences were observed between the groups of treatment, and both therapies led to significant improvements of the investigated clinical parameters.

In contrast to these studies, a flap surgery and use of an Er:YAG laser (160 mJ, 10 Hz) in comparison to the use of ultrasonics in conjunction with surgical treatment showed at six months after treatment that both therapies led to significant improvements of the clinical parameters. The Er:YAG laser may represent a suitable alternative for root surface and defect debridement in conjunction with periodontal surgery (Sculean et al. 2004b).

Additional studies showed positive effect using the Er,Cr:YSGG laser in the treatment of intrabony defects associated with chronic periodontitis and minimal invasive nonsurgical (closed) procedure. Specifically, the study was performed by Al-Falaki et al. (2016) and showed significant reduction in intrabony defect depth but no change in suprabony bone height. More than half (9 of 15) of the examined defects presented more than 50% bone fill. The Er,Cr:YSGG laser was used with a 14 mm 500 μm radial firing periodontal tip (RFTP5, Biolase, Irvine, CA, USA) and 1.5 W power, 30 Hz frequency, and 20 : 11% (water: air) ratio. The tip was placed parallel to the long axis of the tooth into the base of the pocket, moving in vertical and horizontal movements as long as granulation tissue was debrided from the pocket. Deepithelization occurred using a 50 Hz frequency outside the periodontal pocket to the level of the mucogingival junction to be able to eliminate the epithelial cells and control the epithelial proliferation (downgrowth).

> The erbium family of lasers may be used for the removal of calculus in a similar way, like ultrasonics, improving the clinical outcomes. The main advantage over ultrasonic use is less sensitivity and discomfort during the cleaning procedure.

In contrast to the previous laser wavelengths, studies showed that the conventional CO_2 laser in the periodontal pocket may lead to alterations in the root surfaces and charring or carbonization. Modifying the pulse duration and using microsecond pulse lengths, Vaderhobli et al. (2010) were able to show histologically in porcine oral mucosa and periodontal tissues no damage of the hard tissues, such as root surface, enamel, and bone during sulcular debridement. In addition, the coagulation zone was less than 100 nm. With the clinically effective ablation of the pocket epithelium, there was not damage of the periodontium or the pulp. This effect is due to the increased tissue relaxation time with the use of microsecond pulses during the laser irradiation.

5.4 Removal of Pocket Epithelium

For about 5% of periodontitis patients it is advisable to make the elimination of plaque easier by removal of the pocket epithelium and the inflamed connective tissue to prevent a recurrence of the lesion. This inflamed tissue can be removed by irradiation of the periodontal pocket walls with an Nd:YAG laser.

Successful results in intraoral soft tissue applications were reported by White et al. (1991), which showed specifically pocket depth reduction, and less postoperative bleeding, inflammation, and pain after the use of the Nd:YAG laser compared to scalpel surgery. Similarly, we demonstrated positive effects of the Nd:YAG laser use in oral soft tissue and periodontal applications (Romanos 1994a). We were able to observe relatively early a slower epithelial migration and proliferation in the periodontal sites in a patient with acute necrotized ulcerative gingivitis (1.75 W and 20 pps on the contact probe) (Romanos 1994b). In comparison to the conventional gingivectomy with the gingivectomy knife, the laser glass fiber removes the sulcular and oral epithelium of the pocket presenting a slower formation and apical migration of the epithelial layers compared to the conventional excision (Romanos 1994b). This was explained due to the delayed wound healing associated with the laser, due to heat transfer. After this observation was made in more clinical cases, we were able to evaluate in vitro the impact of the laser on the epithelial proliferation.

The lack of pocket epithelium immediately after laser curettage was also histologically proven in a study by Gold and Vilardi (1994). Specifically, in patients with moderate periodontal pockets, a Nd:YAG laser was used with a frequency of 20 Hz, pulse duration of 150 μs, power of 1.25, and 1.75 W (representing the energy density of 70 and 120 J/cm^2 with the use of a fiber 320 μm in diameter) and treatment duration of two to three minutes per tooth. With both implemented powers, biopsies of the soft tissues (taken immediately after irradiation) showed that the pocket epithelium could be completely removed without causing detectable damage (at the light microscopical level) of the underlying connective tissues.

New studies using an Nd:YAG laser with water-cooling compared short-term effects of the pulsed Nd:YAG laser as an adjunct to SRP in the treatment of periodontitis. The clinical improvement was significantly higher in the lased group, and samples of gingival crevicular fluid (GCF) showed specifically a significant reduction of IL-1b and MMP-8 after the use of the pulsed Nd:YAG laser (average power: 4 W; energy: 80 mJ/pulse; frequency: 50 Hz; fiber diameter: 600 μm) compared to SRP alone (Qadri et al. 2010). The authors cannot easily explain the reason for improvement of the periodontal status after the use of the laser glass fiber in the periodontal tissues but discuss the significance of the partial removal of the pocket epithelial lining as a contributing factor for the decrease of periodontal inflammation and less discomfort for patients in these sites (Qadri et al. 2010). In addition, the long-term effects (after 20 months) of the single application of an Nd:YAG laser in combination with SRP had positive effects on periodontal health compared to treatment by SRP alone (Qadri et al. 2011).

Additional studies in animal in vitro models using the glass fiber (300 μm) of a 980 nm diode laser for soft tissue curettage have been used in comparison to conventional curettes (Figure 5.3). The study showed a complete removal of the epithelium (Figure 5.3a–c) within the pocket after use of a 980 nm diode laser (2 W, CW) but no epithelial removal after the use of hand

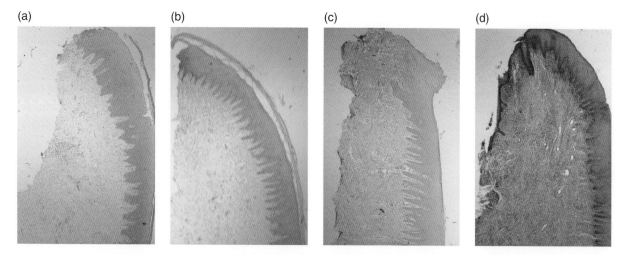

Figure 5.3 Removal of the long junctional epithelium in ex vivo conditions in the bovine periodontium (treatment provided by [a] a clinician with complete training in periodontology and oral surgery; [b] an oral surgeon; [c] a general dentist); (d) control debridement with a curette shows still presence of the long junctional epithelium. *Source:* Dr. Georgios E Romanos.

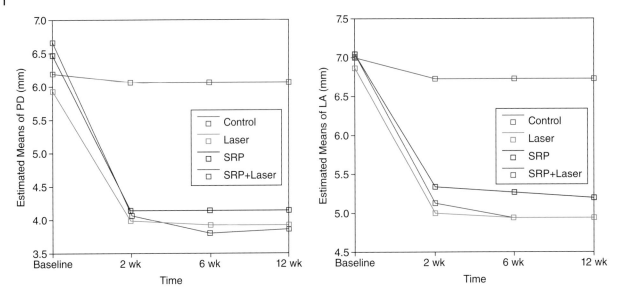

Figure 5.4 Mean PPD over time and mean CAL over time. Clinical parameters after the use of a 980 nm diode laser in the periodontal pocket in aggressive periodontitis patients. The laser-assisted SRP reduced significantly the PPD and the loss of attachment (Kamma et al. 2009).

instruments (Figure 5.3d). This epithelial removal was achieved in all cases with the laser and independent of the experience level of the clinicians (Romanos et al. 2004).

Clinical studies using a 980 nm diode laser as an adjunct tool to SRP showed a moderate qualitative improvement over traditional treatment in the clinical indices with significant reduction of sensitivity and less discomfort during treatment (Borrajo et al. 2004). In addition, no detectable surface alterations and no signs of thermal side effects in any of the treated teeth were observed (Castro et al. 2006).

A significant contribution in the literature is the clinical and microbiological study performed by Kamma et al. (2009), who showed a significant reduction of periodonto-pathogenic bacteria in patients with aggressive periodontitis using a 980 nm continuous wave laser and 2 W average power (Figure 5.4).

Due to the effects of laser decontamination and laser coagulation, the vascularization of the periodontal tissues will be reduced, the water content will be reduced, and the tissue becomes firm and less vascularized. Like the Nd:YAG laser, the diode lasers have a relatively high affinity for chromophores in pigmented tissues, which results in good hemostasis. In addition, there is higher penetration in the tissue and higher resorption by black-pigmented bacteria compared to the Er:YAG and CO_2 lasers. Therefore, irradiation using these wavelengths is more selective to the periodonto-pathogenic bacteria and removal of the epithelial lining in the pocket.

Retrospective analysis of clinical cases after the use of laser-assisted nonsurgical periodontal therapy after 10 years in deep periodontal pockets with more than 6 mm PPD was published by Roncati et al. (2017). The application of an 810 nm pulsed diode laser with 1 W power (mean: 0.5 W; 10 Hz; fiber 320 μm) or a 980 nm pulsed diode laser with 2.5 W power (mean: 0.75 W; 15 kHz; fiber 400 μm) had a significant improvement of the periodontal clinical parameters over the long term.

Also, in a high number of clinical cases (2683 patients in a multicenter study), the microbial profiling of the periodontal pockets was evaluated after the use of an Nd:YAG laser. This recent study demonstrates for the first time the efficacy of the laser-assisted periodontal therapy based on the microbial response of the tissue to the laser therapy (Martelli et al. 2016).

Nevertheless, more research is necessary to prove that the removal of inflamed granulation tissue from osseous periodontal defects is also possible without simultaneous damage to the surrounding healthy periodontal structures due to the deep tissue penetration. This applies particularly to the treatment of deep vertical and furcation defects.

The following protocol is suggested for removal of pocket epithelium and inflamed periodontal tissues:

After the initial phase of periodontal therapy (hygiene phase) and evaluation of the clinical condition, scaling and root planing will be performed to establish a smooth cementum, free of biofilm and calculus, in order to achieve a new attachment.

Laser-assisted SRP will be performed according to the following protocol:

1) Topical anesthesia, low power laser irradiation (1 W for pulsed Nd:YAG and maximum 2 W for diode lasers in a continuous mode) or pulsed mode using the 300–400 μm glass fiber in order to enlarge the pocket for better access. An initiated tip allows excision of the soft tissue (ablation of the inner part of the pocket epithelium will be accomplished).

2) The next step includes corono-apical movements within the pocket in a depth of approximately 3 mm. Laser coagulation during irradiation and decontamination can be achieved at the same time.

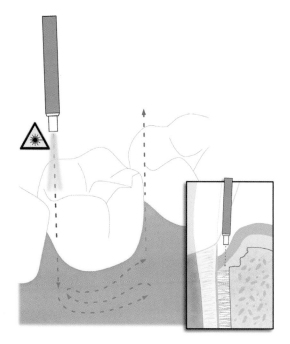

Figure 5.5 Schematic illustration of the laser fiber movement within the pocket for coagulation and decontamination.

In case of sensitivity or pain, local anesthesia is indicated. A noninitiated tip allows diffused energy transfer into the connective tissue to reduce bacteria and exudation.

3) Removal of calculus with an Er:YAG laser or ultrasonics in conjunction with hand instruments (scalers and curettes) for root planing. Due to instrumentation, spontaneous bleeding is initiated.

4) The final step of the treatment is irradiation and coagulation (bleeding control) with the fiber using corono-apical movements in simultaneous mesio-distal orientation (Figure 5.5) using 1.5–2 W average power with a frequency of 50–70 Hz for the pulsed Nd:YAG (fiber 300–400 μm), or 2–3 W (CW) or 4 W (pulsed mode, 50 Hz) for the diode laser (fiber 400 μm), after initiation (with an articulating paper). If the fiber is coated with debris, the fiber has to be cleaved and recalibrated. This laser procedure will be done in the maximum depth (based on PPD measurement), reduced 1–2 mm with the glass fiber in the pocket.

At this final step, removal of the epithelium migrating into the pocket, the so-called sulcular epithelium, will be performed, as well as stabilization of the blood clot within the pocket using the laser. This clot represents a biological barrier in the wound, which does not allow migration of the epithelium in the wound (Figure 5.6). For pockets more than 4–5 mm deep, a removal of the oral epithelium (outer surface of the pocket is also recommended (deepithelialization). This will be done only in deep pockets and should not be utilized in every pocket.

5) During laser irradiation the fiber will be kept in contact with soft tissues (laser curettage) and in parallel position to the root surface. In case of the CO_2 laser application, the perio-tip will be positioned in a similar way within the pocket (Figure 5.7).

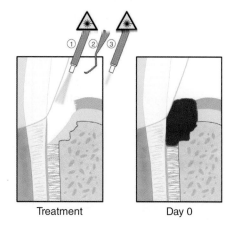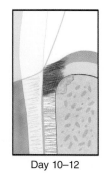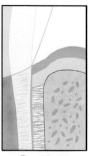

| Treatment | Day 0 | Day 10–12 | Day 30–60 |

Figure 5.6 Schematic illustration of the periodontal wound healing after laser irradiation of the pocket.

The Er:YAG laser sapphire, chisel-type tip is used in contact with the root surface also performing calculus removal and simultaneously root planing (Figure 5.8).

For localized deep pockets (advanced periodontal lesions) a deepithelialization should be performed every 7–10 days (see also Section 5.5) or a flap surgery in conjunction with laser treatment may be indicated. In case of nonsurgical laser-assisted therapy, the deepithelialization should be performed without inserting the fiber in the newly formed sulcus. Only the oral epithelium should be ablated with the laser at this time.

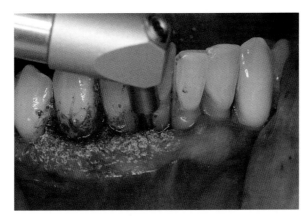

Figure 5.7 CO_2 laser irradiation in the pocket as well as deepithelialization technique. *Source:* Dr. Georgios E Romanos.

7) Routine postoperative instructions, such as rinsing with salt water as well as careful toothbrushing with a soft toothbrush using gentle pressure, are recommended. Interdental flossing is indicated with special care to avoid tissue irritation for the first four to seven days of healing. Analgesics will be used as needed. Avoidance of crunchy food that could irritate the tissue and jeopardize the healing is advised. Mouthwashes may be used as well.

The role of the initiated and noninitiated tips is fundamental, every clinician must have a clear understanding of the laser effects and must be proficient in reading laser-tissue interactions (Smith 2011).

> *CLINICAL TIP: For areas with thin tissue bio(pheno) type, a faster movement of the fiber, moving within and without the pocket and with relatively low energy, may control possible side effects due to overheating.*

Modification of this technique was described by Gregg and McCarthy (1998) using the PerioLase pulsed Nd:YAG dental laser for laser curettage with the name laser periodontal therapy (LPT). This technique was developed based on the master's thesis of M. E. Neill (1997) and a previous study published by Neill and Mellonig (1997) from University of San Antonio, TX,

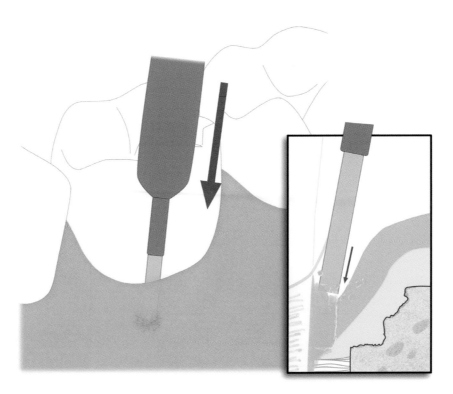

Figure 5.8 Schematic illustration of the laser tip within the pocket for removal of calculus.

who evaluated the effects of the pulsed Nd:YAG laser using the PulseMaster 1000 Dental Laser. This study showed improvement of the clinical parameters after the use of a low power Nd:YAG laser in conjunction with scaling root planing and 2 W power (80 mJ energy and 25 Hz frequency) for an average of two minutes of tooth irradiation. In addition, the impact of this laser irradiation was positive on the bacteria (specifically on the *Porphyromonas gingivalis* and *Prevotella intermedia)* reduction.

Modifying this method, using the LPT with the PerioLase digital laser, the initial pocket debridement occurs with a 6 W true pulse free running (FR) Nd:YAG laser (PerioLase MVP-7) and 100–150 µs pulse duration to remove the pocket epithelium and periodontal pathogens. After use of ultrasonics and hand instruments for removal of calculus the pulse duration will be increased from 450 to 650 µs in order to create a blood clot and clot stability in the pocket. The promoters of the technique recommend occlusal adjustment after laser therapy.

Further data from the use of this technique seem to show no significant differences between the surgical periodontal therapy and the LPT in private practice, providing benefits for patients who do not like to undergo surgical treatment (Harris et al. 2002).

The first report presenting histologic results in humans following a laser-assisted new attachment procedure (LANAP) for the treatment of periodontal pockets was published by Yukna et al. (2007). All teeth were scaled and root planed with ultrasonic and hand scalers. One of each pair of teeth received treatment of the inner pocket wall with a free-running pulsed Nd:YAG-laser to remove the pocket epithelium, and the test pockets were lased a second time to seal the pocket. The clinical parameters showed better PPD and CAL compared to the control teeth. After three months, all treated teeth were removed *en bloc* for histologic processing. All laser-assisted treated specimens showed formation of new cementum and connective tissue attachment and occasionally coronal to the notch, whereas five of the six control teeth had a long junctional epithelium with no evidence of new attachment or regeneration.

Recent studies also showed that this technique may induce periodontal regeneration, but there is need for further investigation with long-term clinical trials to compare the stability of clinical results to conventional therapy (Nevins et al. 2012). In this histological report five from ten examined teeth were evaluated histologically presenting evidence of some degree of periodontal regeneration with new cementum, periodontal ligament, and alveolar bone.

5.5 Retardation of the Epithelial Downgrowth

The retardation, or delay, of epithelial downgrowth is a basic concept for potential gain of new connective tissue attachment in periodontal tissues. With the use of the CO_2 laser a removal of pocket epithelium is possible without damage of the underlying connective tissue (Rossmann et al. 1987). In experimental studies with monkeys, it was proved that using the CO_2 laser inside and outside the pocket, the sulcular and oral epithelium was removed to the level of the mucogingival junction, and therefore epithelial cells were absent in the periodontal apparatus. Since epithelium was absent, a long junctional epithelium formation within the pocket is impossible if ablation of the newly formed epithelium (out of the pocket) was removed every 7–10 days. Therefore, a delay of the epithelial downgrowth of approximately 14 days was achieved (Istael et al. 1992). Another study with two patients having hopeless teeth also showed a delay of epithelial migration according to formation of a new connective tissue attachment instead of long junctional epithelium.

Based on this concept, the oral epithelium was removed with a CO_2 laser on the day of the surgical intervention as well as 10, 20, and 30 days postsurgically. In order to confirm the complete removal of the epithelial cells, a wet gauze soaked with saline will be used (Figure 5.9) in a similar manner as previously described in the ablation of leukoplakia (see also Chapter 3). Clinical case series with two- to three-wall intrabony defects were published, presenting an improvement of bone fill and the clinical parameters (with or without osseous grafting) in conjunction with the deepithelialization technique (Rossmann and Israel 2000).

Further studies showed that direct irradiation of root surfaces using a defocused CO_2 laser induces fibroblast attachment without melting and deleterious changes of the root surface. This is the result of in vitro studies (Barone et al. 2002; Crespi et al. 2002) based on animal preclinical experiments demonstrating the positive effects of the CO_2 laser irradiation in periodontal tissues and the improvement of periodontal regeneration after irradiation (Crespi et al. 1997). Specifically, class III furcation defects in beagle dogs were treated with a defocused, pulsed CO_2 laser (with 2 W power). This treatment induced the formation of new periodontal ligament, cementum, and bone.

Recent clinical case series demonstrated the clinical protocol of the CO_2 laser irradiation on the root surface in conjunction with the deepithelialization technique to

(a)

(b)

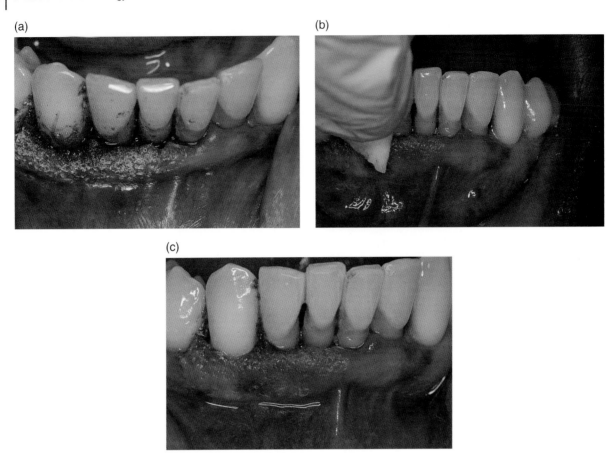

(c)

Figure 5.9 Removal of the oral epithelium after CO_2 laser irradiation (a) using a wet gauze (b) in order to produce bleeding from the underlying connective tissue and final hemostasis (c). *Source:* Dr. Georgios E Romanos.

improve bone regeneration (Crespi et al. 2004). The predictability of the CO_2 laser-assisted technique in comparison to the traditional Widman flap procedure was published recently after 15 years of follow-up (Crespi et al. 2011).

Since this laser-assisted procedure aims to remove specific types of cells, control cell proliferation, and promote the healing of other types of cells, we named this surgical treatment concept *laser-assisted guided tissue regeneration (LA-GTR)*, which can be used within the periodontal pocket (Figure 5.10) but also in other areas and indications in surgical procedures. Specifically, this technique has been applied to increase the width of keratinized tissues instead of harvest a gingival graft from the palate (FGG), with predictable long-term results (see also Figure 5.17).

CLINICAL TIP: *Using the glass fiber of a pulsed Nd:YAG laser or diode laser, it is possible to remove the inflamed epithelium of the pocket, the soft tissues can be reshaped, and the oral epithelium will be ablated for further control of the epithelial downgrowth. During this clinical procedure, excessive debris of granulation*

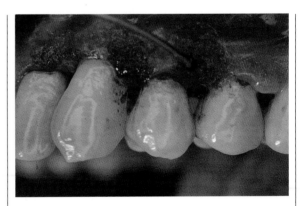

Figure 5.10 Laser-assisted guided tissue regeneration (LA-GTR) for pocket reduction or elimination. The laser glass fiber (here) removes the oral epithelium to the mucogingival line level. This procedure will be repeated once every 7–10 days for a period of six weeks to establish a new connective tissue attachment. *Source:* Dr. Georgios E Romanos.

*tissue may stay in the fiber and has to be periodically wiped from the fiber tip with moistened gauze to avoid thermal side effects due to scattering (*Figure 5.10*).*

The glass fiber during irradiation has to be inspected carefully to avoid side effects, such as breakage and undetected exposures of energy to the surrounding tissues.

A cleaving of the fiber means a 90-degree surface at the terminal end of the fiber which can be achieved with special cleaving tools, such as ceramic scissors or glass-cutting pens. An optimal cleave with a well-defined solid circular appearance of the laser light is a prerequisite for a high-quality laser irradiation with maximum energy delivery in the target tissues.

Clinical Case

Pocket Elimination with the Nd:YAG Laser

A 59-year-old patient was referred by her general dentist for a systematic periodontal treatment. The patient was informed about the advantages and effects of laser treatment, and she requested a laser-assisted periodontal treatment. After informed consent was signed describing the different options of treatment, the initial phase (hygiene phase) took place (motivation, instruction, measurements of the periodontal pockets) and then the periodontal pockets were scaled conventionally with curettes under local anesthesia. The area demonstrated a deep periodontal pocket of 7 mm at #4 distally (Figure 5.11a), which was treated with this procedure. The exact protocol was described above using a pulsed Nd:YAG laser (1.5 W power setting, 50 Hz frequency) and using the 400 µm contact glass fiber. A root planing occurred afterwards with conventional curettes and finally the inflamed pocket epithelium (contact fiber) was removed.

A deepithelialization of the oral epithelium was performed lastly (noncontact ablative mode) with the Nd:YAG laser using 2 W power and 20 Hz frequency. The oral and sulcular epithelium was removed only at this site every four to five days for a period of six weeks (Figure 5.11b). For this procedure, only topical anesthesia was required. After six months, a periodontal pocket depth of 3 mm was found. A recession of the gingival margin was not observed; therefore, an attachment gain of 4 mm was demonstrated (Figure 5.11c). The result was stable for three years (Figure 5.11d) and five years (Figure 5.11e) following conventional recall visits every five to six months.

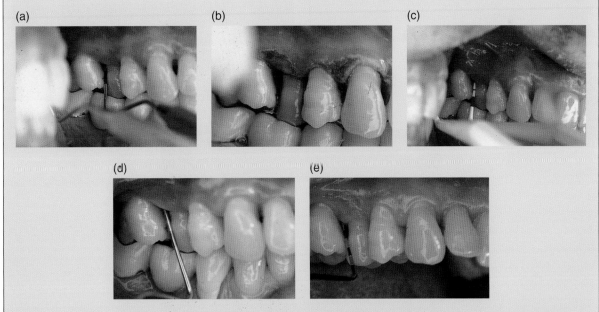

Figure 5.11 Deep periodontal pocket of 7 mm (a), which was treated with this procedure. The pulsed Nd:YAG laser (1.5 W power setting, 50 Hz frequency) using the 400 µm contact glass fiber removed the pocket epithelium and oral epithelium (b) and demonstrates a predictable clinical outcome without gingival recession after six months (c), three years (d) and five years (e). *Source:* Dr. Georgios E Romanos.

5.6   Laser Application in Gingivectomy and Gingivoplasty

The most common laser application in the field of periodontology is soft tissue surgery (Pick and Colvard 1993), especially using the CO_2 laser. A good indication for laser use is the removal of drug-induced gingival hyperplasia, which is associated with a spontaneous bleeding during conventional surgical excision. The laser can be used after the initial periodontal therapy including SRP as part of the surgical procedure removing all hyper-plastic tissues. As a complication from this procedure, superficial damage of the teeth from accidental laser irradiation on the enamel should be discussed. To prevent this, the teeth may be protected in the surgical field with matte metal foils or metal matrix bands (Magid and Strauss 2007).

Nevertheless, a definitive recommendation for the practitioner cannot be given, because more research is necessary to define the safety margin which allows laser application without undesirable side effects under the usual conditions in the private practice.

Clinical Case

Removal of a Drug-Induced Gingival Hyperplasia

A 24-year-old epileptic patient was referred by his physician because of advanced gingiva hyperplasia caused by a hydantoin medication (Figure 5.12a). The gingivectomy was carried out under local anesthesia with the CO_2 laser (average power: 8 W, continuous beam) in combination with curettes. A marking of the probing pocket depth was initially performed and transferred then apically for a submarginal incision (Figure 5.12b). Soft and hard deposits, such as plaque and calculus, were removed from the teeth, and the roots were

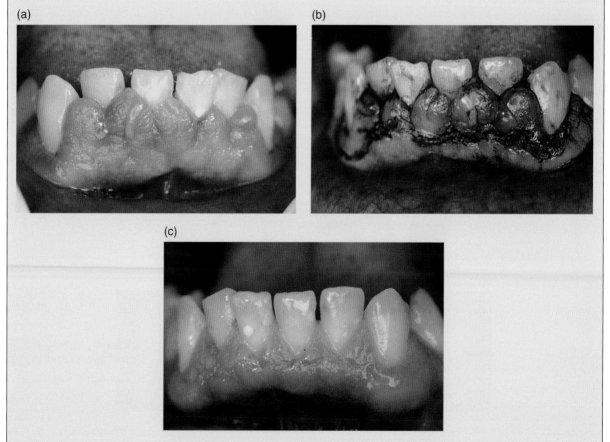

(a)   (b)   (c)

Figure 5.12   Advanced gingiva hyperplasia caused by a hydantoin medication (a). The gingivectomy was carried out with the CO_2 laser (average power: 8 W, continuous beam) in combination with curettes (b). Six months after surgery the patient presented a good soft tissue condition (c). *Source:* Dr. Georgios E Romanos.

conventionally planed. The underlying remaining tissue was ablated with the defocused beam at the end of the procedure for adequate hemostasis.

A periodontal pack was not required. After 10 days a slight redness in the marginal gingiva could be observed as a result of the formation of the first capillaries. One month later, uneventful healing was observed, which remained stable for six months, in spite of the further intake of the responsible medication (Figure 5.12c). Reevaluations were carried out every six months, and local recurrences were further treated with the CO_2 laser, in terms of gingivoplasty.

Gingivectomy with CO_2 Laser in a Patient Due to Combination Therapy of Medications

A 64-year-old female patient was introduced with a severe gingival hyperplasia associated with cyclosporin-A (CyS-A) and nifedipine medications (Figure 5.13a). She had undergone kidney transplantation approximately 15 months before, and the daily medication of Sandimmune® (Sandoz, Basel, Switzerland) 50 mg (three times daily) was indicated. The patient was also taking nifedipine against hypertension. After the probing pocket depths were recorded and the oral hygiene instruction and prophylaxis visit was completed, a submarginal incision was performed with conventional gingivectomy knifes under local anesthesia. After excision (Figure 5.13b), all hyperplastic tissues were removed with curettes, and a CO_2 laser (continuous mode, 6 W) was utilized for hemostasis (Figure 5.13c). Wound healing completed without complications. Postoperative bleeding did not occur providing an excellent clinical result after four weeks (Figure 5.13d).

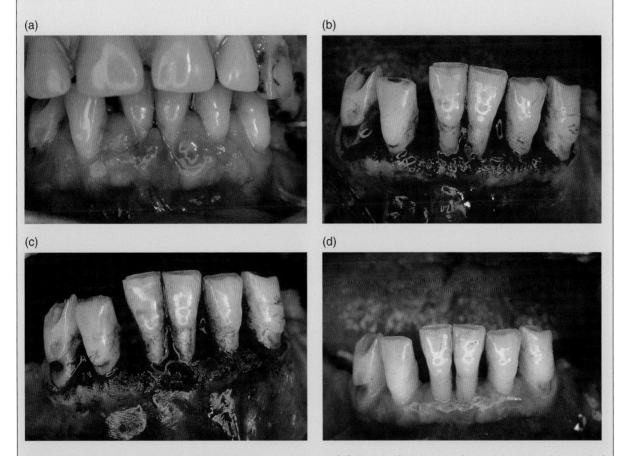

Figure 5.13 Gingival hyperplasia associated with cyclosporin-A (CyS-A) and nifedipine (a); after excision (b) and removal of the hyperplastic tissues, the CO_2-laser was utilized for hemostasis (c); an excellent final clinical outcome after four weeks (d). *Source:* Dr. Georgios E Romanos.

5.7 Laser-Assisted Hemostasis in Periodontics

Patients with coagulopathies are relatively frequent patients in every dental office. However, general practitioners very often make the decision to refer those patients to a specialist or to a hospital or university clinic. The laser wavelengths, which provide a good and adequate hemostasis due to high absorption from chromophores, such as Nd:YAG and diode lasers, can be used beneficially in conjunction with conventional nonsurgical, periodontal treatment (Figure 5.14). Additional discussions with the patient's physician are indicated in order to implement the treatment plan and the maintenance visits using the laser as a tool for adequate hemostasis. This may control use of blood transfusions and other systemic medical treatments (sometimes in conjunction with hospitalization). Therefore, the treatment costs can be decreased significantly for the patient as well as the medical insurance, allowing more frequent and noncomplicated dental visits improving general oral health, and leading to socioeconomic benefits.

Further laser applications in the oral cavity may be the hemostasis at the donor site of free gingival grafts (Figure 5.15), coagulation of extraction sockets, as well as other areas for required hemostasis in patients with bleeding disorders (i.e. mild to moderate hemophilia) or on anticoagulants (Grasser and Ackermann 1977; Chellappah and Loh 1990; Chrysikopoulos et al. 2006). For these indications, the most efficient laser wavelengths are the CO_2 or the noncontact Nd:YAG and the diode lasers. Even though a recent clinical report does not see the use of the Nd:YAG laser to be superior for cardiac patients taking coumarin medications compared to conventional local hemostatic measures (Deppe et al. 2013), there is a need in the future for a clinical prospective study of patients with different bleeding disorders to evaluate the benefits of the laser-assisted hemostasis.

(a)   (b)

(c)   (d)

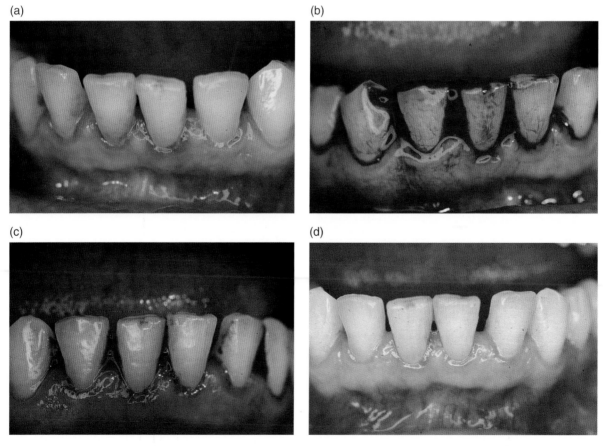

Figure 5.14 Periodontal nonsurgical therapy in a patient with stage 1 periodontitis (a) and bleeding disorder (thrombasthenia Glantzmann) (a); scaling was performed in the conventional way without blood transfusion. The clinical photos demonstrate the bleeding during the procedure (b); adequate hemostasis with a dental pulsed Nd:YAG laser (c), and uneventful clinical outcome after two weeks (d). *Source:* Dr. Georgios E Romanos.

(a)　　　　　　　　　　(b)

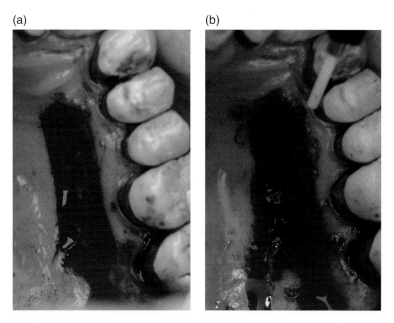

Figure 5.15 Donor site of a free keratinized gingival graft (a) and adequate hemostasis using a CO_2 laser (b). *Source:* Dr. Georgios E Romanos.

Clinical Case

Nonsurgical Periodontal Therapy in a Patient with Bleeding Disorder

A patient presented for scaling and root planing with Factor VII deficiency. After discussion with the physician, a conventional laser-assisted SRP was utilized with a 980 nm diode laser without preoperative plasma transfusions. Benzocaine topical was applied, and conventional local infiltration anesthesia with lidocaine HCl 2% with epinephrine (1 : 100 000) was administered.

(a)　　　　　　　　　　(b)

(c)　　　　　　　　　　(d)

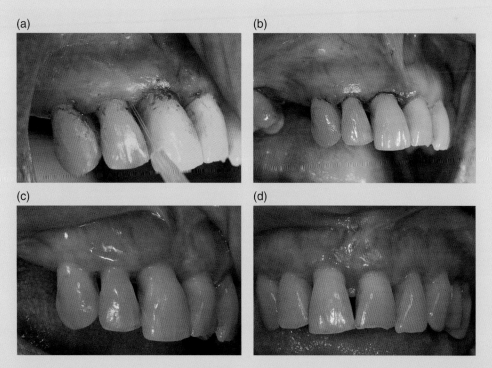

Figure 5.16 Pulsed diode laser 2 W for laser-assisted SRP (a); noncontact diode pulsed laser with 2.5 W utilized for sufficient coagulation without blood transfusion (b); eight weeks after treatment good clinical outcome without bleeding on probing (c, d) (Treatment provided with the periodontal resident: Dr. Nathan Estrin, Stony Brook). *Source:* Dr. Georgios E Romanos.

The pulsed diode laser 2 W was utilized initially in the pockets to remove the sulcular epithelium. Scaling and root planing was achieved with ultrasonic (Cavitron) and no hand instruments. Diode pulsed laser 2.5 W in noncontact mode was utilized to coagulate sufficiently the pockets. Intraoral photographs were taken at this appoint-ment. Oral hygiene instructions were reinforced. Patient was advised that her home care is crucial to the success of periodontal therapy. Advised patient to control minor bleeding by applying pressure with salt and gauze. Wound healing was uneventful without postoperative discomfort and bleeding (Figure 5.16).

5.8 Photodynamic Therapy in Periodontology

Photodynamic therapy (PDT) and its effects in periodontology are described in the Chapter 7. The reader will be able to get comprehensive information about the concept of PDT and the impact of this treatment on the periodontal tissues.

Clinical Case

Combined Frenectomy and Vestibuloplasty for Improvement of Keratinized Tissue Width

A 21-year-old female patient was referred for the surgical removal of multiple lip frenula in the anterior region of the mandible. Excellent plaque control was not possible in this area because of constant soft tissue irritation and injuries during toothbrushing. The unfavorable anatomical relations encouraged the deposition of soft and hard deposits in the area of the marginal gingiva of the mandibular incisors leading to recurrent inflammations (Figure 5.17a). A frenectomy was performed under local anesthesia with the CO_2 laser in the continuous mode (CW) and a power of 4–5 W. In addition, an incision was done in the vestibule, between keratinized and not keratinized mucosa, to enlarge the width of the keratinized gingiva (it was narrower than 2 mm) (Figure 5.17b). The laser ablation was longer (high power was emitted in the tissue) in the deeper part of the vestibule in

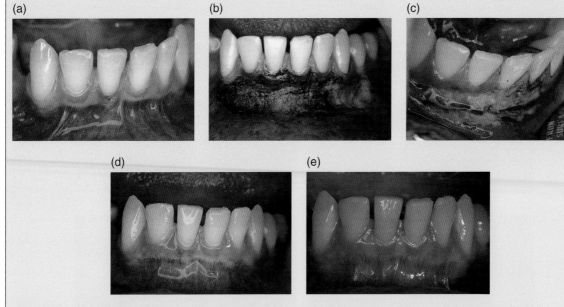

Figure 5.17 Insufficient vestibule depth (a); frenectomy performed with a CO_2 laser in the continuous mode (CW) and a power of 4–5 W (b); fibrin layer was observed three days after surgery (c); no pathological findings were observed after one month (d); the result was stable after eight years demonstrating good vestibule depth and sufficient width of keratinized tissue (e). *Source:* Dr. Georgios E Romanos.

order to create more thermal transfer. The carbonized tissue closed to the mucogingival junction (incision area) was removed immediately after laser irradiation with wet gauze. Therefore, a better cell proliferation and apical migration of the keratinized mucosa was achieved. Special postsurgical instructions were not required. Wound healing was completed without complications. Fibrin layer was observed three days after surgery (Figure 5.17c). The clinical situation did not demonstrate any pathological findings after one month (Figure 5.17d), and the local plaque control improved significantly. The result after eight years was stable, and a distinctive enlargement of the keratinized tissue width was observed (Figure 5.17e).

Removal of a Gingival Tumor during Pregnancy Using a Diode Laser

A 28-year-old female patient demonstrated a gingival tumor at #28–29 for the last two months of her pregnancy (Figure 5.18a). The general periodontal condi-

tion was very good and the plaque control optimal. Under local anesthesia and use of a 980 nm diode laser (Ceralas15, Biolitec, Jena, Germany) with 5 W power setting in continuous mode (contact glass fiber: 400 μm), the soft tissue tumor was excised (Figure 5.18b). The hemostasis was excellent. An additional SRP was performed with conventional curettes, and the diode laser was utilized to coagulate the pockets at the final stage with 2 W (CW) in an ablative noncontact mode. The soft tissue tumor was sent to an oral and maxillofacial pathologist for confirmation of the clinical diagnosis (Figure 5.18c). The diagnosis was epulis granulomatosa. The follow up examination after 10 days showed uneventful wound healing (Figure 5.18d).

Crown Lengthening with the Nd:YAG Laser

A 67-year old patient was referred with the request of crown lengthening of tooth #20. The clinical situation revealed:

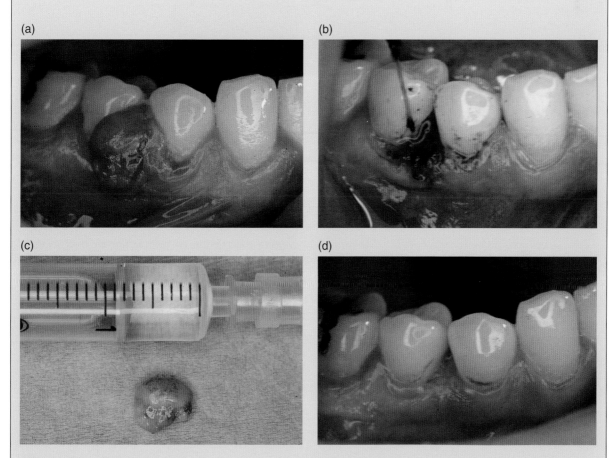

(a)   (b)

(c)   (d)

Figure 5.18 Gingival tumor in a pregnant patient (a); the diode laser excised the soft tissue tumor and in conjunction with SRP (b, c); the hemostasis was excellent. Ten days after surgery uneventful wound healing was observed (d). *Source:* Dr. Georgios E Romanos.

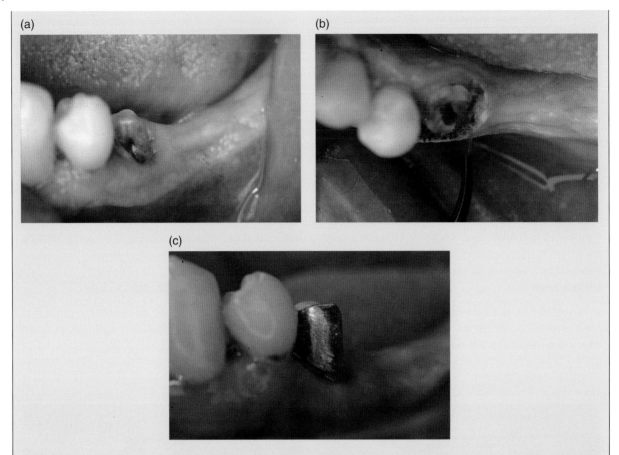

Figure 5.19 Crown lengthening procedure (a) with the pulsed Nd:YAG laser (b); six weeks after surgery a post and core was delivered (c). *Source:* Dr. Georgios E Romanos.

- Probing pocket depth: buccally 4 mm, distally: 6 mm, lingually: 2 mm, mesially: 5 mm
- Width of the keratinized gingiva: 5–6 mm.

The tooth was destroyed disto-buccally, and the treatment plan was to make a post and core after the crown lengthening procedure and finally a metalo-ceramic crown (Figure 5.19a). A gingivectomy was carried out under topical anesthesia and with a power of 3 W with the pulsed Nd:YAG laser (Figure 5.19b) and a 400 μm contact glass fiber. After healing of six weeks, the post and core were fabricated and cemented without complications (Figure 5.19c).

Crown Lengthening with the CO_2 Laser

A 37-year old female patient presented with the chief complaint that she "does not like spaces between her anterior teeth and wishes also white teeth." The medical history was unremarkable. The comprehensive dental and periodontal examination presented healthy teeth and healthy periodontal tissues. Radiographically, no pathological signs were found. Different orthodontic and restorative options were discussed with the patient, but she immediately declined the orthodontic therapy due to the length. A diagnostic composite mock-up was performed, and the dental technicians created an ideal functional diagnostic wax-up and a soft tissue surgical guide.

Using the surgical guide in situ, the soft tissue was removed and then the bone where the probing was less than 3 mm to reestablish biological width. The teeth were prepared under local anesthesia, and the zenith of the teeth was shifted 1 mm mesially and 1.5 mm apically. The CO_2 laser (DEKA, Ultraspeed) was used with the perio tip and 3 W power setting and 100 Hz frequency (noncontact) to incise and scallop the tissue precisely for appropriate gingival contour. Immediately after surgery, impressions were taken and provisional restorations were fabricated. No antibiotics or pain medications were prescribed postoperatively. The final veneer restorations were placed and cemented 2.5 weeks later. The final esthetic outcome was impressive, and this would not be possible to accomplish without the laser-assisted approach, especially in such a short period of time (Figure 5.20).

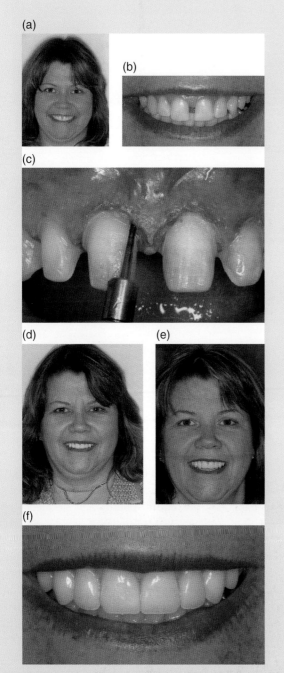

Figure 5.20 Diastema in the anterior maxilla before treatment (a, b); soft tissue removal (c) before bone removal to reestablish biological width (supracrestal connective tissues). Immediately after surgery, impressions were taken and provisional restorations were fabricated (d); the final veneer restorations were placed and cemented 2.5 weeks later (e); the final esthetic outcome was impressive (f) (From: Sweeny and Romanos 2006).

Crown Lengthening with Osseous Recontouring

A gingivectomy procedure was performed using an Er:YAG laser to improve esthetics. Tooth #9 presented a shorter clinical crown compared to the adjacent tooth #8. The patient was interested in improving the esthetic result. Under local anesthesia, we evaluated the pocket depth, and we found healthy periodontal tissues with a probing of 3 mm (Figure 5.21a and b). Therefore, an excision was performed under air/water supply using the Er:YAG laser (120 mj/10 Hz) and a contact tip (focused beam). The bleeding control was achieved in noncontact tip and defocused mode (100 mJ energy; frequency of 20 Hz). Finally, osseous removal was performed without flap elevation and parameters of 300 mJ energy and frequency of 2 Hz using water/air supply. The laser tip was placed parallel to the tooth within the sulcus in order to remove only the bone crest (Figure 5.21c and d). The final result was significantly improved after four months without recurrence (Figure 5.21e).

Crown Lengthening in the Anterior Teeth to Improve Esthetics

A 57-year old male Caucasian patient was referred to the Department of Periodontology for esthetic crown lengthening using the closed laser-assisted crown lengthening technique. The treatment objective was to establish a new supracrestal tissue and create a more esthetically pleasing crown width to length ratio of 8 : 10 at the maxillary anterior teeth based on the esthetic guidelines. The treatment area was anesthetized with benzocaine 20% as topical anesthetic and 2% lidocaine HCL with epinephrine 1 : 100000 (Henry Schein, Melville, NY, USA) using local infiltration technique below the mucogingival junction. Patient presented for gingivectomy in conjunction with ostectomy using an Er:YAG laser for upper right side. The rationale for surgery was that the patient presented with delayed passive eruption of anterior teeth #7–9. The goals of surgery were to uncover the clinical crowns of teeth #7, #8, and #9 for esthetic purposes, removing the excess of crestal bone present at the CEJ of these teeth, and to create a new supracrestal tissue dimension (previously called "biologic width"). A guide was fabricated using alginate impressions followed by a master cast and a diagnostic wax-up based on the ideal esthetic guidelines. The guide was placed in the correct position, and after evaluation was trimmed accordingly to esthetic parameters.

Soft Tissue Laser Parameters: Gingivectomy was performed using Er:YAG laser with an energy of 120 mJ and frequency of 10 Hz using a contact tip (focused

(a)

(b)

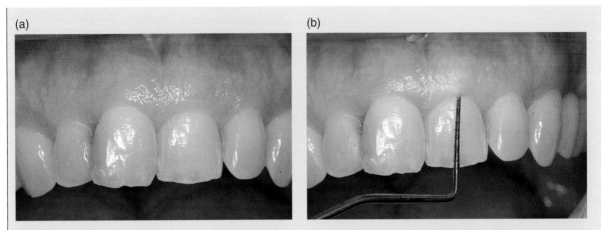

Figure 5.21a and b Periodontal condition before treatment and probing of the periodontal pocket. *Source:* Dr. Georgios E Romanos.

(c)

(d)

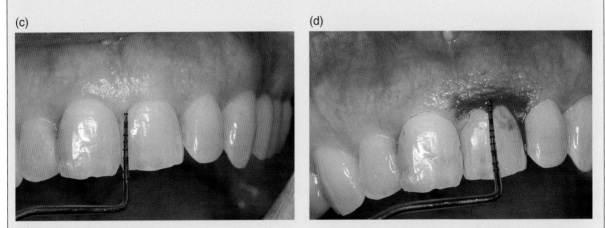

Figure 5.21c and d Probing and soft tissue coagulation after osseous recontouring with the Er:YAG laser. *Source:* Dr. Georgios E Romanos.

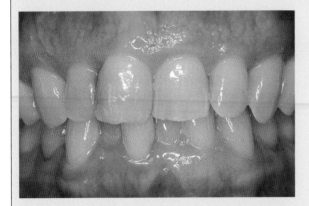

Figure 5.21e Clinical outcome four months after surgery demonstrating excellent clinical outcome without recurrence. *Source:* Dr. Georgios E Romanos.

beam) under water/air supply. In addition, a frenectomy at # 8 and 9 was performed using the same parameters. The laser tip was placed perpendicular to the gingival tissue until bone contact. The soft tissue collar was removed using a Rhodes back action instrument.

Ostectomy Parameters: Osseous removal was performed without flap elevation using the Er:YAG laser and parameters of 300 mJ energy and frequency of 10 Hz and sufficient water flow for adequate cooling of the tissues. The laser tip was placed parallel to the tooth within the sulcus in order to remove only the crest of bone. In order to have sufficient bleeding control and stabilization of the blood clot, coagulation parameters of 160 mJ energy and frequency of 10 Hz were used in the surgical area and frenectomy site (Figure 5.22).

Since the procedure was done with minimal visualization, frequent evaluations of the depth and shape of recontouring were required. Any irregularities were smoothed up with a curette after the bone recontouring to optimize the esthetic result.

The patient exhibited normal, uneventful postoperative healing without any discomfort or pain. No

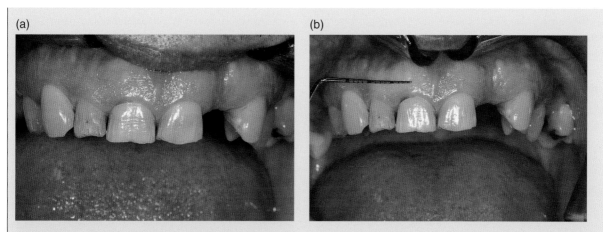

Figure 5.22a and b Pre-op clinical condition (a) and marking of the exact level of gingival excision (b). *Source:* Dr. Georgios E Romanos.

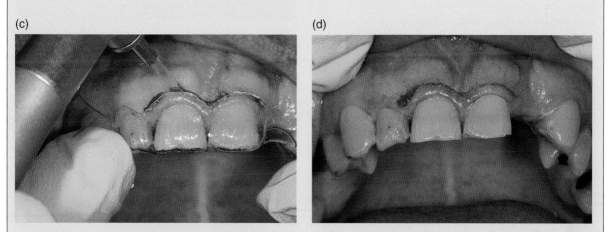

Figure 5.22c and d Gingivectomy using the guide (c) and submarginal laser-assisted incision (d). *Source:* Dr. Georgios E Romanos.

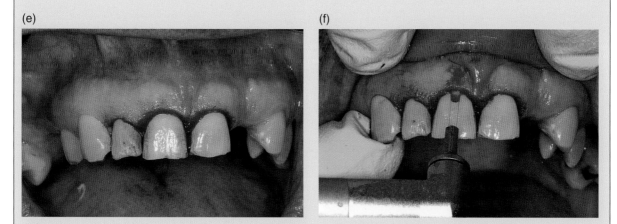

Figure 5.22e and f Gingival margin after gingivectomy (e); laser-assisted osseous recontouring (f). *Source:* Dr. Georgios E Romanos.

antibiotics or analgesics were prescribed postoperatively. The patient was very satisfied with the final esthetic outcome. Of special consideration is that the patient was very happy with the length of time it took to complete these two surgical procedures, which would not have been possible using conventional surgical protocol.

The patient exhibited 10 mm of clinical crown length at the central incisors (6 months after surgery) and was totally pleased with the esthetic clinical outcome. The periodontal probing depths were within normal limits with probing depths of 2–3 mm (Figure 5.22h).

Similarly, the mandibular anterior teeth were also treated (Figure 5.23).

Mandible

A gingivoplasty was performed at mandibular incisors using energy 160 mJ and a frequency of 20 Hz and final hemostasis of the gingiva in noncontact tip and a defocused mode was performed using parameters, such as 100 mJ energy and a frequency of 20 Hz.

Case was treated together with the resident Dr. James Ramos (Dept. of Periodontology, Stony Brook University, Stony Brook, NY).

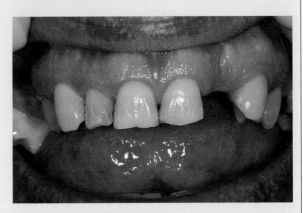

Figure 5.22h Two-month postoperative clinical photo. *Source:* Dr. Georgios E Romanos.

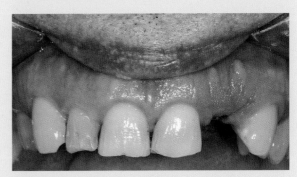

Figure 5.22i Six-month postoperative clinical photo. An implant at #10 was placed at this time. *Source:* Dr. Georgios E Romanos.

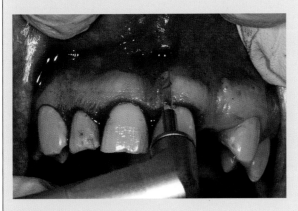

Figure 5.22g Laser-assisted frenectomy. *Source:* Dr. Georgios E Romanos.

(a)

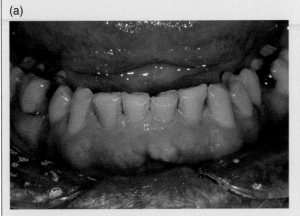

(b)

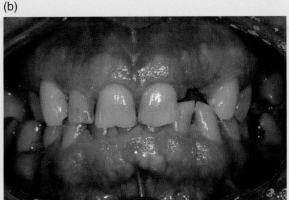

Figure 5.23a and b Mandibular teeth pre-op. *Source:* Dr. Georgios E Romanos.

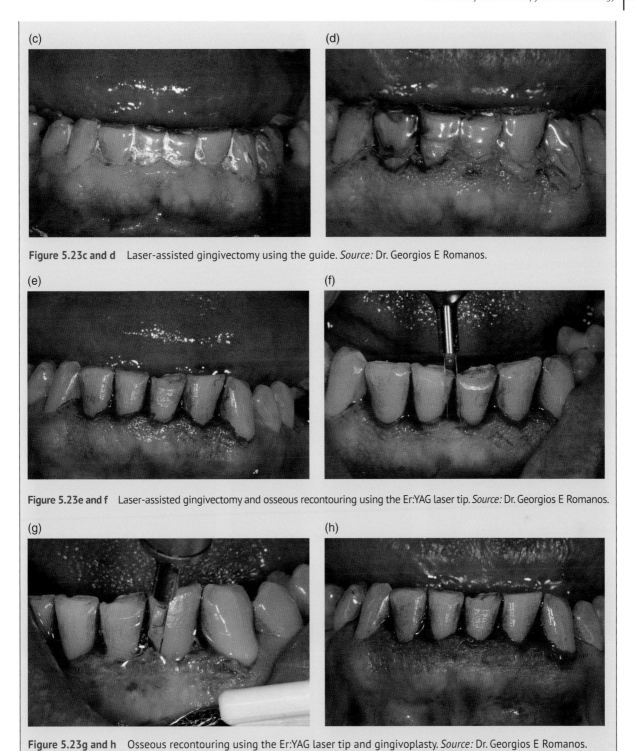

Figure 5.23c and d Laser-assisted gingivectomy using the guide. *Source:* Dr. Georgios E Romanos.

Figure 5.23e and f Laser-assisted gingivectomy and osseous recontouring using the Er:YAG laser tip. *Source:* Dr. Georgios E Romanos.

Figure 5.23g and h Osseous recontouring using the Er:YAG laser tip and gingivoplasty. *Source:* Dr. Georgios E Romanos.

Crown Lengthening in the Maxillary Arch for Esthetic Purposes

Clinical case series have been published using this minimally invasive surgical technique by different authors showing different advantages. Some authors state that this minimally invasive procedure decreases the time needed to establish the gingival margin necessary for definitive restoration (Chen et al. 2017). Also, other authors recommended the use of an Er,Cr:YSGG laser for this kind of clinical indication following from beneficial clinical results (Fekrazad

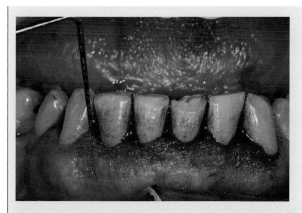

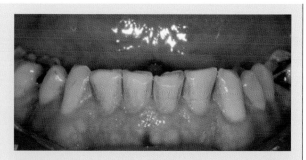

Figure 5.23j Final result 4 months after surgery. *Source:* Dr. Georgios E Romanos.

Figure 5.23i Probing depths of 3 mm establish proper supra-crestal soft tissues (biological width). *Source:* Dr. Georgios E Romanos.

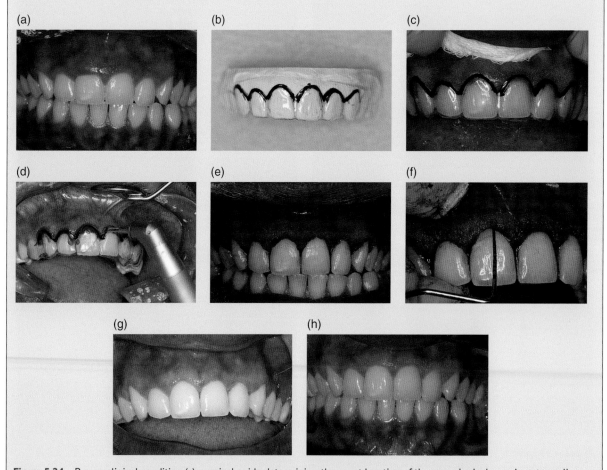

Figure 5.24 Pre-op clinical condition (a); surgical guide determining the exact location of the new gingival margin extraorally (b) and in situ (c); laser excision with the Er:YAG laser (d) and new gingival margin after hemostasis (e); determining the supracrestal attached tissues (f); excellent clinical outcome after two weeks of healing (g) and nine months after surgery (h). Case was treated together with the resident Dr. Alex Zusin (Stony Brook University, Stony Brook, NY). *Source:* Dr. Georgios E Romanos.

et al. 2018). Even other authors recommend this procedure in periodontology, the potential damage of the root surface during the minimally invasive laser-assisted crown lengthening procedure has been discussed (McGuire and Scheyer 2011). However, the used protocol and the relatively high power of the used beam for soft tissue removal perpendicularly to the tooth root may cause this kind of root damage.

Therefore, in order to evaluate the literature at the appropriate level, it is recommended to read carefully the protocol used by the authors in the different studies.

5.9 Gingival Troughing for Prosthetic Restorations

In daily restorative practice there is a need to enlarge the gingival sulcus in order to identify the exact restorative margin of a tooth preparation. Clinical conditions sometimes require the use of electrosurgical excisions or laser excision. The electrosurgical method has a high risk of tooth damage and is associated with pain and tissue shrinkage as well as scar tissue formation (Srivastava and Lossin 1976; Krejci et al. 1982; Pearlman et al. 1991; Visser et al. 1994; Romanos et al. 1998a, b).

The clinical case in Figure 5.25 presents a patient who had multiple impressions due to lack of bleeding control at the placement of retraction cords. Therefore, soft tissue excision was performed using a diode 980 nm dental laser allowing a good quality of a digital

impression (Figure 5.25a–c). The follow-up after delivery of the prosthesis (three months after healing) presented an esthetic clinical outcome (Figure 5.25d).

5.10 Fractional Photothermolysis in Periodontology

The concept of fractional photothermolysis seems to be of great interest with potentially beneficial effects in the periodontal tissues. The technique has so far been applied in limited clinical case series to improve:

- Soft tissue quality and increase of attached gingiva/mucosa around teeth and implants.
- The method also seems to improve the bone formation in conjunction with flap procedure (or no) around teeth and/or implants and should be systematically studied in the future (Figures 5.26 and 5.27).

For the treatment of these periodontal lesions, an intrasulcular irradiation with mean power of 1.5 W (pulsed mode; 20 Hz frequency, 5% duty cycle) in conjunction with

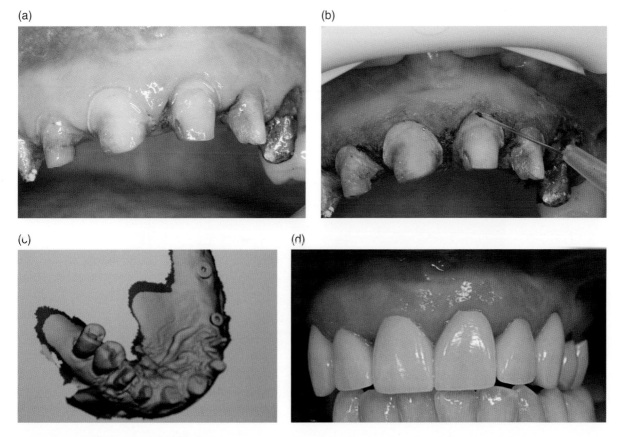

(a)

(b)

(c)

(d)

Figure 5.25 Clinical periodontal condition before digital impression (a); the diode laser (980 nm) was used in contact to excise the soft tissue margins (b) in order to present good access to the tooth preparation margins for a digital impression (c); final restorations after two months of healing (d) (prosthetic restoration: by M. Callahan, DDS and R. Reiner, DMD). *Source:* Dr. Georgios E Romanos.

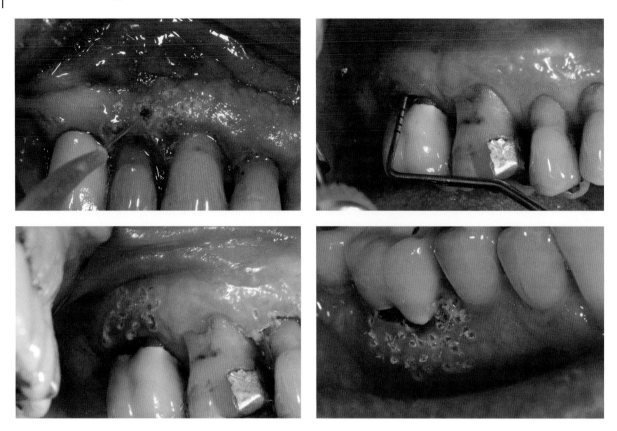

Figure 5.26 Fractional photothermolysis using glass fiber of a 980 nm diode laser to improve connective tissue attachment. *Source:* Dr. Laura Braswell (Atlanta, GA).

(a) (b)

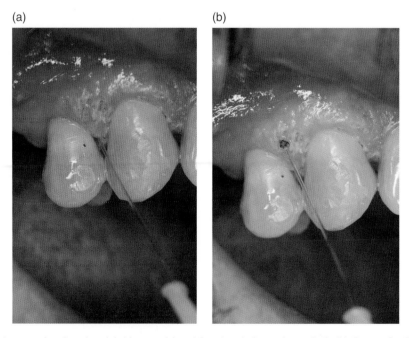

Figure 5.27 Diode laser-assisted pocket debridement (a) and fractional photo-thermolysis (b). *Source:* Dr. Georgios E Romanos.

an SRP using ultrasonics was used, and later (in the same visit) fractional photo-thermolysis using pulsed mode (pulse width: 150 ms) with a maximum power of 24.8 W, frequency of 330 Hz and 99% duty cycle. The cases demonstrate an excellent bone regeneration without the use of bone grafting or flap elevation (Figures 5.28 and 5.29).

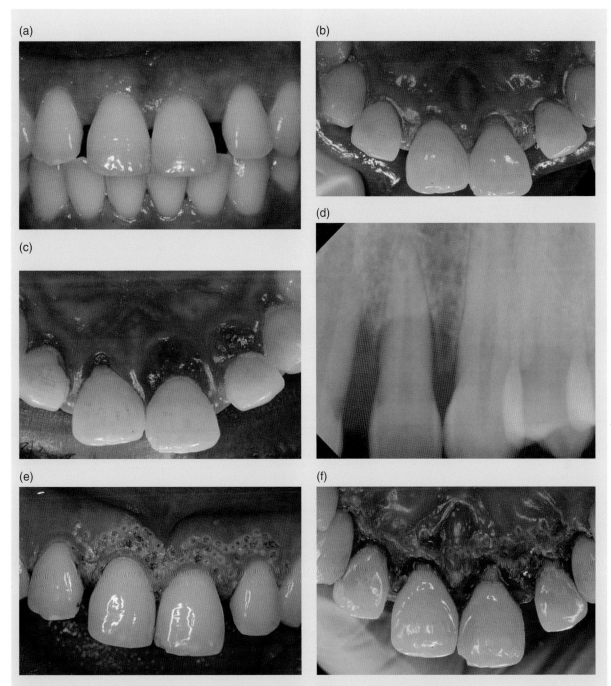

Figure 5.28a–f Preoperative clinical (a–c) and radiological condition (d) with fractional photothermolysis and laser-assisted debridement (e, f). *Source:* Dr. Laura Braswell (Atlanta, GA).

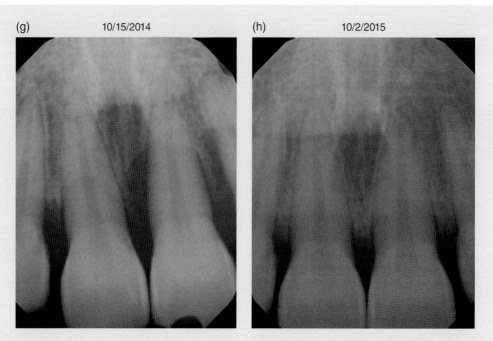

(g) 10/15/2014 (h) 10/2/2015

Figure 5.28g and h Preoperative radiological condition (#9) with severe bone loss (g) and follow-up after one year showing significant bone growth (h). *Source:* Dr. Laura Braswell (Atlanta, GA).

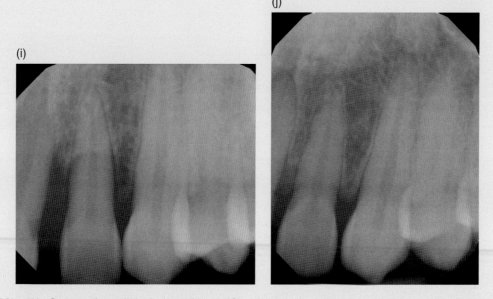

(j)

(i)

Figure 5.28i and j Preoperative radiological condition (#10) with severe bone loss (i) and follow-up after one year showing bone growth (j). *Source:* Dr. Laura Braswell (Atlanta, GA).

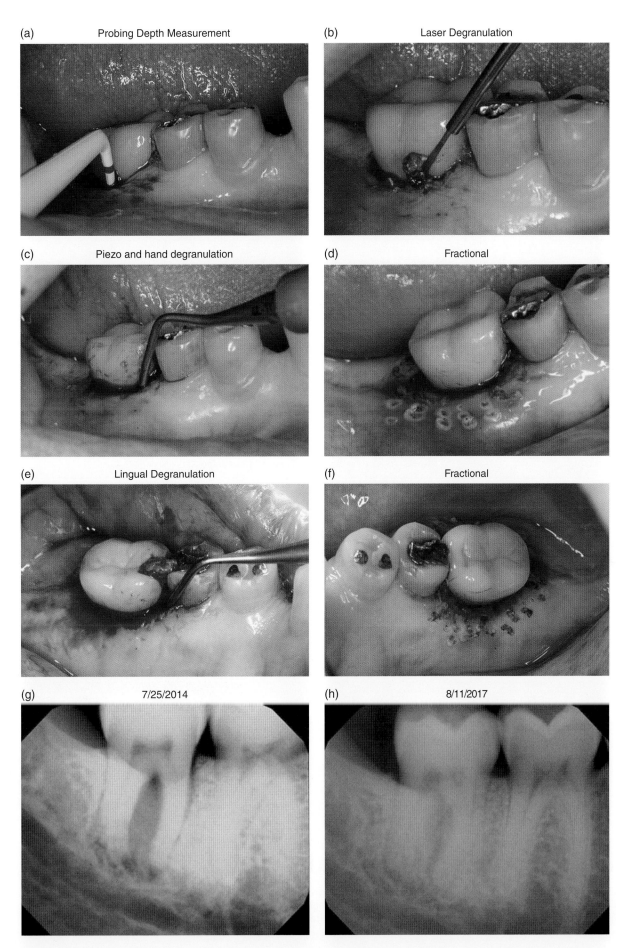

Figure 5.29 Preoperative condition with severe attachment loss (a), with laser-assisted degranulation (b) and using hand instruments (c); fractional photothermolysis (d–f); new bone formation after two years using diode laser-assisted pocket debridement and fractional photothermolysis (g, h). *Source:* Dr. Laura Braswell (Atlanta, GA).

(a) (b)

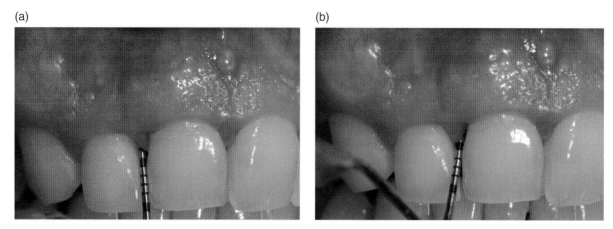

Figure 5.30a and b 8 mm initial probing depth on the mesial aspect of the right maxillary lateral incisor (a) and 9 mm on the distal aspect of the right maxillary central incisor (b). *Source:* Dr. Marisa Roncati (Ferrara, Italy).

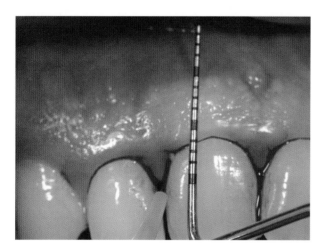

Figure 5.30c Cause-related laser-assisted nonsurgical periodontal therapy was scheduled, with the adjunctive use of a 980 nm diode laser (Wiser 2, Doctor Smile, Lambda S.p.A.,Vi, Italy), with following parameters:

- Wavelength: 980 nm
- Power: 2.5 W – mean 0.7 W – 10 kHz
- Modality: pulsed (pw) ton = 30 µs, toff = 70 µs
- Fluence: 120 j/cm^2
- Time: 30 seconds/pockets
- Fiber: 400 nm

This specific type of diode laser works in a superpulsed mode, with a T on, of 30 µs, and a T off, of 70 µs, with an average output power of 0.7 W, and peak of power at 2.5 W. The treatment in each site takes 30 seconds, preceded and followed by hydrogen peroxide 3% or 10 volumes irrigation. The same procedure was replicated in each pocket three times. Each compromised periodontal site must receive a minimum of 90 seconds of treatment, in total, but always alternated to the comprehensive nonsurgical periodontal debridement, using manual and ultrasonic instruments.

(d) (e)

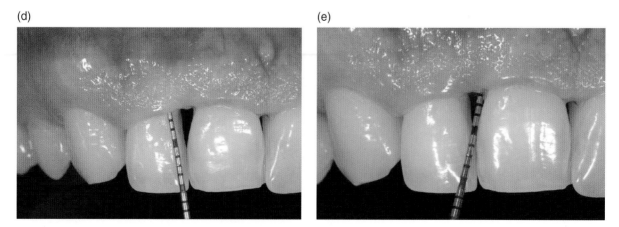

Figure 5.30d and e Clinical aspect of the case at one year follow-up recall appointment. The periodontal probe detects 2 mm probing depth, in the absence of bleeding, both on the mesial aspect of the maxillary right lateral incisor and on the distal aspect of the central incisor. *Source:* Dr. Marisa Roncati (Ferrara, Italy).

(f)

(g)

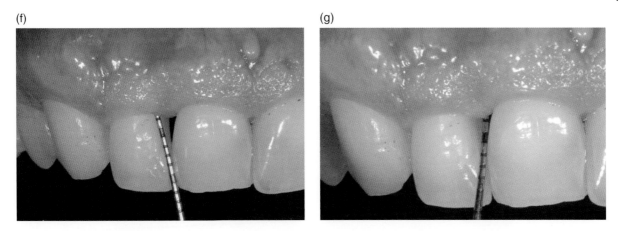

Figure 5.30f and g At eight-year follow-up recall appointment, the probing readings are maintained within normal values, 3 mm in the absence of bleeding, but an improvement of the interproximal papilla, is appreciated in a highly esthetic area. *Source:* Dr. Marisa Roncati (Ferrara, Italy).

(h)

(i)

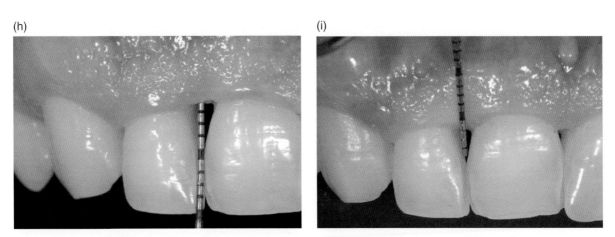

Figure 5.30h and i Comparative clinical images one year (h) and eight years (i) after the laser-assisted nonsurgical periodontal treatment. An esthetic improvement of the interdental papilla can be observed. The distance from the interproximal contact area to the gingival margin, from 5 mm (h) has been reduced to 3 mm (i). *Source:* Dr. Marisa Roncati (Ferrara, Italy).

Figure 5.30j and k Comparative periapical radiographs, made at baseline (j) and after eight years of follow-up (k). Bone remodeling is appreciated, associated with the presence of a more represented lamina dura (k). *Source:* Dr. Marisa Roncati (Ferrara, Italy).

(j)

(k)

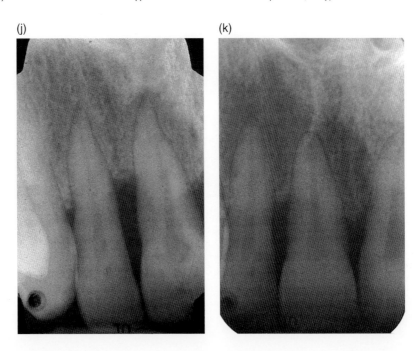

(a)   (b)

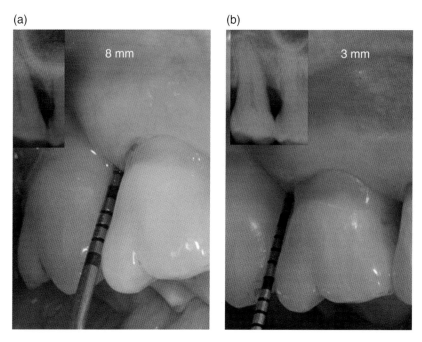

Figure 5.31a and b Clinical aspect pre- (a) and six years post- (b) from cause-related laser-assisted nonsurgical periodontal therapy. The periodontal probe detected 8 mm initial probing depths (a) and 3 mm PPD (b) at six-year follow-up recall appointment. *Source:* Dr. Marisa Roncati (Ferrara, Italy).

(c)   (d)

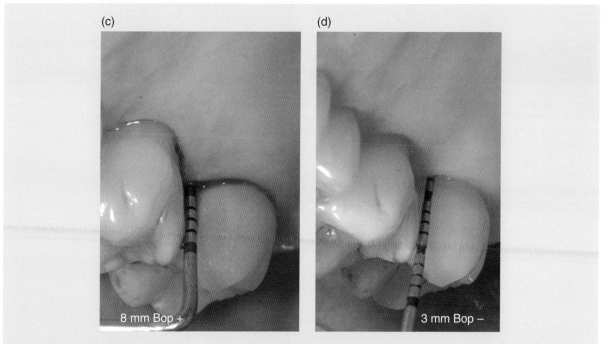

Figure 5.31c and d Clinical aspect pre- (c) and six years post- (d) from cause-related laser-assisted nonsurgical periodontal therapy. The periodontal probe detected 9 mm initial probing depths (c) at mesial-palatal site and 3 mm PPD (d) at six-year follow-up recall appointment. *Source:* Dr. Marisa Roncati (Ferrara, Italy).

(e)   (f)

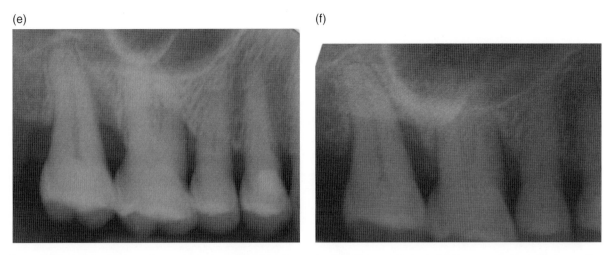

Figure 5.31e and f Comparative periapical radiographs taken at baseline (e) and at six year follow-up recall appointment (f). *Source:* Dr. Marisa Roncati (Ferrara, Italy).

(g)   (h)

(i)

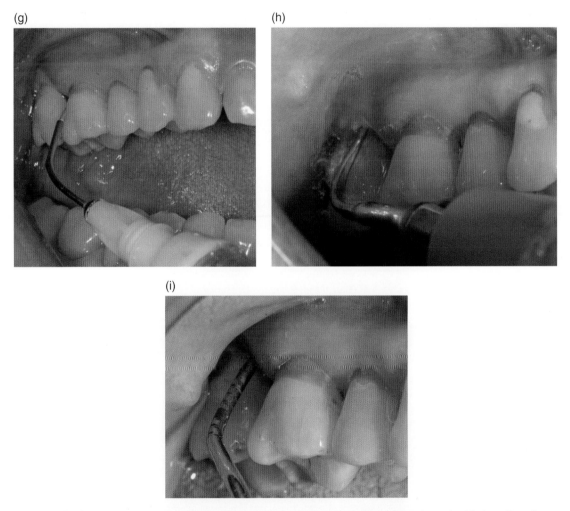

Figure 5.31g–i Cause-related laser-assisted nonsurgical periodontal therapy was performed, with the adjunctive use of a 980 nm diode laser (g) (Wiser 2, Doctor Smile, Lambda S.p.A.,Vi, Italy), with the following parameters

- Wavelength: 980 nm; Power: 2.5 W – mean 0.7 W – 10 kHz; Modality: pulsed (pw) ton = 30 µs, toff = 70 µs; Fluence: 120 j/cm^2; Time: 30 seconds/pockets; fiber: 400 nm.

Comprehensive nonsurgical periodontal debridement was accomplished using both mechanical (h) and manual (i) instrumentation

(j) (k)

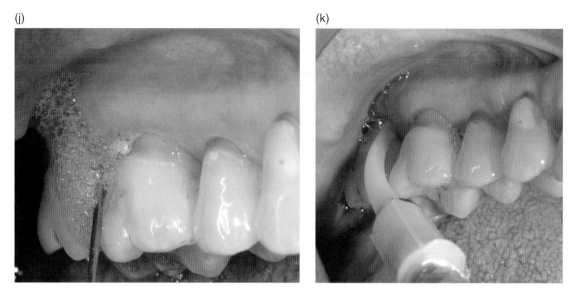

Figure 5.31j and k The treatment in each site takes 30 seconds, preceded and followed by hydrogen peroxide 3% or 10 volumes irrigation (j). The same procedure is replicated in each pocket three times (k). *Source:* Dr. Marisa Roncati (Ferrara, Italy).

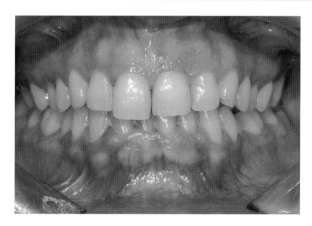

Figure 5.32a Initial clinical aspect. *Source:* Dr. Marisa Roncati (Ferrara, Italy).

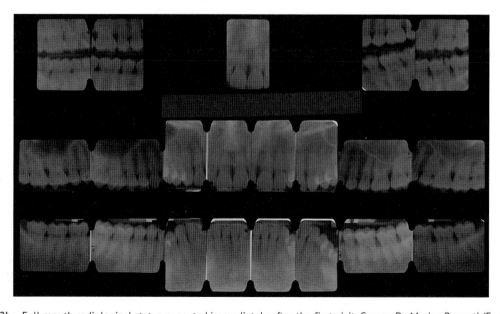

Figure 5.32b Full mouth radiological status, executed immediately after the first visit. *Source:* Dr. Marisa Roncati (Ferrara, Italy).

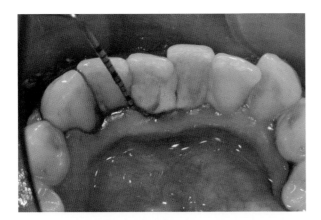

Figure 5.32c On the lingual appearance of the mandibular incisors, abundant calcified deposits are present. The probing values are slightly deeper than normal, but associated with particularly pronounced bleeding. *Source:* Dr. Marisa Roncati (Ferrara, Italy).

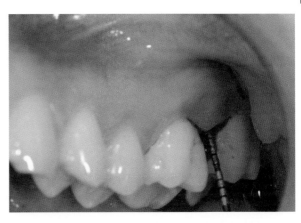

Figure 5.32d At the first visit, the biometric periodontal indexes are collected, including periodontal probing and bleeding index, which in this case was 94%. The most critical areas occur in the maxillary molars, with ≥ 6 mm initial probing depth (see also figures 5.32k and 32t). *Source:* Dr. Marisa Roncati (Ferrara, Italy).

The presence of calcified deposits, in such a generous amount, justifies the extent of the plaque-induced inflammatory reaction. It is also a "positive prognostic factor" because, if properly removed, it will lead to a clinical improvement, influenced by effective nonsurgical periodontal instrumentation and the patient's compliance with daily oral hygiene recommendations.

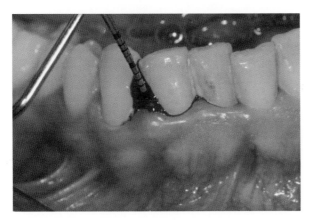

Figure 5.32e On the distal aspect of the mandibular right lateral incisor, a 4 mm probing is detected, associated with profuse bleeding. *Source:* Dr. Marisa Roncati (Ferrara, Italy).

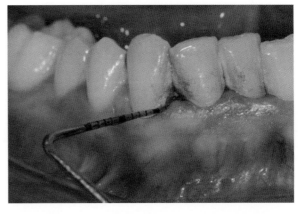

Figure 5.32f The periodontal probe, kept oblique to the vertical axis of the tooth, detects abundant subgingival calcified deposits. *Source:* Dr. Marisa Roncati (Ferrara, Italy).

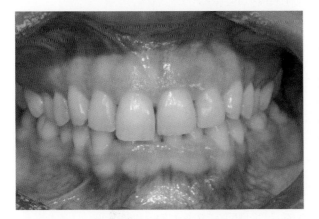

Figure 5.32g Clinical aspect of the case following comprehensive nonsurgical periodontal debridement session. The second appointment is scheduled a few days after the previous one. An improved general condition is already appreciated. *Source:* Dr. Marisa Roncati (Ferrara, Italy).

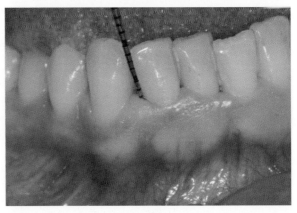

Figure 5.32h With only one professional oral hygiene session, it was possible to improve the periodontal biometric parameters in most sites with initial probing depths 4–5 mm. *Source:* Dr. Marisa Roncati (Ferrara, Italy).

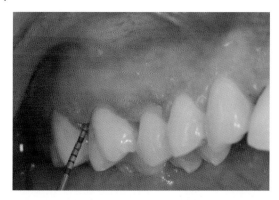

Figure 5.32i On the distal aspect of the right maxillary first molar, 7 mm probing depth was detected, associated with bleeding. Cause-related laser-assisted nonsurgical periodontal therapy is scheduled. *Source:* Dr. Marisa Roncati (Ferrara, Italy).

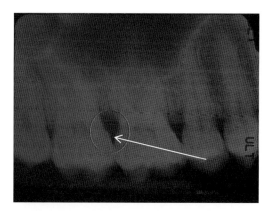

Figure 5.32j In the periapical radiograph, a calculus spicola on the mesial aspect of the second right maxillary molar is observed. If the calcified deposits are visible radiographically, it means that it is present in conspicuous proportions. The radiographic identification facilitates the subsequent clinical detection and nonsurgical instrumentation. *Source:* Dr. Marisa Roncati (Ferrara, Italy).

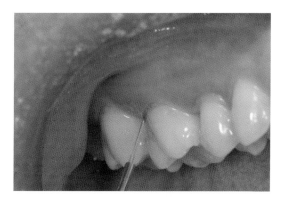

Figure 5.32k Considering the probing depth ⩾ 6mm, the use of a diode laser is recommended, prior to non-surgical periodontal instrumentation, which remains essential and necessary. *Source:* Dr. Marisa Roncati (Ferrara, Italy).

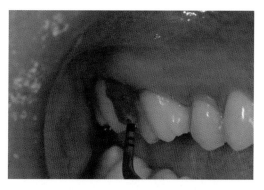

Figure 5.32l Nonsurgical periodontal instrumentation with universal curette (Universal Curette, ENACARE, Micerium, Avegno (Ge) Italy), using vertical movements. It is recommended that the manual instrument is always dipped in 3%, 10 volume, hydrogen peroxide. *Source:* Dr. Marisa Roncati (Ferrara, Italy).

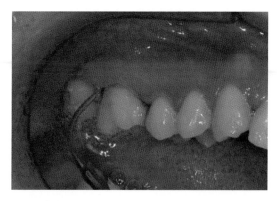

Figure 5.32m Ultrasonic instrumentation (Combi, Mectron S.p.A., Ge, Italy) is always complemented by manual instrumentation (Fig. 5.32l). *Source:* Dr. Marisa Roncati (Ferrara, Italy).

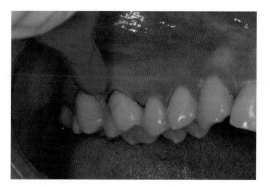

Figure 5.32n Etiological therapy essentially consists of two main phases: nonsurgical periodontal instrumentation (see figures 5.32k-m) and evaluation of the patient's standard of home care and oral hygiene skills. It is important to make the patient aware that interdental cleaning is crucial for long-term maintenance. It is the responsibility of the oral health-care professional to make certain that the patient can master oral hygiene skills required for disease prevention. (Interdental Brush, Enacare, Micerium, Avegno, GE, Italy). *Source:* Dr. Marisa Roncati (Ferrara, Italy).

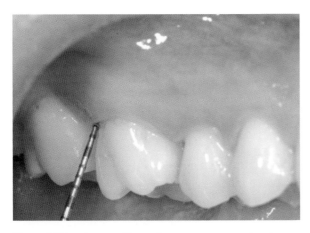

Figure 5.32o At a recall appointment, one year after the initial cause-related laser-assisted nonsurgical periodontal therapy, 2mm probing depth is detected with no bleeding. *Source:* Dr. Marisa Roncati (Ferrara, Italy).

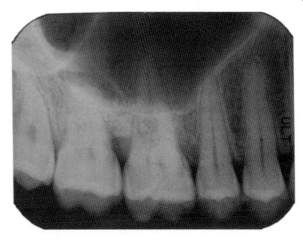

Figure 5.32p A periapical radiograph is taken to confirm a condition of clinical stability. *Source:* Dr. Marisa Roncati (Ferrara, Italy).

Consequently, in this site, presenting an initial 7 mm probing depth (see figure 5.32i), the surgical treatment, which seemed indicated in the first visit, following initial therapy re-evaluation, is no longer necessary at least in the immediate future. It will be advisable to monitor the area over time to intercept any relapses.

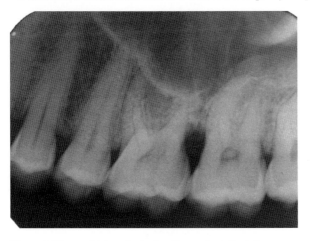

Figure 5.32q Initial periapical radiograph at the left maxillary molars. A localized bone loss is observed in the interproximal space between the first and second molars. *Source:* Dr. Marisa Roncati (Ferrara, Italy).

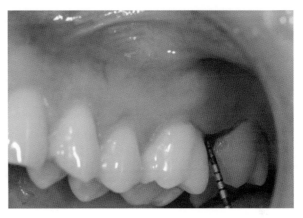

Figure 5.32r The periodontal probe detects 7mm on the distal aspect of the left maxillary first molar, at the time of the first visit. *Source:* Dr. Marisa Roncati (Ferrara, Italy).

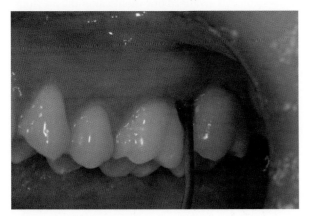

Figure 5.32s Also, in this site, as in the contralateral site (see figure 5.32m), it is recommended to use a diode laser (980 nm, Wiser, Doctor Smile, Lambda S.p.A., Vi, Italy), to facilitate the subsequent comprehensive nonsurgical periodontal debridement and for the bactericidal effect. *Source:* Dr. Marisa Roncati (Ferrara, Italy).

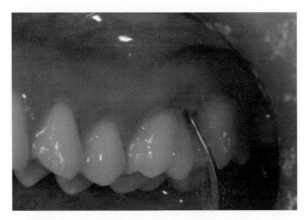

Figure 5.32t Nonsurgical periodontal instrumentation remains absolutely essential, both with ultrasonic instruments (Multipiezo, Mectron S.p.A., Carasco, GE, Italy) and with manual ones (see figure 5.32u). *Source:* Dr. Marisa Roncati (Ferrara, Italy).

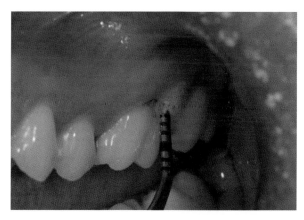

Figure 5.32u A universal curette (Universal curette, ENACARE, Micerium, Avegno (Ge) Italy) is used on the distal aspect of the first maxillary molar on the left, associated with hydrogen peroxide at 3%, 10 volumes. *Source:* Dr. Marisa Roncati (Ferrara, Italy).

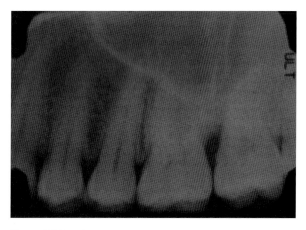

Figure 5.32v Periapical radiograph of, taken one year after Figure 5-32r radiograph, showing improved bone mineralization. *Source:* Dr. Marisa Roncati (Ferrara, Italy).

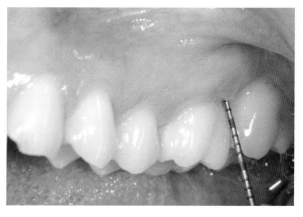

Figure 5.32w At a recall appointment one year after the cause-related laser-assisted nonsurgical periodontal therapy, 2mm probing depth is detected by the periodontal probe. *Source:* Dr. Marisa Roncati (Ferrara, Italy).

Following diagnosis of generalized mild to moderate and localized moderate to severe periodontal disease, cause-related laser-assisted nonsurgical periodontal therapy was executed in two closely scheduled sessions, within a week, with the additional use of a diode laser. A third session was arranged one month after the previous ones, then the patient was treated quarterly for the first year.

At one-year follow-up recall appointment, all indexes were recorded again in the periodontal chart. An overall improvement was observed, associated with a satisfactory home care performance, enhancing the case prognosis, managed only with the nonsurgical approach. The patient was very satisfied as no immediate surgical treatment was proposed, but above all she understood the need for scrupulous monitoring to maintain the clinical stability of the case. *Source:Dr. Marisa Roncati (Ferrara, Italy).*

5.11 Education and Future of Lasers in Periodontal Therapy

The use of laser devices is not usually part of the basic curriculum in dental education and can be learned at the postgraduate education level. Like in medicine (for example in dermatology), the requirement is at least a concentrated, focused, theoretical, and practical education for several days. The education should contain basic instruction in the theoretical and practical levels as well as advanced training in all the different techniques with various laser wavelengths, delivery systems, and laser safety protocols.

The used parameters for the laser-assisted SRP, the removal of granulation tissue in conjunction with a flap procedure, and the deepithelialization technique using the pulsed Nd:YAG, diode (810–980 nm) lasers, CO_2 and Er:YAG laser are presented in Table 5.4.

Table 5.4 Suggested laser parameters for periodontal procedures.

Laser	Procedure	Power (W)	Frequency (Hz)	Energy (mJ)	Fiber (µm)
Nd:YAG	Curettage	1.5–2.8	50–70	30–40	300–400
	Deepithelialization	1.7–2.0	20–25	75–100	400
	Bacteria reduction	1.0–1.5	10–15	100	400
	Gingivectomy	2.0–3.0	30–70	100	300–400
	Gingivoplasty	2.0	25–30	50–75	400
Diode	Curettage	2.0	CW		
		2.5–4.0	50	80	400
	De-epithelialization	3.0–4.0	CW		400
	Bacteria reduction	2.0–3.0	CW		400
	Gingivectomy	3.0–4.0	CW		400
	Gingivoplasty	3.0	CW		400
CO₂	Curettage	3–4	CW		0.35 metal tip
		3–4	50	60–80	0.8 ceramic tip
	Deepithelialization	4–6	CW		0.8 ceramic tip
	Bacteria reduction	4	CW		0.8 ceramic tip
	Gingivectomy	4	CW		400
		4–6	20	200–300	0.8 ceramic tip
	Gingivoplasty	4–6	CW		0.8 ceramic tip
	Root modification	2	20	100	0.8 ceramic tip
Er:YAG	Calculus removal. tip (+water)	2.4–3.0	30	80–100	chisel type
	Osseous contouring	3.0	1–2	200–300	400 (+water)
	Curettage	1.4–1.6	10	140–160	chisel type tip
	De-epithelialization	1.5–3.0	50	30–60	400–600
	Bacteria reduction	1.0–1.8	10–15	100–120	chisel type tip
	Gingivectomy	1.5–3.0	20–50	75–80	400–600
	Gingivoplasty	1.5–3.0	50	30–60	600
Er,Cr:YSGG	Calculus removal	0.75–2.5	50		600 (7–11%water/60–100% air) - Z6 tip
	Osseous contouring	3.0	2		600 (50% water/60% air)
	Curettage	1.0–1.5	50mj/pulse		500 30 (short pulses: 60µsec; H mode) (50%water/40%air) RFTP5 tip
	Deepithelialization	1.5			500 50 (short pulses: 60µsec; H mode) (20%water/11%air) – RFTP5 tip
	Gingivectomy	max. 4	20		600 (0% water/0% air) G-/T-/C6 or C3-chisel type tip
	Gingivoplasty	max. 4	20		600 (0% water/0% air) with G-/T-/ C6 or C3-tip

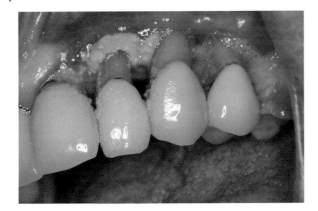

Figure 5.33 Advanced periodontal necrosis due to severe overheating using the Nd:YAG laser (LANAP). The use of this laser wavelength utilized without to control penetration depth especially when tissues are inflamed.

The exact protocols can be explained in consideration with the laser-tissue interactions, the use of the specific laser wavelength, the goals of periodontal therapy, the soft tissue biotype (phenotype), and the available laser devices in the dental office.

The knowledge of the laser-tissue interactions and the advanced training of laser applications are very important in order to avoid complications in clinical practice. Tissue damage due to overheating should be controlled, and only low powers should be used when susceptible tissues, like the periodontal apparatus, have to be treated. Uncontrolled laser energy levels and tissue irradiation for long periods may damage the tissues and can lead to unexpected side effects with potential legal consequences (Figure 5.33).

The use of laser wavelengths which do not have deep penetration depth in the tissues, such as CO_2 and Er:YAG lasers, may be the future of lasers for laser-assisted periodontal therapy. Short pulse durations (in micro-, pico- or femtoseconds) are fundamental in order to reduce those risks.

The developments of the last few years, such as the new technology and delivery systems for CO_2 lasers, have already led to an improved "handling" of these laser devices. Nevertheless, concerning the beneficial effects of the CO_2 laser irradiation on the root surfaces, and the removal of the inflamed pocket epithelium and connective tissue, there is a need for further studies in order to improve the technique of deepithelialization and to establish new regenerative clinical protocols in daily practice.

The companies manufacturing laser devices should be involved in clinical trials in order to provide strong evidence of lasers in periodontal therapy. Only then, the lasers can replace beneficially conventional treatment approaches and have an impact on saving teeth, reducing the costs of therapy to patients, insurance policy makers, and tax payers.

In summary, the effects of different laser wavelengths on the periodontal tissues are demonstrated in the schematic drawings (Figure 5.34).

Also, incision quality, carbonization effect, and hemostatic properties are dependent on the laser wavelength besides selected laser parameters and tissue condition (Figure 5.35).

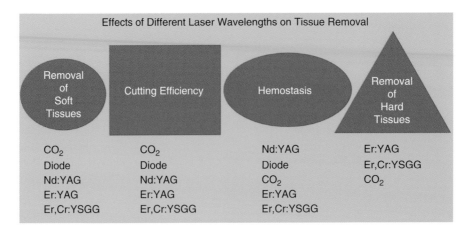

Figure 5.34 Effects of different laser wavelengths on the tissues.

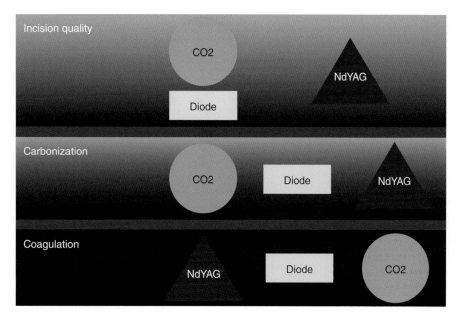

Figure 5.35 Laser wavelengths and tissue effects.

References

Al-Falaki, R., Hughes, F., Wadia, R. et al. (2016). The effect of an Er,Cr:YSGG laser in the management of intrabony defects associated with chronic periodontitis using minimally invasive closed flap procedure. A case series. *Laser Ther. 25*: 131–139.

Ando, Y., Aoki, A., Watanabe, H., and Ishikawa, I. (1996). Bactericidal effect of erbium:YAG laser on periodontopathic bacteria. *Lasers Surg. Med. 19*: 190–200.

Aoki, A., Ando, Y., Watanabe, H., and Ishikawa, I. (1994). In vitro studies on laser scaling of subgingival calculus with an erbium:YAG laser. *J. Periodontol. 65*: 1097–1106.

Barone, A., Covani, U., Crespi, R., and Romanos, G.E. (2002). Root surface morphological changes after focused versus defocused CO_2 laser irradiation. a scanning electron microscopy analysis. *J. Periodontol. 73*: 370–373.

Ben Hatit, Y., Blum, R., Severin, C. et al. (1996). The effects of a pulsed Nd:YAG laser on subgingival bacterial flora and on cementum: an in vivo study. *J. Clin. Laser Med. Surg. 14*: 137–143.

Borrajo, J.L., Varela, L.G., Castro, G.L. et al. (2004). Diode laser (980 nm) as adjunct to scaling and root planing. *Photomed. Laser Surg. 22*: 509–512.

Caffesse, R.G. and Quiñones, C.R. (1993). Outcome studies of periodontal treatment modalities. *Curr. Opin. Periodontol.*: 170–177.

Castro, G.L., Gallas, M., Núñez, I.R. et al. (2006). Histological evaluation of the use of diode laser as an adjunct to traditional periodontal treatment. *Photomed. Laser Surg. 24*: 64–68.

Caton, J.G. and Nyman, S. (1980). Histometric evaluation of periodontal surgery. I. The modified Widman flap procedure. *J. Clin. Periodontol. 7*: 212–223.

Caton, J.G. and Zander, H. (1979). The attachment between tooth and gingival tissues after periodic root planing and soft tissue curettage. *J. Periodontol. 50*: 462–466.

Caton, J.G., Nyman, S., and Zander, H. (1980). Histometric evaluation of periodontal surgery. II. Connective tissue attachment levels after four regenerative procedures. *J. Clin. Periodontol. 7*: 224–231.

Chellappah, N.K. and Loh, H.S. (1990). Laser therapy for a haemophiliac. Case report. *Aust. Dent. J. 35*: 121–124.

Chen, C.K., Wu, Y.T., Chang, N.J. et al. (2017). Er:YAG laser for surgical crown lengthening: a 6-month clinical study. *Int. J. Periodont. Rest. Dent. 37*: e149–e153.

Chrysikopoulos, S., Papaspyridakos, P., and Eleftheriades, E. (2006). Laser-assisted oral and maxillofacial surgery for patients on anticoagulant therapy in daily practice. *J. Oral Laser Appl. 6*: 79–88.

Claffey, N. and Egelberg, J. (1995). Clinical indicators of probing attachment loss following initial periodontal treatment in advanced periodontitis patients. *J. Clin. Periodontol. 22*: 690–696.

Cobb, C.M. (1996). Non-surgical periodontal therapy: mechanical. *Ann. Periodontol. 1*: 443–490.

Cobb, C.M. (2006). Lasers in periodontics: a review of the literature. *J. Periodontol. 77*: 545–564.

Cobb, C.M., Mccawley, T.K., and Killoy, W.J. (1992). A preliminary study on the effects of the Nd:YAG laser on root surfaces and subgingival microflora in vivo. *J. Periodontol. 63*: 701–707.

Coffelt, D.W., Cobb, C.M., MacNeill, S. et al. (1997). Determination of energy density threshold for laser ablation of bacteria. An in vitro study. *J. Clin. Periodontol. 24*: 1–7.

Crespi, R., Covani, U., Margarone, J.E., and Andreana, S. (1997). Periodontal tissue regeneration in beagle dogs after laser therapy. *Lasers Surg. Med. 21*: 395–402.

Crespi, R., Barone, A., Covani, U. et al. (2002). Effects of CO_2 laser treatment on fibroblast attachment to root surfaces. A scanning electron microscopy analysis. *J. Periodontol. 73*: 1308–1312.

Crespi, R., Covani, U., Romanos, G.E., and Barone, A. (2004). CO_2 laser effects on root surface in periodontal therapy. Case reports. *J. Oral Laser Appl. 4*: 109–117.

Crespi, R., Cappare, P., Gherlone, E., and Romanos, G.E. (2011). Comparison of modified Widman and coronally advanced flap surgery combined with CO_2 laser root irradiation in periodontal therapy. A 15-year follow-up. *Int. J. Periodontics Restorative Dent. 31*: 641–651.

Deppe, H., Muecke, T., Auer-Bahrs, J. et al. (2013). Bleeding complications following Nd:YAG laser-assisted oral surgery vs conventional treatment in cardiac risk patients: a clinical retrospective comparative study. *Quintessence Int. 44*: 513–520.

Eriksson, A.R. and Albrektsson, T. (1983). Temperature threshold levels for heat induced bone tissue injury: a vital microscopic study in the rabbit. *J. Prosthet. Dent. 50*: 101–107.

Fekrazad, R., Moharrami, M., and Chiniforush, N. (2018). The esthetic crown lengthening by Er,Cr:YSGG laser: a case series. *J. Laser Med. Sci. 9*: 283–287.

Folwaczny, M., Thiele, L., Mehl, A., and Hickel, R. (2001). The effect of working tip angulation on root substance removal using Er:YAG laser radiation: an in vitro study. *J Clin Periodontol. 28* (3): 220–226.

Frentzen, M., Koort, H.J., and Thiensiri, I. (1992). Excimer lasers in dentistry: future possibilities with advanced technology. *Quintessence Int. 23* (2): 117–133.

Frentzen, M., Braun, A., and Aniol, D. (2002). Er:YAG laser scaling of diseased root surfaces. *J. Periodontol. 73*: 524–530.

Gokhale, S.R., Padhye, A.M., Byakod, G. et al. (2012). A comparative evaluation of the efficacy of diode laser as an adjunct to mechanical debridement versus conventional mechanical debridement in periodontal flap surgery: a clinical and microbiological study. *Photomed. Laser Surg. 30*: 598–603.

Gold, S.I. and Vilardi, M.A. (1994). Pulsed laser beam effects on gingiva. *J. Clin. Periodontol. 21*: 391–396.

Grasser, H. and Ackermann, K. (1977). Possibilities for the use of lasers in dental surgery. *Dtsch. Zahnaerztl. Z. 32*: 512–515. (German).

Gregg, R. and McCarthy, D.K. (1998). Laser ENAP for periodontal bone regeneration. *Dent. Today 17*: 88–91.

Harris, D.M., Gregg, R.H., Mc Carthy, D.K. et al. (2002). Sulcular debridement with pulsed Nd:YAG. Laser periodontal therapy™ in private practice. *Proc. SPIE 4610* (6): 49–58.

Ishikawa, I. and Sculean, A. (2007). Laser dentistry in periodontics. In: *Proceedings of the 1st International Workshop of Evidence Based Dentistry on Lasers in Dentistry* (ed. N. Gutknecht), 115–128. Berlin: Quintessence Publ.

Israel, M., Rossmann, J.A., and Froum, S.J. (1995). Use of the carbon dioxide laser in retarding epithelial migration: a pilot histological human study utilizing case reports. *J. Periodontol. 66*: 197–204.

Kamma, J., Romanos, G.E., and Vasdekis, V. (2009). The effect of diode laser (980nm) treatment on aggressive periodontitis. Evaluation of microbial and clinical parameters. Photomed. *Laser Surg. 27*: 11–19.

Keller U, Hibst R. Experimental removal of subgingival calculus with an Er:YAG laser. Lasers in Dentistry SPIE 1995;2623:189–198.

Komatsu, Y., Morozumi, T., Abe, D. et al. (2012). Effects of erbium-doped:yttrium aluminum garnet (Er:YAG) laser on bacteremia due to scaling and root planing. *J. Lasers Med. Sci. 3*: 175–184.

Krejci, R.F., Reinhardt, R.A., Wentz, F.M. et al. (1982). Effects of electrosurgery on dog pulps under cervical metallic restorations. *Oral Surg. Oral Med. Oral Pathol. 54*: 575–582.

Liu, C.M., Hou, L.T., Wong, M.Y., and Lan, W.H. (1999). Comparison of Nd:YAG laser versus scaling and root planing in periodontal therapy. *J. Periodontol. 70*: 1276–1282.

Magid, K.S. and Strauss, R.A. (2007). Laser use for esthetic soft tissue modification. *Dent. Clin. N. Am. 51*: 525–545.

Manor, A., Lebendiger, M., Shiffer, A., and Tovel, H. (1984). Bacterial invasion of periodontal tissues in advanced periodontitis in humans. *J. Periodontol. 55*: 567–573.

Martelli, F.S., Fanti, E., Rosati, C. et al. (2016). Long-term efficacy of microbiology-driven periodontal laser-assisted therapy. *Eur. J. Clin. Microbiol. Infect. Dis. 35*: 423–431.

McGuire, M.K. and Scheyer, E.T. (2011). Laser-assisted flapless crown lengthening: a case series. *Int. J. Periodontics Restorative Dent. 31*: 357–364.

Morlock, B.J., Pippin, D.J., Cobb, C.M. et al. (1992). The effect of Nd:YAG laser exposure on root surfaces when used as an adjunct to root planing: an in vitro study. *J. Periodontol. 63*: 637–641.

Needleman, I.G., Worthington, H.V., Giedrys-Leeper, E., and Tucker, R.J. (2006). Guided tissue regeneration for periodontal infrabony defects. *Cochrane Database Syst. Rev. 19*: CD001724.

Neill ME. Sulcular debridement and bacterial reduction with the Pulse Master Dental Laser: Clinical Evaluation of the effects of pulsed Nd:YAG laser on periodontitis and periodontal pathogens. M.S. Thesis, University of Texas Graduate School of Biomedical Sciences at San Antonio, April 1997.

Neill, M.E. and Mellonig, J.T. (1997). Clinical efficacy of the Nd:YAG laser for combination periodontitis therapy. *Pract. Periodontics Aesthet. Dent. 9* (6 Suppl): 1–5.

Nevins, M.L., Camelo, M., Schupbach, P. et al. (2012). Human clinical and histologic evaluation of laser-assisted new attachment procedure. *Int. J. Periodontics Restorative Dent. 32*: 497–507.

Pearlman, N.W., Stiegmann, G.V., Vance, V. et al. (1991). A prospective study of incisional time, blood loss, pain, and healing with carbon dioxide laser, scalpel, and electrosurgery. *Arch. Surg. 126* (8): 1018–1020.

Pick, R.M. and Colvard, M.D. (1993). Current status of lasers in soft tissue dental surgery. *J. Periodontol. 64*: 589–602.

Purucker, P., Ertl, T., Uhlmann, G., and Bernimoulin, J.-P. (1994). Das Wachstum von *Porphyromonas gingivalis* und *Prevotella intermedia* nach Bestrahlung mittels Excimer-Laser. *Dtsch. Zahnarztl. Z. 49*: 412–414, (German).

Qadri, T., Poddani, P., Javed, F. et al. (2010). A short-term evaluation of Nd:YAG laser as an adjunct to scaling and root planing in the treatment of periodontal inflammation. *J. Periodontol. 81*: 1161–1166.

Qadri, T., Javed, F., Poddani, P. et al. (2011). Long-term effects of a single application of a water-cooled pulsed Nd:YAG laser in supplement to scaling and root planing in patients with periodontal inflammation. *Lasers Med. Sci. 26*: 763–766.

Radvar, M., Crean, S.L., Gilmour, W.H. et al. (1995). An evaluation of the effects of an Nd:YAG laser on subgingival calculus, dentin and cementum. *J. Clin. Periodontol. 22*: 71–77.

Ramfjord, S.P., Caffesse, R.G., Morrison, E.C. et al. (1987). 4 modalities of periodontal treatment compared over 5 years. *J. Clin. Periodontol. 14*: 445–452.

Rechmann P, Henning T. Selective ablation of subgingival calculus. In: Loh HS. (ed.): 4th International Congress on Lasers in Dentistry, Bologna 1995, Monduzzi Editore, pp. 159–162.

Romanos, G.E. (1994a). Clinical applications of the Nd:YAG laser in oral soft tissue surgery and periodontology. *J. Clin. Laser Med. Surg. 12*: 103–108.

Romanos, G.E. (1994b). Chirurgische Therapie der akuten nekrotisierenden, ulzerierenden Gingivitis mit Hilfe des Nd:YAG-Lasers. *Parodontologie 5*: 53–60. (German).

Romanos, G., Purucker, P., and Renner, P.J. (1998a). Laseranwendung in der Parodontologie. Aktueller Stand. *Parodontologie 9*: 299–312. (German).

Romanos, G.E., Altmann, M., Pelekanos, S., and Strub, J.R. (1998b). Klinische und histologische Untersuchung der Wundheilung nach der Anwendung von Laser- und HF-Präparation an der Rattenhaut. *ZWR 107*: 274–279. (German).

Romanos, G.E., Henze, M., Banihashemi, S. et al. (2004). Removal of epithelium in periodontal pockets following diode (980nm) laser application in the animal model: an in vitro study. *Photomed. Laser Surg. 22*: 177–183.

Roncati, M., Gariffo, A., Barbieri, C., and Vescovi, P. (2017). Ten-year nonsurgical periodontal treatment protocol with adjunctive use of diode laser monitoring clinical outcomes in ≥ 6mm pockets: a retrospective controlled case series. *Int. J. Periodontics Restorative Dent. 37*: 647–654.

Rossmann, J.A. and Israel, M. (2000). Laser de-epithelialization for enhanced guided tissue regeneration. A paradigm shift? In: Convissar RA (ed.). *Dental Clin North Am 44*: 793–809.

Rossmann, J.A., Gottlieb, S., Koudelka, B.M., and McQuade, M.J. (1987). Effects of CO_2 laser irradiation on gingiva. *J. Periodontol. 58*: 423–425.

Rossmann, J.A., McQuade, M.J., and Turunen, D.E. (1992). Retardation of epithelial migration in monkeys using a carbon dioxide laser: an animal study. *J. Periodontol. 63*: 902–907.

Saunders, E.M. (1990). In vivo findings associated with heat generation during thermomechanical compaction of gutta-percha. 1. Temperature levels at the external surface of the root. 2. Histological response to temperature elevation on the external surface of the root. *Int. Endodont. J. 23*: 263–274.

Schoenly, J.E., Seka, W., and Rechmann, P. (2010). Investigation into the optimum beam shape and fluence for selective ablation of dental calculus at $\lambda = 400$ nm. *Lasers Surg. Med. 42*: 51–61.

Schoenly JE, Seka W, Romanos GE, Rechmann P. The efficacy of selective calculus ablation at 400nm: comparison to conventional calculus removal methods. Proc Soc Photo Opt Instrum Eng (SPIE) 2013; (in press).

Schwarz, F., Sculean, A., Berakdar, M. et al. (2003). Periodontal treatment with an Er:YAG laser or scaling and root planing. A 2-year follow-up split-mouth study. *J. Periodontol. 74*: 590–596.

Sculean, A., Schwarz, F., Berakdar, M. et al. (2004a). Periodontal treatment with an Er:YAG laser compared to ultrasonic instrumentation: a pilot study. *J. Periodontol. 75*: 966–973.

Sculean, A., Schwarz, F., Berakdar, M. et al. (2004b). Healing of intrabony defects following surgical treatment with or without an Er:YAG laser. *J. Clin. Periodontol. 31*: 604–608.

Smith, M.L. (2011). Laser-assisted non-surgical periodontal therapy. In: *Principles and Practice of Laser Dentistry*, (2nd ed. R. A. Convissar). St. Louis, MO: Elsevier.

Srivastava, C.M. and Lossin, C. (1976). A comparative study of the healing of wounds made by scalpel and electrosurgery in rabbits. *Aust. Dent. J. 21*: 252–257.

Sweeny, S. and Romanos, G.E. (2006). Laser-assisted soft tissue management in esthetic dentistry. *J. Oral Laser Appl. 6*: 133–139.

Thomas, M. and Shafer, K. (2011). Insufficient evidence that pulsed Nd:YAG laser treatment is superior to conventional nonsurgical therapy in the treatment of periodontal disease. *J. Am. Dent. Assoc. 142*: 194–195.

Thomas, D., Rapley, J., Cobb, C. et al. (1994). Effects of the Nd:YAG laser and combined treatments on in vitro fibroblast attachment to root surfaces. *J. Clin. Periodontol. l21*: 38–44.

Trylovich, D.J., Cobb, C.M., Pippin, D.J. et al. (1992). The effects of the Nd:YAG laser on in vitro fibroblast attachment to endotoxin-treated root surfaces. *J. Periodontol. 63*: 626–663.

Tseng, P., Gilkeson, C.F., Pearlman, B., and Liew, V. (1991a). The effect of Nd:YAG laser treatment on subgingival calculus in vitro. *J. Dent. Res. 70*: 657, Abstract No. 62.

Tseng, P., Gilkeson, C.F., Palmer, J., and Liew, V. (1991b). The bactericidal effect of a Nd:YAG laser in vitro. *J. Dent. Res. 70*: 650, Abstract No. 7.

Vaderhobli, R.M., White, J.M., Le, C. et al. (2010). In vitro study of the soft tissue effects of microsecond-pulsed CO_2 laser parameters during soft tissue incision and sulcular debridement. *Laser Surg. Med. 42*: 257–263.

Visser, H., Mausberg, R., Fastenmeier, K., and Lohr, G. (1994). High-frequency dental surgery near metal reconstructions. *Schweiz. Monatsschr. Zahnmed. 104*: 278–283. (German).

White, J.M., Goodis, H.E., and Rose, C.L. (1991). Use of the pulsed Nd:YAG laser for intraoral soft tissue surgery. *Lasers Surg. Med. 11*: 455–461.

White, J.M., Goodis, H.E., Horton, J., and Gold, S. (1994). Current status of lasers in soft tissue dental surgery. *J. Periodontol. 65*: 733–735.

Wilder-Smith, P., Arrastia, A.M., Schell, M.J. et al. (1995). Effect of Nd:YAG laser irradiation and root planing on the root surface: structural and thermal effects. *J. Periodontol. 66*: 1032–1039.

Yukna, R.A. (1976). A clinical and histologic study of healing following the excisional new attachment procedure in rhesus monkeys. *J. Periodontol. 47*: 701–709.

Yukna, R.A., Bowers, G.M., Lawrence, J.J., and Fedi, P.F. Jr. (1976). A clinical study of healing in humans following the excisional new attachment procedure. *J. Periodontol. 47*: 696–700.

Yukna, R.A., Carr, R.L., and Evans, G.H. (2007). Histologic evaluation of an Nd:YAG laser-assisted new attachment procedure in humans. *Int J Periodontics Restorative Dent 27*: 577–587.

6

Lasers and Implants
Georgios E. Romanos

Stony Brook University, School of Dental Medicine, Stony Brook, NY, USA

6.1 Introduction

In modern clinical dentistry, the application scope of lasers has also been extended to the field of oral implantology. Different laser systems have various indications in the multiple phases of implant treatment and for the management of complications. These clinical options include today:

- soft tissue surgery before implant placement or at the stage of implant uncovering (second stage surgery),
- during the loading phase,
- for the treatment of peri-implantitis,
- for implant removal and,
- for implant placement.

The different indications of laser use for clinicians using dental implants are described extensively in the literature. The reader is advised here to study these papers to understand better the interactions between lasers and titanium surfaces and also to evaluate the scope of practice, as a standard of care, when lasers are involved in implant dentistry (Romanos et al. 2009a, 2013).

This chapter presents clinical applications, including step-by-step illustrations, where different laser systems are used in various stages of treatment with dental implants.

6.2 Laser-Assisted Surgery Before Implant Placement and Implant Exposure

Before implant surgery, the implant bed may be modified using different laser systems. Specifically, areas with high attachment of muscles (i.e. frenum), insufficient width of keratinized mucosa, reduced depth of the vestibulum, presence of soft tissue benign tumors (e.g. fibromas, papillomas), and leukoplakia and other oral mucosal conditions (e.g. lichen planus) should be treated before implant placement (see also Chapter 3).

For the surgical exposure of endosseous (two-staged) submerged healed dental implants, the use of the CO_2 laser is recommended (Catone 1997). The implant surface can reflect the beam; therefore, a temperature increase of the implant body and the peri-implant hard and soft tissues does not take immediately place. For the protection of the adjacent soft tissues, use of instruments (e.g. metal spatula and matrices) is recommended.

Another alternative seems to be the Er:YAG laser (Arnabat-Domínguez et al. 2003), but the Er,Cr:YSGG laser also provides advantages and superior esthetic benefits compared to the scalpel (Arnabat-Domínguez et al. 2010). This laser can uncover implants and allows apical position of the tissue, increasing the width of attached mucosa.

In vitro studies showed that the irradiation of different implant surfaces with the CO_2 laser does not change the surface characteristics of the implant (Romanos et al. 1997). Previous morphological studies using a scanning electron microscopy (SEM) showed that the CO_2 laser irradiation of machined, sandblasted, and titanium plasma-sprayed (TPS) and hydroxyapatite (HA)-coated implants does not cause damage to the implant surface, using different power settings (2–4 W) in the continuous (Figure 6.1) as well as pulsed mode. However, in the superpulsed mode, oxidation-related discolorations of the implant surface were reported, as well as extensive melting (Deppe et al. 1998). Recent studies by Park et al. (2012) showed no changes on titanium (Ti) surfaces after CO_2 laser irradiation, compared to irradiation with the Er,Cr:YSGG and Er:YAG laser. The latter presented surface changes on Ti disks according to the power output. The CO_2 laser irradiation did not affect the surface of Ti disks, irrespective of the power output.

Advanced Laser Surgery in Dentistry, First Edition. Georgios E. Romanos.
© 2021 John Wiley & Sons, Inc. Published 2021 by John Wiley & Sons, Inc.

In contrast to the use of CO_2 laser, the application of a pulsed Nd:YAG laser led to severe damage of implant surfaces. Block et al. (1992) reported irreversible changes in HA-coated implants. Extensive melting, porosity alterations, cracks, and ruptures of the HA-coating of IMZ implants, as well as on sandblasted and Ti- plasma-sprayed implants were shown (Figure 6.2).

However, SEM studies demonstrated changes (Figure 6.3) in the surface pattern of implants when they were irradiated with a diode 810 nm laser (unpublished data) compared to a diode 980 nm laser (Romanos et al. 2000). Therefore, more studies in this field with specific parameters should be performed to evaluate the power settings of diode lasers in implant dentistry to avoid postoperative complications. In another in vitro study, it was found out that strong absorption of the Nd:YAG laser lead to a biologically, not tolerant temperature rise (Romanos et al. 1996).

Therefore, the use of the Nd:YAG laser is recommended with caution for surgical exposure (uncovering) of implants or peri-implant soft tissue conditioning due to the high risk of overheating.

Similarly, the temperature can be clinically unacceptable when the continuous wave mode is used for diode lasers (810 or 980 nm) over an irradiation period of 15–20 seconds. Therefore, professional advanced training and exact knowledge about the power settings for the use of diode lasers is very important to avoid

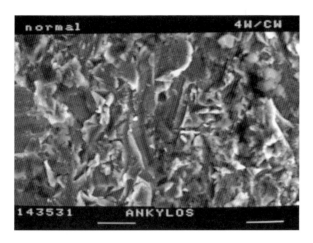

Figure 6.1 Scanning electron microscopic analysis of sandblasted implant surface (Ankylos implant system; left) and after 4 W continuous mode of CO_2 laser irradiation (right). *Source:* Dr. Georgios E. Romanos.

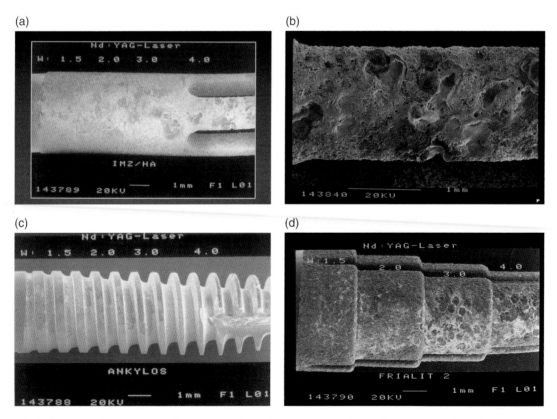

Figure 6.2 Extensive melting, porosity alterations, cracks, and ruptures of the HA-coating of IMZ implants (a, b) as well as sandblasted Ankylos® dental implant (c) and Ti-plasma-sprayed Frialit-2® -implant (d) after irradiation with a dental, pulsed Nd:YAG laser. *Source:* Dr. Georgios E. Romanos.

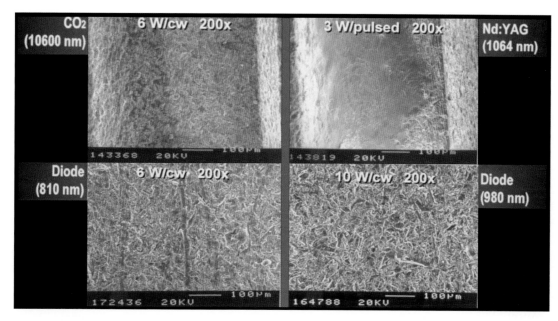

Figure 6.3 Morphological studies on implant surface analysis after laser irradiation using a scanning electron microscope demonstrated changes in the surface pattern of implants, when they were irradiated with a pulsed Nd:YAG laser or a continuous wave diode 810 nm laser compared to a continuous wave diode 980 nm or a CO_2 laser. *Source:* Dr. Georgios E. Romanos.

complications in the final clinical outcome (Geminiani et al. 2012; Leja et al. 2013).

> Clinicians who use diode lasers should be well informed about the limitations and risks of these wavelengths in relation to dental implants. The risk of overheating and possible changes of the implant surface pattern may be the main reasons to develop new diode lasers in implant dentistry in order to use them in routine daily practice without risks of complications.

In contrast to that, recent studies with thermo-elements showed that during laser surgery using the CO_2 laser in the continuous mode, the temperature rises. For example, in a few seconds a temperature rise of 20 °C can be reached, when it is used the continuous mode with a power of 4–6 W. Using the pulsed mode of CO_2 lasers, no significant overheating of the implant is caused at an output power of up to 6 W (Ganz 1994; Geminiani et al. 2012; Leja et al. 2012).

The coagulation of soft tissues using laser-assisted implant exposure is very good. The incision is carried out in the middle of the alveolar crest or in the area where the implant was placed according to the surgical (prosthetic) guide. The use of a punch for removal of the peri-implant mucosa with the CO_2 laser is no longer recommended because this method leads to loss of tissue especially keratinized mucosa. Abutments (sulcus formers) are then connected with the implant after surgical exposure.

Usually, impressions for the completion of the prosthetic restoration can be carried out after 10 days.

> It is from clinical significance that the CO_2 laser is applied in daily practice around implants in continuous mode using the defocused beam and in the pulsed mode in the focused beam.

The use of the Er:YAG family of lasers may be used near metal surfaces and especially dental implants. However, the use of air and water is important to control the temperature rise. The parameters of the Er:YAG laser application seems to be sensitive and may have dramatic effects on the temperature levels (Geminiani et al. 2011; Leja et al. 2012). The recommendations for clinicians who use the Er:YAG or the Er,Cr:YSGG lasers are to follow strictly the manufacturer guidelines but also to study the current literature.

6.3 Laser Application During Function

The most frequent problem in implant dentistry during the functional phase is the growth of peri-implant gingival hyperplasia, of unknown etiology, especially in cases with removable implant-supported restorations, which can affect the long-term prognosis of implants (Adell et al. 1981, 1986; Lekholm et al. 1986; Engquist et al. 1988). In this field, the CO_2 laser, as well as the diode laser, can be applied successfully. Hyperplasia is usually removed with the continuous laser beam of the

CO_2 laser and output power of approximately maximum 4W. Peri-implant soft tissues will be ablated to create a smooth, tissue morphology (gingivoplasty). This surgical treatment needs sometimes to be carried out in several sessions. For diode lasers, a significantly lower power of 2–3W (with initiator) is usually sufficient for soft tissue excisions.

Other surgical corrections of the peri-implant soft tissues may be necessary during implant loading, such as removal of muscular attachments (frenectomy) and vestibuloplasty (Figure 6.4; see also Chapter 3). In such surgical interventions, additional suturing is not necessary. Wound healing succeeds usually without complications. The charring may serve as a wound dressing, and it is more common in the application of the CO_2 laser.

6.4 Laser Applications in Peri-implantitis Treatment

Peri-implant diseases have increased in the last few years. Studies by Zitzmann and Berglundh (2008) presented peri-implant inflammatory reactions over 50%

for peri-implant mucositis and a maximum of 43% for peri-implantitis. However, peri-implantitis has been defined recently as a peri-implant infection with bleeding on probing, suppuration, and a progressive crestal bone loss. Other signs of inflammation (i.e. pain) may be included (Albrektsson et al. 2012a). Based on this definition and the recent analysis of the literature, the frequency of peri-implantitis and implant failures are commonly less than 5% over 10 years of follow-up for modern implants using established protocols (Albrektsson et al. 2012b).

Laser use in the field of the peri-implantitis treatment does not seem to be an evidence-based approach. One reason for that is that there is no possibility of having randomized-controlled split-mouth clinical trials on the treatment of peri-implant diseases. Many case series and clinical reports present the application of various laser wavelengths for the decontamination of failing implants. Early case reports showed the effects of the use of a diode laser for the decontamination of implant surfaces with an output power of 1W and 20 seconds application period (under noncontact fiber). Specifically, a

(a) (b)

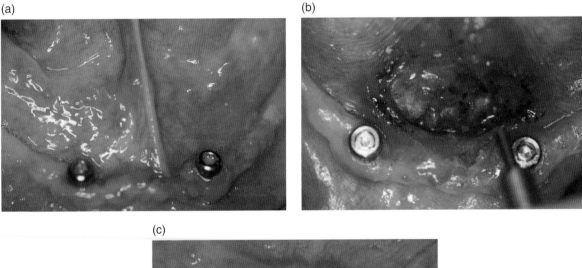

(c)

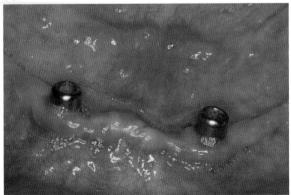

Figure 6.4 Lingual frenum, which does not allow optimal stability of the prosthesis (a) excised with a noncontact CO_2 laser (4W) (b); wound healing completed in six weeks without any scar tissue. *Source:* Dr. Georgios E. Romanos.

significant reduction of the pathogenic bacteria (*Porphyromonas gingivalis and fusobacteria*) was observed (Hartmann and Bach 1997).

Other microbiological studies showed bacteria (especially *Bacillus subtilis*) reduction on implant surfaces with various surface patterns, after Nd:YAG laser irradiation. Only one output power up to 3 W was studied. However, the risk of metal overheating should be taken into consideration. An absolute bacteria elimination (i.e. sterilization) could not be observed (Block et al. 1992). For this reason, and also because of the severe damage of the implant surface after irradiation with the Nd:YAG laser, the use of this laser might be avoided in peri-implantitis therapy.

In contrast to the Nd:YAG laser, it was confirmed in another in vitro study that, after contamination of implant surfaces with pathogenic bacteria (*Porphyromonas gingivalis*), the bacteria can be reduced by the CO_2 laser irradiation (Purucker et al. 1998). A significant reduction of bacteria was observed in samples of irradiated surfaces, in comparison to the nonirradiated titanium surfaces (Figures 6.5 and 6.6).

Some animal experiments and clinical studies showed that the use of the CO_2 laser can be promising for the peri-implantitis therapy (Figure 6.7). Based on an animal study in dogs, the progression of the inflammatory osseous reduction can be prevented around the implant, without leaving thermal damages in the osseous bed, when implants are irradiated with the CO_2 laser. Of particular interest is the new bone formation on peri-implant osseous defects after decontamination with the CO_2 laser (Figure 6.8) in close contact with the implant surface (re-osseointegration). Furthermore, implant surfaces could be decontaminated using appropriate

parameters, without changes of the surface pattern (Deppe et al. 1998).

In contrast to the use of the CO_2 laser for implant surface decontamination, Schmage et al. (2012) also

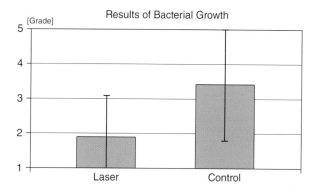

Figure 6.6 Bacterial growth after the CO_2 laser irradiation presents reduction of bacteria after laser irradiation.

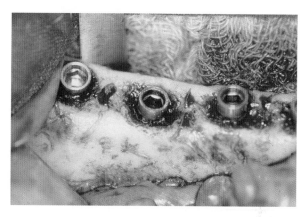

Figure 6.7 Ligature-induced peri-implant defects in dog irradiated with the CO_2 laser. *Source:* Dr. H. Deppe, Munich, Germany.

Figure 6.5 Bacterial reduction after CO_2 laser irradiation. Left slide: test group after laser irradiation. Right slide: bacteria without CO_2 laser irradiation. *Source:* Dr. Georgios E. Romanos.

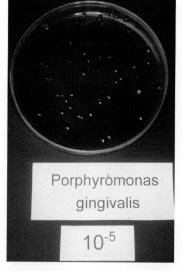

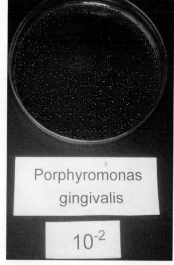

showed inefficient cleaning of implant surfaces using an Er:YAG laser (Key Laser 3, KaVo Dental, Biberach, Germany). Another study also stated that surface alterations may occur with the Er:YAG laser (Kreisler et al. 2002). Compared to numerous studies by the group of Schwarz et al. (2005, 2006), who promoted the use of Er:YAG laser in the treatment of peri-implant diseases (Schwarz et al. 2005, 2006), there is evidence that the radiological bone fill after decontamination of failing implants with the Er:YAG laser is not predictable,

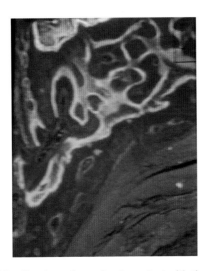

Figure 6.8 New bone formation in contact with the implant surface after CO_2 laser irradiation of the peri-implant defect. *Source:* Dr. H. Deppe, Munich, Germany.

especially when the peri-implant lesions are advanced (Schmage et al. 2012; Schwarz et al. 2012).

In contrast to that, the use of CO_2 laser for decontamination of peri-implant infrabony defects (before bone augmentation) seems to be a predictable method with a long-term success, also when these lesions are advanced (Romanos and Nentwig 2008; Romanos et al. 2009a, b).

Also, of significant importance is the improvement of corrosion resistance of laser-irradiated titanium surfaces due to surface melting and rutile (TiO_2) formation. Studies indicate that rutile particles are less bioreactive than titanium particles (wear-related debris from the implant surface) and, therefore, higher biocompatibility of titanium-based implants modified with an outer surface layer of rutile is expected (Vallés et al. 2006). This was also tested in human osteoblast cultures as well (Vallés et al. 2008), promoting this surface modification of implants due to the modulation of secretion of mediators associated with bone resorption, such as interleukin 6 (IL-6) and prostaglandin (PGE-2).

In contrast to the use of CO_2 lasers, pulsed Nd:YAG lasers were used to modify the surface of hydroxyapatite-coated dental implants and showed changes of the coating, alterations of the surface phase composition, as well as the morphology. These changes were not acceptable for biomedical applications. However, repetitive passes with the pulsed laser did not help to seal the cracks that formed (Cheang et al. 1996).

Clinical Cases

Uncovering of Two-Staged Implants

This case concerns a 72-year-old patient with three endosseous implants, which were exposed with the 445 nm (blue light) diode laser with initiated tip. The incision was carried out in the exact location of the placed implants (using as a guide the surgical guide) under topical anesthesia. Bleeding was not observed (Figure 6.9a). The healing was without complications, and after one week the clinical situation presented an excellent clinical condition (Figure 6.9b).

Uncovering of Two-Staged Implants

Similar to the above clinical case, a second stage surgery was performed using topical anesthesia to expose a submerged dental implant with platform switching (Figure 6.10a). The CO_2 laser with a noncon-tact defocused beam and ceramic tip was used with a power of 4W (Figure 6.10b). The cover screw was removed and a sulcus former was placed based on the manufacturer guidelines. The wound healing was uneventful and after one week the soft tissue was excellent (Figure 6.10c).

Excision of Peri-implant Gingival Hyperplasia

A patient's peri-implant gingival hyperplasia made oral hygiene difficult so that the long-term prognosis of the implants would have been affected (Figure 6.11a). The hyperplasic tissues were removed using the focused beam of the CO_2 laser and a power of 6W (continuous wave) for excision (Figure 6.11b) and sufficient coagulation in an ablative mode (Figure 6.11c). The clinical situation has significantly improved, and after a repeated laser-supported

(a)

(b)

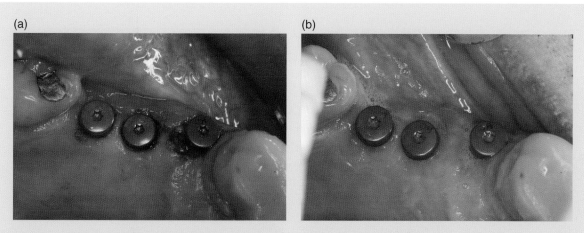

Figure 6.9 Soft tissue incision with a CO_2 laser for implant uncovering; an excellent hemostasis was provided (a); one week postoperatively, excellent wound healing after abutment connection (b). *Source:* Dr. Georgios E. Romanos.

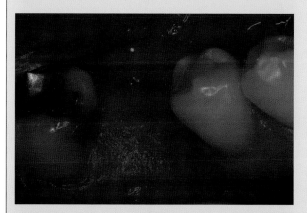

Figure 6.10a Clinical condition of a submerged implant system before uncovering. *Source:* Dr. Georgios E. Romanos

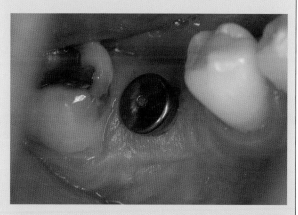

Figure 6.10c One week after implant uncovering presents an excellent peri-implant soft tissue condition. *Source:* Dr. Georgios E. Romanos.

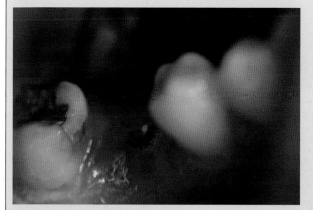

Figure 6.10b Second stage surgery with a focused beam of a CO_2 laser (4W, CW). *Source:* Dr. Georgios E. Romanos

gingivoplasty, the peri-implant mucosa was free of inflammation (Figure 6.11d). Plaque control was possible without any difficulties for the patient.

Soft Tissue Management Around Implants with the Pulsed Diode Laser

A 62-year-old patient with two endosseous implants in the lower jaw introduced himself to us before the making of a prosthetic bar-supported restoration. The peri-implant mucosa was free of inflammation, and a hyperplasic change of the soft tissue was seen (Figure 6.12a). The peri-implant proliferation was removed with the 980 nm diode laser (Ceralas® Biolitek AG, Bonn, Germany), and the entire soft tissue was reshaped to create a smooth surface. The surgical intervention was carried out under topical anesthesia after tip initiation and without bleeding (Figure 6.12b). The clinical situation after four weeks presented excellent healing, without complications, and hyperplasia was not clinically visible.

(a)
(b)
(c)
(d)

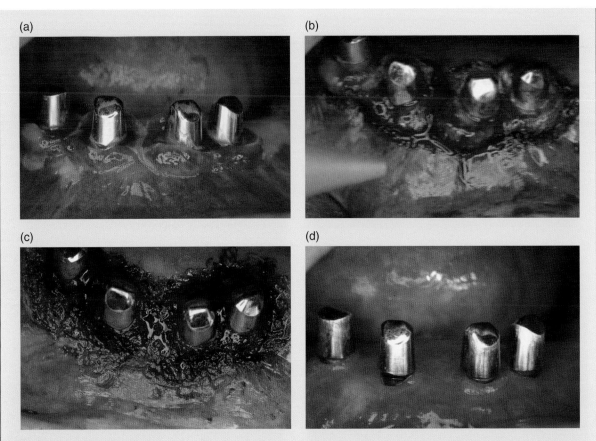

Figure 6.11 Peri-implant hyperplasia before surgery (a); using noncontact focused beam of the CO_2 laser (b); sufficient coagulation and superficial blood clot stabilization using a defocused beam (c); follow up after one year (d). *Source:* Dr. Georgios E. Romanos.

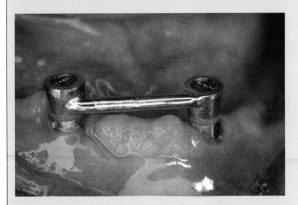

Figure 6.12a Peri-implant hyperplastic mucosa demonstrating difficulties in plaque control. *Source:* Dr. Georgios E. Romanos.

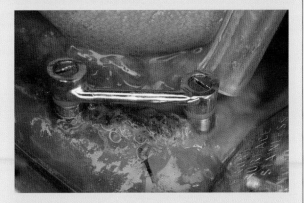

Figure 6.12b Removal of the peri-implant hyperplastic tissues with a 980 nm diode laser under topical anesthesia and fiber initiation. An excellent coagulation occurs in noncontact mode. *Source:* Dr. Georgios E. Romanos.

Soft Tissue Management Around Implants with the CO_2 Laser

A 68-year-old medically compromised patient with four endosseous implants in the mandible and a

bar-implant supported restoration presented hyperplastic tissue around the implants at the left mandibular side (Figure 6.13a).

The peri-implant soft tissues were removed after removal of the bar (Figure 6.13b) with the CO_2 laser in

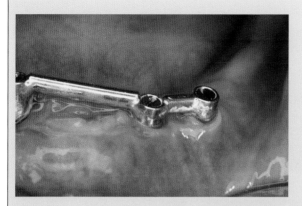

Figure 6.13a Peri-implant hyperplasia underneath a bar-retained implant supported prosthesis. *Source:* Dr. Georgios E. Romanos.

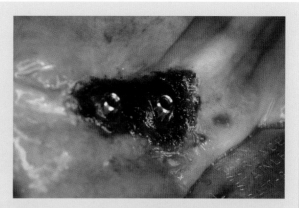

Figure 6.13c Excision and sufficient coagulation after CO_2 laser irradiation. *Source:* Dr. Georgios E. Romanos.

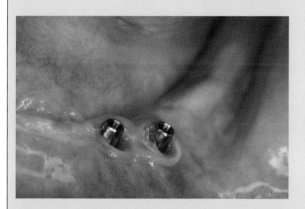

Figure 6.13b Hyperplastic tissues before laser excision after removal of the bar restoration. *Source:* Dr. Georgios E. Romanos.

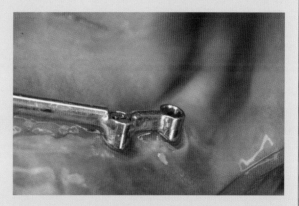

Figure 6.13d Two weeks postoperative clinical condition presents an improvement of the peri-implant tissues. *Source:* Dr. Georgios E. Romanos.

a focused beam and to coagulate in a defocused beam (Figure 6.13c). The soft tissues already demonstrated better condition two weeks later (Figure 6.13d).

Laser-Supported Treatment of Peri-implantitis

The treatment of the peri-implant lesions in the area #19–21 was performed after removal of the restoration (Figure 6.14a), periosteal flap elevation under local anesthesia, degranulation with curettes (Figure 6.14b), and decontamination with a pulsed mode CO_2 laser (4 W, non-contact). The blood clot was stabilized in the defects (Figure 6.14c) and was preserved during the bone augmentation with bovine mineral bone grafting material (Figure 6.14d). A collagen membrane covered the defects and was immobilized with titanium tags (Figure 6.14e). The flap was closed with conventional interrupted sutures. Wound healing

was uneventful, and new bone formation around the implants was shown after two years (Figure 6.14f). No other clinical findings were presented.

Peri-implantitis Treatment Before Functional Loading

The case presents peri-implantitis before delivery of the final prosthesis. The patient complained of acute pain and swelling in the mesial implant (#21 area). After irrigation with chlorhexidine solution to clean up the acute infection, a mucoperiosteal flap was elevated and the peri-implant bony defect was degranulated with curettes. The maximum depth of the infrabony defect was 12 mm. The decontamination with a CO_2 laser (4 W; pulsed mode) was performed, and the entire defect was irradiated in an ablative mode. Bone grafting with bovine mineral was finally

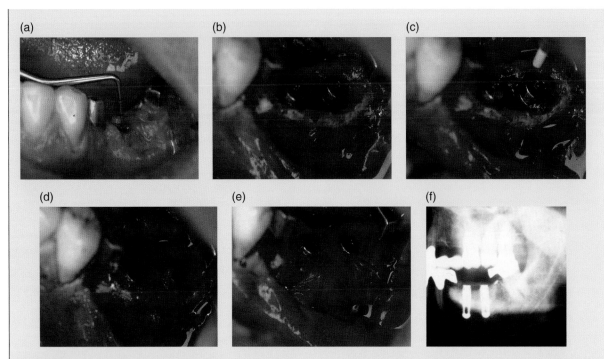

Figure 6.14 Peri-implant lesions in the area #19–21 after removal of the restoration (a); defect after degranulation with curettes (b); decontamination with a pulsed mode CO_2 laser (4W, noncontact) providing blood clot stabilization in the defects (c); bone augmentation with bovine mineral (d); collagen membrane coverage of the defect immobilized with titanium tacks (e); new bone fill, around implants after two years (f). *Source:* Dr. Georgios E. Romanos.

used to fill the defect, and a collagen membrane covered the augmented site. The healing was uneventful, and the clinical and radiological condition improved over the three-years of follow-up (Figure 6.15).

Peri-implantitis Treatment with Autogenous Bone Grafting Material

This case showed an advanced peri-implant bony defect with symptoms of peri-implantitis and no implant mobility. The patient was interested to maintain this implant and asked for surgical treatment. A flap elevation and a meticulous degranulation of the defect were initially performed. The decontamination of the defect was performed with a CO_2 laser (4W, pulsed mode, noncontact) and final bone augmentation with autogenous bone harvested from the chin region (particulate with a bone mill). Coverage of the augmentation site with a collagen membrane stabilized the particulate bone and condensed within the defect. The flap was closed with conventional sutures. The bone regeneration occurred in the next few months and showed an excellent crestal bone after four months when the implants were restored prosthetically (Figure 6.16).

Laser-Supported Treatment of Peri-implantitis

A 55-year-old patient was diagnosed with peri-implant inflammation (Figure 6.17a) associated with pain and suppuration and presented radiological findings of an advanced peri-implant osseous lesion (Figure 6.17b). The implant prosthesis was a screw-retained restoration, which was fabricated 10 years ago. The prosthesis and the abutment of the failing implant were removed. Under local anesthesia, a mucoperiosteal flap was elevated, the peri-implant granulation tissue was conventionally removed with plastic curettes (Figure 6.17c), and subsequently the implant surface and the surrounding bone were decontaminated with the CO_2 laser (average power: 4W, CW). The laser-assisted decontamination permitted a good hemostasis (Figure 6.17d). The osseous defect was filled with bovine mineral bone grafting material (Figure 6.17e) and covered with an absorbable collagen membrane, based on the principles of guided bone regeneration (GBR) for submerged healing (Figure 6.17f). After four months the implant was uncovered, the previous abutment was placed in the same position, and the older prosthesis was delivered. Healing succeeded with no complications, and after four months the clinical situation (as well as

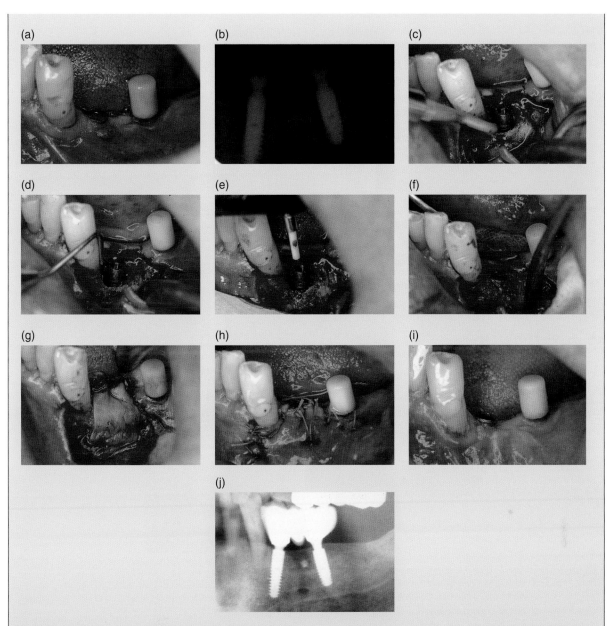

Figure 6.15 Peri-implantitis diagnosed immediately before delivery of the final prosthesis associated with pain and suppuration (a, b); scaling of the defect with plastic curette (c) and measurement intraoperatively with a periodontal probe showing a depth of 12 mm (d); decontamination with a CO_2 laser (e); bone grafting with a bovine mineral (f); collagen membrane covered the augmented site (g); flap closure (h); uneventful healing after three months (i); radiological condition presenting bone fill after three years (j). *Source:* Dr. Georgios E. Romanos.

the radiological examination) showed excellent peri-implant conditions. The clinical situation was stable for four years (Figure 6.17g and h). However, 13 years later the patient decided to replace the bridge for esthetic reasons and mesial migration of the anterior teeth. The peri-implant condition showed after 21 years stability of the peri-implant bone, proof of the long-term success of the peri-implantitis treatment concept (Figure 6.17i, j, k).

Peri-implantitis Treatment with a Diode Laser

This clinical case presents a female patient with endosseous dental implants placed almost four years ago and loaded with a fixed prosthesis (Figure 6.18a). The patient complained about subacute pain, especially during toothbrushing. The clinical examination showed bleeding on probing and suppuration in conjunction with peri-implant intrabony defects at #19–20 (Figure 6.18b). After

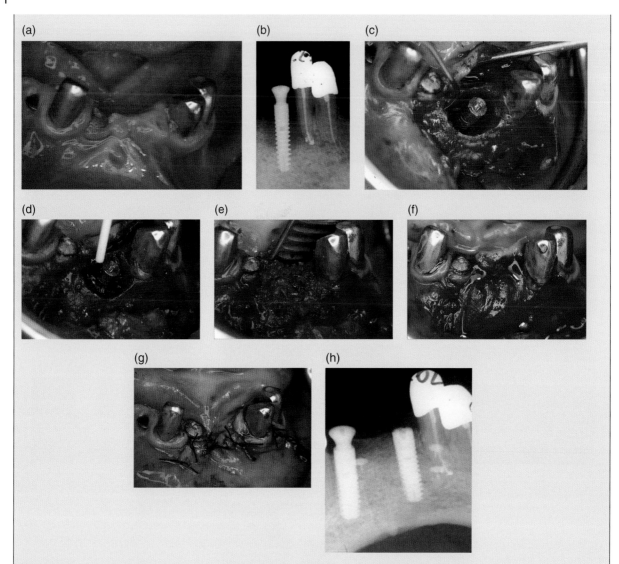

Figure 6.16 Advanced peri-implant bony defect with symptoms of peri-implantitis and no implant mobility (a, b); after flap elevation and meticulous degranulation of the defect (c); decontamination of the defect with a CO_2 laser (d); bone augmentation with autogenous particulate bone (e); coverage of the augmentation site with a collagen membrane (f); flap closure (g); excellent bone crest after four months (h). *Source:* Dr. Georgios E. Romanos.

local anesthesia and mucoperiosteal flap elevation with meticulous degranulation of the peri-implant defects (Figure 6.18c), a 980 nm diode laser with a 300 μm glass fiber was used, in a noncontact mode and 2 W power settings for a 3 × 20 seconds irradiation period. The fiber was activated with an initiator, a red-colored occlusal paper (Figure 6.18d).

Autogenous, particulate bone grafting material was used (patient decision) to fill the defects (Figure 6.18e), and a collagen membrane was applied and fixated with titanium tacks (Figure 6.18f). The flap was closed with interrupted silk sutures. The sutures were removed after one week. Healing was uneventful, and after one year the clinical and radiological evaluation (Figure 6.18g, h) showed a significant increase of the bone fill around the failing implants and no clinical symptoms of inflammation.

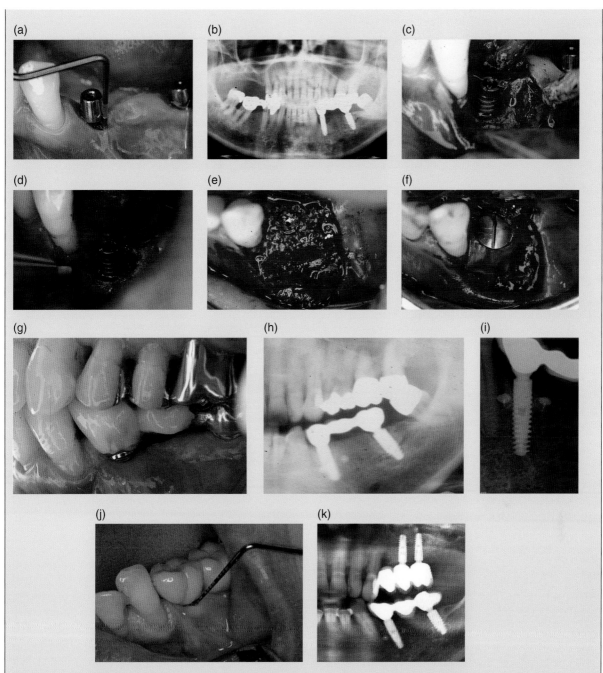

Figure 6.17 Peri-implant bone loss associated with pain and suppuration (a); radiological findings of an advanced peri-implant osseous lesion (b); demonstration of the defect after degranulation (c); decontamination with the CO_2 laser (d); bovine mineral bone grafting material (e) and coverage with a collagen membrane (f); clinical and radiographic evaluation after four years (g, h); the peri-implant condition showed after 21 years stability of the peri-implant bone without periodontal pocket (i, j, k). *Source:* Dr. Georgios E. Romanos.

Peri-implantitis Treatment Associated with Postoperative Complications

This clinical case presents an advanced peri-implant bony defect around the splinted implants #13 and 14. The implant prognosis was "questionable" to "hope-less"; the crowns were cemented with permanent cement material, and the probing pocket depth measurements were between 8 and 15 mm (Figure 6.19a, b). The removal of the implants as an alternative treatment was considered, but in order to avoid the

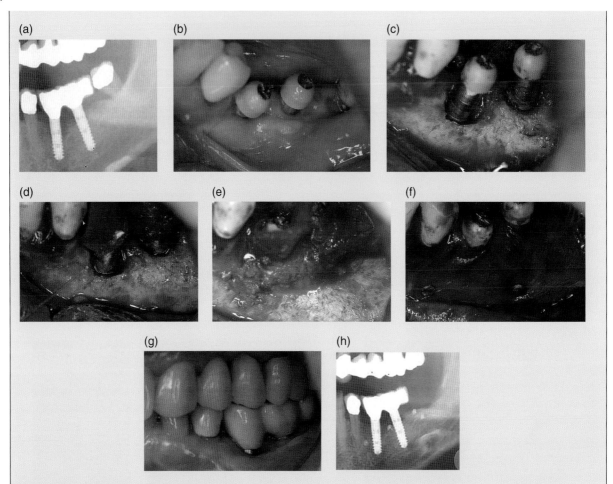

Figure 6.18 Peri-implant infrabony defects at #19–20 (a, b); meticulous degranulation of the peri-implant defects (c); a 980 nm diode laser was used to irradiate the defects (d); autogenous, particulate bone grafting material was used to fill the defects (e); a collagen membrane was fixated around the augmentation area (f); clinical and radiological evaluation (g); bone fill around the failing implants one year after grafting (h). *Source:* Dr. Georgios E. Romanos.

oro-antral communication in the #14 (after implant removal), the treatment plan was modified. The main goal was to treat the peri-implant lesions with meticulous degranulation (Figure 6.19c, d, e), decontamination of the implant surfaces, and bone augmentation. A diode laser with a wavelength of 810 nm was used (2 W, pulsed mode) for this purpose (Figure 6.19f). Due to the size of the defects, the irradiation period was relatively long but not calculated. After decontamination, the lesions were augmented using a composite graft with autogenous bone (harvested from the tuberosity, distal of #16) and bovine mineral grafting material (BioOss®, Geistlich, Wolhusen, Switzerland) (Figure 6.19g). A collagen membrane (Biomed Extend®,

Zimmer, Carlsbad, CA) was applied over the grafted sites around the implant margins of the prostheses very carefully in order to condense the grafting material over the implant surfaces. The membrane was fixated with titanium tacks (Salvin Dental Specialties Inc., Charlotte, NC) (Figure 6.19h). The mucoperiosteal flap was advanced coronally and was secured in place with 4-0 silk interrupted sutures. Postoperative instructions were given and healing was uneventful for the next 2–3 months. The patient came back after five months of healing for clinical and radiological reevaluation. The clinical condition was excellent. A healthy tissue surrounded both implants. Unfortunately, the radiological examination presented

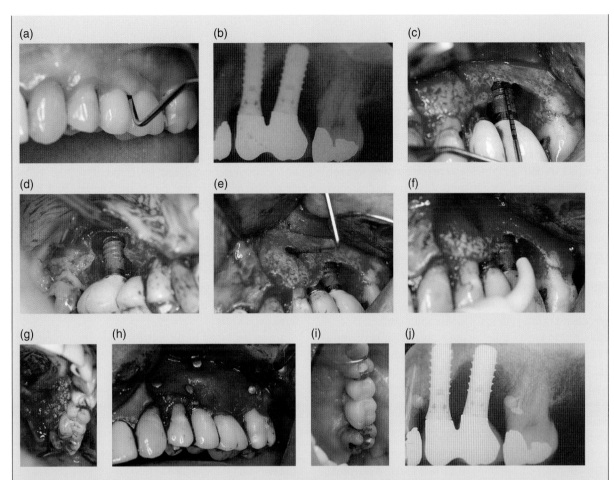

Figure 6.19 Advanced peri-implant bony defect around splinted implants #13 and 14 (a, b); defect morphology after meticulous degranulation (c, d, e); decontamination of the implant surfaces with a diode laser with a wavelength of 810 nm (f); augmentation using a composite graft with autogenous bone and bovine mineral (g); collagen membrane over the grafted sites and fixation with titanium tacks (h); clinical and reevaluation five months of healing presented good soft tissue morphology (i); radiological examination presented a bone radiolucency and insufficient bone fill (j). *Source:* Dr. Georgios E. Romanos.

a bone radiolucency and insufficient bone fill. The patient had not complained, but the unsuccessful result was the primary goal for further investigation.

The results of this analysis were studied and published later (Geminiani et al. 2011; Leja et al. 2013; Romanos et al. 2019).

6.5 Recent Laser Research on Implants

An in vitro model comparative to a clinical presentation of peri-implantitis was created via placement of a 3.5×11 mm titanium alloy dental implant into artificial type II bovine bone, and an irregular 3×5 mm osseous segment was removed to create an infrabony defect. Diode laser systems of varying wavelengths (810, 940, 975, and 980 nm) were subjected to different initiator pigments (uninitiated, blue, red, and cork) and beam types (continuous wave or pulsed mode) prior to surface irradiation. Axial implant surfaces were debrided at 1 W or 2 W mean power for 15 trials/group that were 30-seconds in duration. Implant surface temperature was monitored via apical and coronal thermocouple devices over these irradiation periods.

The results showed that the critical biologic thermal safety threshold for osseous necrosis ($\Delta + 10\,°C$) was commonly surpassed in continuous wave trials regardless of initiator or power condition. Initiated fibers achieved significantly faster changes in temperature than noninitiated fibers. Coronal implant surfaces demonstrated significantly greater temperature increases than that of apical portions, with no apical readings surpassing the critical biologic thermal safety threshold. Different initiating pigments were preferred to best control thermal climb for different wavelength diode systems. Therefore, the mean power settings for implant surface debridement should be less than manufacture recommendations to minimize risks of overheating and consequential implant failure.

Utilization of pulsed modes and wavelength-specific initiators are necessary for thermal protection of implant titanium alloy surfaces and supporting bony structures during clinical decontamination.

Recent in vitro studies in our research lab have evaluated temperature changes during irradiation of the implant with a peri-implant defect (peri-implantitis) and showed that the defect morphology is important. Specifically, five separate defects (circumferential, one-walled, two-walled, three-walled, or horizontal defect) were created around dental implants that were placed into a synthetic (bovine) bone analog that mimics type II quality bone. Each implant surface and the surrounding bone were irradiated by a noncontact CO_2 laser (2 W power in continuous and pulsed mode, defocused beam) for 30 and 60 seconds. Apical and coronal thermocouples placed in contact with implants were used to evaluate ΔT at 30 and 60 seconds. Statistical comparison was performed using statistical software.

The most substantial pulse setting–induced temperature differences (30s) of the apical thermocouple were observed in the two- and three-wall defect. This was also seen at the 60s irradiation period. Similar temperature changes were not observed at the apical thermocouple of the circumferential, one-wall, and horizontal defects using the pulse setting. ΔT at the coronal part of the implant during pulsed laser irradiation recorded less than 10 °C. In contrast, the continuous mode was associated with ΔT over 10 °C for circumferential, three-walled, and two-walled defects during 30 seconds of irradiation and over the critical threshold within 60 seconds of irradiation. In the apical area, the continuous mode created ΔT over 10 °C in the three-wall or circumferential defects.

According to the results of this study, the morphology of the peri-implant defect appears to affect the resultant heat dissemination of CO_2 laser irradiation on an implant. The architecture of the peri-implant defect should influence the protocol with the CO_2 laser treatment modality. Pulsed mode setting is ideal for all laser-assisted peri-implant decontamination (Romanos and Rexha 2019). However, it is important to consider that circumferential and two- and three-walled defects may have a greater risk for heat-induced implant failure, and therefore irradiation should be kept within 30 sec-bursts (Figures 6.20–6.23).

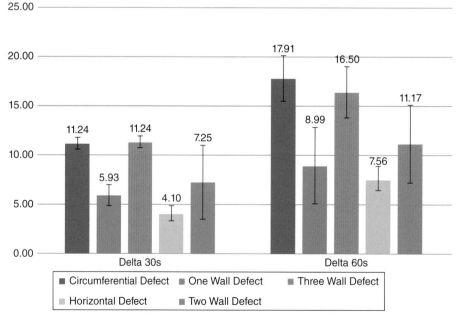

Figure 6.20 Bar chart of means of coronal (continuous) by group over time.

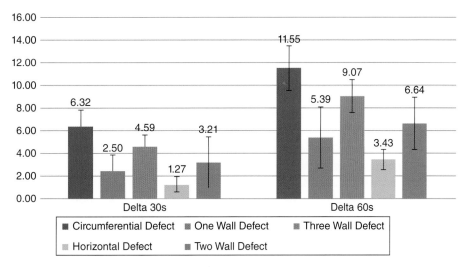

Figure 6.21 Bar chart of means of apical (continuous) by group over time.

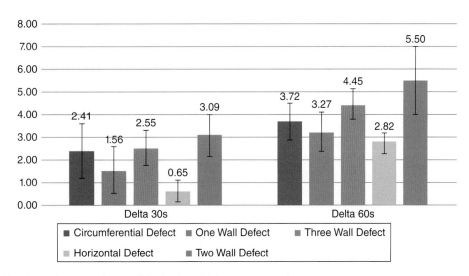

Figure 6.22 Bar chart of means of coronal (pulsed mode) by group over time.

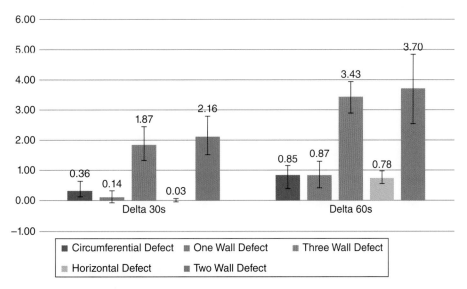

Figure 6.23 Bar chart of means of apical (pulsed mode) by group over time.

Using a similar protocol, implants and the surrounding bone were irradiated by a noncontact Er,Cr:YSGG laser (2 W power; free-running pulsed) for 30 and 60 seconds. Although none of the defects resulted in a temperature change greater than the 10 °C threshold, circumferential and two- and three-walled defects may have a greater risk for overheating using the Er,Cr:YSGG laser (Rexha et al. 2019).

The impact of initiators in the use of diode lasers (940, 975, and 980 nm) for treatment of peri-implantitis was also evaluated in vitro (Romanos et al. 2019).

In our lab, a 940 nm diode laser (EPIC 10, Biolase, Irvine, CA, USA), a 975 nm diode laser (Alta, Walpole, MA, USA), and a 980 nm diode laser (KaVo, GENTLEray, Biberach, Germany) were used. The pulse widths for the 940, 975, and 980 nm were 20, 25, and 25 ms, respectively.

Specifically, unlike the 980 nm diode laser, the average temperature increase and the amount of time (in seconds) that it took to yield the critical temperature threshold of 10 °C was not statistically significant ($p > 0.05$) at the coronal level for the 940 and 975 nm diode lasers (Figure 6.24).

For the 980 nm diode laser, the blue-initiated tip had the highest temperature increase (22.4 °C), followed by the cork (18.8 °C) and the noninitiated tip (17.3 °C) in the coronal area (Figures 6.25 and 6.26).

The average temperature change at the apical level (t = 30 seconds) were observed in Figure 6.25.

The critical threshold at the coronal portion for the 980 nm laser was reached in 11.5, 8.79, and 6.46 seconds for the blue paper, cork, and noninitiated tips, respectively (Figure 6.26).

In comparison with the 940 nm diode laser, both the 975 and 980 nm diode lasers had average temperature increases that were not statistically significant ($p > 0.05$) among the blue paper, cork, and noninitiated tips at the apical level.

Within the limitations of the study, NIR diode laser-initiated tips may overheat the coronal portion of an implant at a faster rate and to a larger extent than noninitiated tips. This should be considered, because initiated tips may pose greater risks when used near titanium implant surfaces, such as inducing necrosis of the surrounding bone and eventual implant failure. However, they have minimal risks at the apical portion of the implant.

Splinted implants with a fixed restoration are under risk if irradiation parameters do not follow the acceptable limits since irradiation on one implant with a peri-implant bony defect can transfer heat to the other implant. This phenomenon occurs due to the material conductivity and must be taken into consideration during laser therapy in association with metals (Figures 6.28 and 6.29) (Romanos et al. 2020, in press).

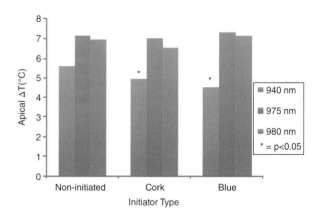

Figure 6.25 Average temperature change at the apical level (t = 30 seconds).

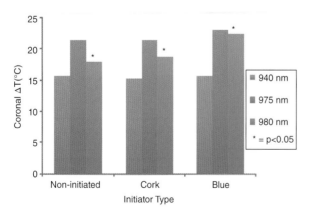

Figure 6.24 Average temperature change at the coronal level (t = 30 seconds).

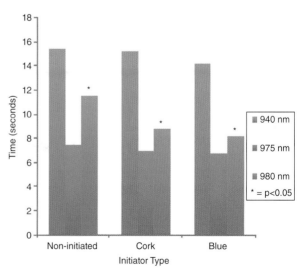

Figure 6.26 Average time to reach critical threshold (Δ10°C) in the coronal area.

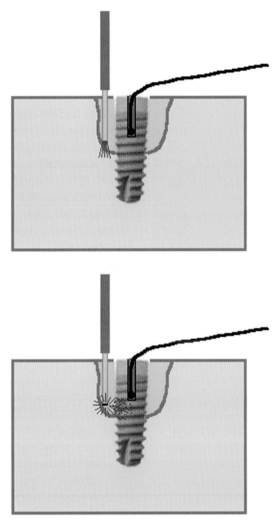

Figure 6.27 Measurement of heat transfer using noninitiated (a) and initiated tips (b) of diode lasers. The initiated tips are associated with higher heat transfer to the implant body.

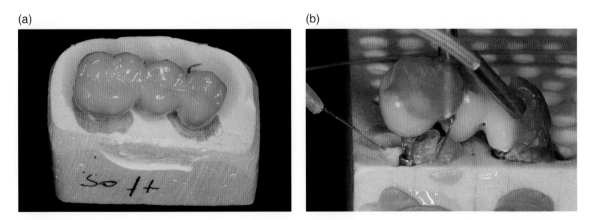

Figure 6.28 Experimental setting to evaluate temperature changes of implants splinted with a fixed implant-supported restoration (a). Irradiation of a peri-implant defect using a diode laser and real time measurement of temperature changes at the irradiation area and the distant implant (coronal and apical sites). The four thermocouples were placed in proper locations (b). *Source:* Dr. Georgios E. Romanos.

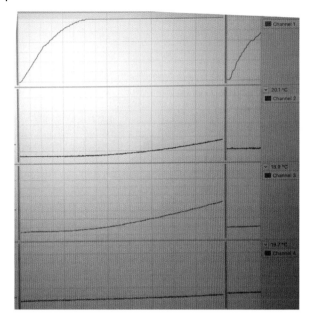

Figure 6.29 Temperature increase during laser irradiation of an implant with peri-implant defect using 2 W power (980 nm diode laser without initiated tip) at the coronal placed thermocouple (channel 1), and at the second distant, "healthy"-implants (splinted with a cemented metalo-ceramic three-unit bridge having a coronal placed thermocouple (channel 3). Channels 2 and 4 demonstrate the temperature changes in the apical area of the implant with the defect and the distant "healthy" implant, respectively. The irradiation period was for 60 seconds. *Source:* Dr. Georgios E. Romanos.

6.6 Implant Removal

Implants placed in prosthetically wrong positions after healing (osseointegration) can be removed with trephines, piezosurgery, or also lasers (see also Chapter 4). The piezosurgery and the laser-assisted surgical removal seem to be more minimally invasive since the osteotomy can be controlled, and it is not necessary to completely remove the bone around an implant (during implant retrieval) (Figure 6.30). There are no data today presenting the laser-assisted implant removal technique, but the Er:YAG laser and the Er,Cr:YSGG lasers are the main laser wavelengths which can be used for this clinical indication (see also Chapter 6). Initial case reports show successful implant removal without complications (Smith and Rose 2010).

6.7 Laser-Assisted Implant Placement

An implant can be placed using a laser-assisted technique with the Er:YAG or the Er,Cr:YSGG laser. Unfortunately, there are not many clinical case series or studies providing histological evidence about this protocol, but pilot data in the rat tibia showed that implant placement with the use of an Er:YAG laser (energy per pulse: 500–1000 mJ; pulse duration: 400 ms; frequency: 10 pps, energy density: 32 J/cm^2) improves significantly the bone-to-implant contact (BIC) percentages compared to the conventional method (Kesler et al. 2006). Specifically, after three weeks of healing the BIC in the laser group was 59.48% vs. 12.85% for the control group. After three months of healing, the laser group showed 73.54% BIC and the control group was 32.65%. These differences were statistically significant (p < 0.001).

Also, it has been proven that the osteotomy for implant placement is associated with platelet-derived growth factor (PDGF) expression in the initial healing stages (Kesler et al. 2011). Maximum power of 8 W, energy per pulse of 700 mJ, and frequency up to 50 Hz was used. The laser was used with external water irrigation, a spot size of 2 mm, energy per pulse of 500–1000 mJ/pulse, and energy density of 32 J/cm^2.

In case of soft tissue incision for implant placement, the Er,Cr:YSGG laser (Waterlase® MD, Biolase Technology Inc., San Clemente, CA, USA) has been used with a light water spray and the parameters of 4 J/cm^2 soft tissue (S) mode, pulsed with a duration of 700 µs and repetition rate of 30 Hz with the MT4 tip. For the osteotomy, the used parameters were: 6 J/cm^2 hard tissue mode (H), (pulsed mode) with a duration of 140 µs and repetition rate of 20 Hz with the MG6 tip (Sohn et al. 2009).

Clinical case series are important to establish this protocol in clinical dentistry. Histological evaluation and multicenter studies are necessary before routine implant placement with the laser beam.

In conclusion, based on the recent literature, the use of lasers appears promising in implant dentistry when correct laser wavelength and power settings for soft and hard tissue are being applied. There is no doubt that extensive knowledge of laser physics in association with laser-tissue interactions and training should be a prerequisite before lasers are used in daily practice. With this knowledge about laser wavelengths, the lasers may be used to treat peri-implantitis, to manage peri-implant inflammatory reactions leading to progressive bone loss with implant failures, and possibly to improve osseointegration.

6.8 Future of Laser Dentistry in Oral Implantology

Recent scientific reports show the potential of laser application for fabrication of dental implants using 3D printing. This interesting technology using the Yb:YAG

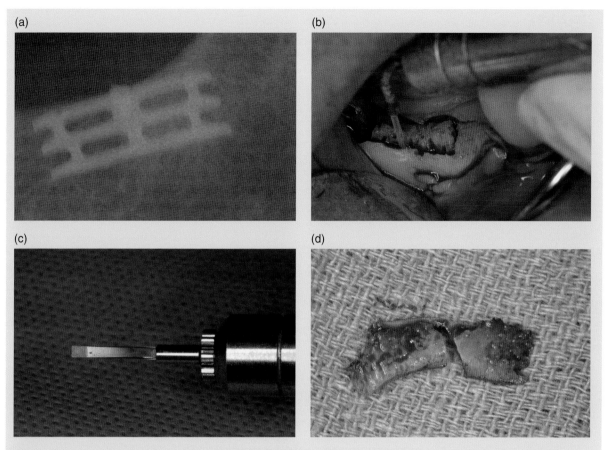

Figure 6.30 Ossseointegrated blade implant removal using an Er:YAG laser (Versawave, Hoya, Tokyo, Japan) (a, b) with a glass tip (c) and 400 mJ pulse energy and frequency of 15 Hz under cooling. The specimen (d) presents good osteotomy quality without complete coagulation. *Source:* Dr. Georgios E. Romanos.

fiber laser (1075 nm) with a maximum output power of 400 W for laser beam melting (LBM) 3D printing may reduce the costs for dental implants and enhance the possibilities of implant dentistry worldwide. Dental implant prototypes (Ti_6Al_4V) with different porous sizes (200, 350, and 500 μm) were used, and cell proliferation tests were performed to demonstrate the biocompatibility of these surfaces. The joint project between Fudan University (Shanghai, China) and the Institute of Photonic Technologies (Erlangen, Germany) concluded that under these circumstances a surface with a porosity of 350 μm provided an optimal potential for improving the mechanical properties of these Ti-alloys. Without doubt, laser technology may be also used for surface modification and other areas in implant dentistry to develop and optimize the clinical outcome (Yang et al. 2017).

In addition, understanding potential risks of metal overheating during irradiation is fundamental to avoid complications of implant integration, and therefore real-time assessment of temperature changes is significant (Montanaro and Romanos 2019). Future technology should be involved to measure these real-time temperature changes.

References

Adell, R., Lekholm, U., Rockier, B., and Branemark, P.I. (1981). A 15-year study of osseointegrated implants in the treatment of the edentulous jaw. *Int. J. Oral Surg.* 10: 387–416.

Adell, R., Lekholm, U., Rockier, B. et al. (1986). Marginal tissue reaction at osseointegrated titanium fixtures (I). A 3-year longitudinal prospective study. *Int. J. Oral Maxillofac. Surg.* 15: 39–52.

Albrektsson, T., Buser, D., Chen, S.T. et al. (2012a). Statements from the Estepona consensus meeting on peri-implantitis, February 2-4, 2012. *Clin. Implant. Dent. Relat. Res.* 14 (6): 781–782.

Albrektsson, T., Buser, D., and Sennerby, L. (2012b). Crestal bone loss and oral implants. *Clin. Implant. Dent. Relat. Res.* 14 (6): 783–791.

Arnabat-Domínguez, J., España-Tost, A.J., Berini-Aytés, L., and Gay-Escoda, C. (2003). Erbium:YAG laser application in the second phase of implant surgery: a pilot study in 20 patients. *Int. J. Oral Maxillofac. Implants* 18 (1): 104–112.

Arnabat-Domínguez, J., Bragado-Novel, M., España-Tost, A.J. et al. (2010). Advantages and esthetic results of erbium, chromium:yttrium-scandium-gallium-garnet laser application in second-stage implant surgery in patients with insufficient gingival attachment: a report of three cases. *Lasers Med. Sci.* 25 (3): 459–464.

Block, C.M., Mayo, J.A., and Evans, J.A. (1992). Effects of the Nd:YAG dental laser on plasma-sprayed and hydroxyapatite-coated titanium dental implants: surface alteration and attempted sterilization. *Int. J. Oral Maxillofac. Implants* 7: 441–449.

Catone, G.A. (1997). Lasers in periodontal surgery. In: *Laser Applications in Oral and Maxillofacial Surgery* (eds. G.A. Catone and C.C. Alling), 181–196. Philadelphia: Saunders.

Cheang, P., Khor, K.A., Teoh, L.L., and Tam, S.C. (1996). Pulsed laser treatment of plasma-sprayed hydroxyapatite coatings. *Biomaterials* 17 (19): 1901–1904.

Deppe, H., Horch, H.H., Hiemer, T. et al. (1998). Zur Wirkung von CO_2-Laserstrahlen an TPS-lmplantaten. *Z. Zahnaerztl. Implantol.* 14: 91–95. (German).

Engquist, B., Bergendal, T., Kallus, T., and Linden, U. (1988). A retrospective multicenter evaluation of osseointegrated implants supporting overdentures. *Int. J. Oral Maxillofac. Implants* 3: 129–134.

Ganz, C.H. (1994). Evaluation of the safety of the carbon dioxide laser used in conjunction with root form implants: a pilot study. *J. Prosthet. Dent.* 71: 27–30.

Geminiani, A., Caton, J.G., and Romanos, G.E. (2011). Temperature increase during CO_2 and Er: YAG irradiation on implant surfaces. *Implant. Dent.* 20 (5): 379–382.

Geminiani, A., Caton, J., and Romanos, G.E. (2012). Temperature change during non-contact diode laser irradiation of implant surfaces. *Lasers Med. Sci.* 27 (2): 339–342.

Hartmann, H.J. and Bach, G. (1997). Diodenlaser-Oberflaechen Dekontamination in der Periimplantitistherapie. Eine Drei-Jahres-Studie. *ZWR* 106: 524–526. (German).

Kesler, G., Romanos, G., and Koren, R. (2006). Use of Er:YAG laser to improve osseointegration of titanium alloy implants-a comparison of bone healing. *Int. J. Oral Maxillofac. Implants* 21 (3): 375–379.

Kesler, G., Shvero, D.K., Tov, Y.S., and Romanos, G. (2011). Platelet-derived growth factor secretion and bone healing after Er:YAG laser bone irradiation. *J. Oral Implantol.* 37 Spec. No:195-204.

Kreisler, M., Götz, H., and Duschner, H. (2002). Effect of Nd:YAG, Ho:YAG, Er:YAG, CO_2, and GaAIAs laser irradiation on surface properties of endosseous dental implants. *Int. J. Oral Maxillofac. Implants* 17 (2): 202–211.

Leja, C., Geminiani, A., Caton, J.G., and Romanos, G.E. (2013). Thermodynamic effects of laser irradiation of implants placed in bone: an in vitro study. *Lasers Med. Sci.* 28: 1435–1440.

Lekholm, U., Adell, R., Lindhe, J. et al. (1986). Marginal tissue reactions at osseointegrated titanium fixtures (II). A cross-sectional retrospective study. *Int. J. Oral Maxillofac. Surg.* 15: 53–61.

Montanaro, N., Romanos, G.E. Optimization of thermal protocols during diode irradiation of dental implants. International Laser Safety Conference of Laser Institute of America, Kissimmee, FL, 2019.

Park, J.H., Heo, S.J., Koak, J.Y. et al. (2012). Effects of laser irradiation on machined and anodized titanium disks. *Int. J. Oral Maxillofac. Implants* 27 (2): 265–272.

Purucker, P., Romanos, G.E., Bernimouin, J.P., and Nentwig, G.H. (1998). Effect of CO_2-laser irradiation on the viability of two pathogenic bacteria covering titanium implants. *J. Dent. Res.* 77: 967, Abstr. No. 2681.

Rexha, E., Hou, W., Zhang, Y., Romanos, G.E. Peri-implant defect morphology and temperature changes during Er,Cr:YSGG-laser decontamination. IADR, Washington DC, March 2020, Abstr. No. 1425.

Romanos, G.E. and Nentwig, G.H. (2008). Regenerative therapy of deep peri-implant infrabony defects after CO_2 laser implant surface decontamination. *Int J Periodontics Restorative Dent* 28 (3): 245–255.

Romanos, G.E., Rexha, E. The safety implications of peri-implant defect morphology on temperature changes during CO_2 laser decontamination. International Laser Safety Conference of Laser Institute of America, Kissimmee, FL, 2019.

Romanos, G.E., Everts, H., and Nentwig, G.H. (2000). Effects of diode and Nd:YAG laser irradiation on titanium discs: a scanning electron microscope examination. *J. Periodontol.* 71 (5): 810–815.

Romanos, G.E., Gutknecht, N., Dieter, S. et al. (2009a). Laser wavelengths and oral Implantology. *Lasers Med. Sci.* 24 (6): 961–970.

Romanos, G.E., Ko, H., Froum, S., and Tarnow, D. (2009b). The use of CO_2 laser in the treatment of periimplantitis. *Photomed. Laser Surg.* 27 (3): 381–386.

Romanos, G.E., Gupta, B., Yunker, M. et al. (2013). Lasers use in dental implantology. *Implant. Dent.* 22 (3): 282–288.

Romanos, G.E., Motwani, S.V., Montanaro, N.J. et al. (2019). Photothermal effects of defocused initiated vs. non-initiated diode implant irradiation. *Photomed. Laser Surg.* 37 (6): 356–361.

Romanos, G.E., Davis R.J, Gallagher, B., Hou, W., Delgado-Ruiz, R. Thermal transfer on splinted implants during diodelaser irradiation in-vitro. *Photomedicine and Laser Surg* 2020 (in press).

Schmage, P., Thielemann, J., Nergiz, I. et al. (2012). Effects of 10 cleaning instruments on four different implant surfaces. *Int. J. Oral Maxillofac. Implants* 27 (2): 308–317.

Schwarz, F., Sculean, A., Rothamel, D. et al. (2005). Clinical evaluation of an Er:YAG laser for nonsurgical treatment of peri-implantitis: a pilot study. *Clin. Oral Implants Res.* 16 (1): 44–52.

Schwarz, F., Jepsen, S., Herten, M. et al. (2006). Influence of different treatment approaches on non-submerged and submerged healing of ligature induced peri-implantitis lesions: an experimental study in dogs. *J. Clin. Periodontol.* 33 (8): 584–595.

Schwarz, F., John, G., Mainusch, S. et al. (2012). Combined surgical therapy of peri-implantitis evaluating two methods of surface debridement and decontamination. A two-year clinical follow up report. *J. Clin. Periodontol.* 39 (8): 789–797.

Smith, L.P. and Rose, T. (2010). Laser explantation of a failing endosseous dental implant. *Aust. Dent. J.* 55 (2): 219–222.

Sohn, D.S., Lee, J.S., An, K.M., and Romanos, G.E. (2009). Erbium,chromium:yttrium-scandium-gallium-garnet laser-assisted sinus graft procedure. *Lasers Med. Sci.* 24 (4): 673–677.

Vallés, G., González-Melendi, P., González-Carrasco, J.L. et al. (2006). Differential inflammatory macrophage response to rutile and titanium particles. *Biomaterials* 27 (30): 5199–5211.

Vallés, G., González-Melendi, P., Saldaña, L. et al. (2008). Rutile and titanium particles differentially affect the production of osteoblastic local factors. *J. Biomed. Mater. Res. A* 84 (2): 324–336.

Yang, F., Chen, C., Zhou, Q.R. et al. (2017). Laser beam printing of Ti_6Al4_V based porous structured dental implants: fabrication, biocompatibility analysis and photoelastic study. *Sci. Rep.* 7: 45360. https://doi.org/10.1038/srep45360.

Zitzmann, N.U. and Berglundh, T. (2008). Definition and prevalence of peri-implant diseases. *J. Clin. Periodontol.* 35 (8 Suppl): 286–291.

7

Photodynamic Therapy in Periodontal and Peri-Implant Treatment

Anton Sculean[1] and Georgios E. Romanos[2]

[1] *School of Dental Medicine, University of Bern, Bern, Switzerland*
[2] *School of Dental Medicine, Stony Brook University, Stony Brook, NY, USA*

7.1 Biological Rationale

Periodontitis is a bacterial biofilm–caused oral disease associated with loss of the supporting tissues (i.e. periodontal ligament and alveolar bone) around the tooth (Page and Kornman 1997). Therefore, the main objective of periodontal therapy is the removal/destruction of the supra- and subgingival biofilm from the root surface to stop or slow down disease progression (Cobb 1996). A plethora of studies have provided evidence for the clinical efficacy of nonsurgical periodontal treatment, and therefore, it is considered to be the key part of cause-related periodontal therapy and maintenance (Badersten et al. 1981; 1984; Lindhe et al. 1984).

Nonsurgical periodontal treatment is usually performed by means of power-driven instruments, curettes, or a combination thereof and, in the great majority of cases, is sufficient to reestablish periodontal health. However, under certain clinical circumstances, such as persistent deep periodontal pockets with or without infrabony defects or pockets located in the furcation area of multirooted teeth, nonsurgical subgingival instrumentation may not be sufficiently effective to adequately eliminate/disrupt the subgingival bacterial biofilm and calculus (Drisko 1998; Adriaens and Adriaens 2004; Umeda et al. 2004). At these sites, mechanical debridement alone is insufficient to eliminate some "key note" pathogens, such as *Aggregatibacter actinomycetemcomitans (A.a.)* (Rudney et al. 2001) and/or *Porphyromonas gingivalis (P.g.)* (Bostanci and Belibasakis 2012), which have been shown to possess the ability to penetrate in the surrounding soft tissues. In such complex clinical situations, in order to optimize the clinical outcomes, topical or systemic antibiotics may be used (Bonito et al. 2006; Keestra et al. 2015a, b).

However, although antibiotics have been shown to be efficient in reducing or eliminating periodontal pathogens, their use may be associated with a number of side effects, including skin rash, itching, oral candidiasis, or gastrointestinal problems such and nausea or vomiting (Gillies et al. 2015) and may comport the risk to increase bacterial resistance, a growing public health issue with substantial economic and social consequences (Rams et al. 2014; Olsen 2015). Thus, there is an obvious need for developing new treatment alternatives with fewer side effects, but with the potential to effectively reduce or eliminate bacterial biofilms (Grzech-Lesniak 2017).

Photodynamic therapy (PDT), also termed photoradiation therapy, phototherapy, photochemotherapy, photo-activated disinfection (PAD), or light-activated disinfection (LAD), was introduced in medical therapy in 1904 as the light-induced inactivation of cells, microorganisms, or molecules and involves the combination of visible light, usually through the use of a diode laser and a photosensitizer (von Tappeiner 1904).

The photosensitizer is a substance that is capable of absorbing light of a specific wavelength and transform it into useful energy. When used alone, neither of the two components (i.e. photosensitizer and light) is harmful. However, when combined they can lead to the production of lethal cytotoxic substances which can selectively destroy bacteria or cells (Sharman et al. 1999). Therefore, PDT has been proposed as a modality to reduce bacterial load or even to eliminate periodontal pathogens (Wilson et al. 1992; Pfitzner et al. 2004).

Most frequently, diode lasers of a wavelength between 635 and 670 nm are used, although in some studies also wavelengths of 808 nm (Dilsiz et al. 2013) and 940 nm have been also tested (Lui et al. 2011).

Advanced Laser Surgery in Dentistry, First Edition. Georgios E. Romanos.
© 2021 John Wiley & Sons, Inc. Published 2021 by John Wiley & Sons, Inc.

The most commonly used photosensitizers in the treatment of periodontal and peri-implant therapy infections are methylene blue (MB) and toluidine blue (TB) (Romanos and Brink 2010; Noro Filho et al. 2012; Bassir et al. 2013; Javed and Romanos 2013; Schär et al. 2013). The two substances have similar chemical and physicochemical characteristics and have been demonstrated to be effective against both Gram-positive and Gram-negative bacteria (Kikuchi et al. 2015; Olsen et al. 2017).

Ideally, following its application, the photosensitizer should remain for a period of 1–5 minutes in the periodontal and peri-implant pockets followed by irradiation with wavelengths between 630 and 660 nm, respectively (Chan and Lai 2003; Kikuchi et al. 2015).

On the other hand, when green-colored photosensitizers such as indocyanine green are used, the irradiation wavelength is 805 nm (Nagahara et al. 2013).

The action mechanism of PDT has been extensively described (Dougherty et al. 1998). Briefly, upon illumination the photosensitizer is excited from the ground state to the triplet state. The longer lifetime of the triplet state enables the interaction of the excited photosensitizer with the surrounding molecules. It is anticipated that the generation of the cytotoxic species produced during PDT occurs while in this state (Moan and Berg 1991; Ochsner 1997).

The cytotoxic product, usually singlet oxygen ($^1O_2$), cannot migrate at a distance of more than 0.02 μm after its formation, thus making it ideal for local application of PDT, without endangering distant molecules, cells, or organs (Moan and Berg 1991).

During the last two decades, a considerable interest has evolved in evaluating the use of PDT in the treatment of periodontal and peri-implant infections.

In patients with untreated periodontitis, treatment with subgingival scaling and root planing (SRP) followed by subsequent application of PDT may lead to statistically significant higher improvements in probing depth (PD) reduction and/or clinical attachment (CAL) gain than following SRP alone (Andersen et al. 2007; Braun et al. 2008; Sigusch et al. 2010; Al-Zahrani and Austah 2011; Dilsiz et al. 2013; Betsy et al. 2014; Alwaeli et al. 2015), while other studies have failed to reveal statistically significant differences in these parameters (Christodoulides et al. 2008; Polansky et al. 2009; Ge et al. 2011; Lui et al. 2011; Theodoro et al. 2012; Balata et al. 2013; Luchesi et al. 2013; Queiroz et al. 2015).

A frequently observed outcome following the use of PDT was additional improvement in terms of bleeding on probing (BOP), thus pointing to the potential effects of this treatment on reducing periodontal inflammation (Christodoulides et al. 2008; Polansky et al. 2009; Ge et al. 2011; Lui et al. 2011; Theodoro et al. 2012; Balata et al. 2013; Luchesi et al. 2013; Queiroz et al. 2015). However, it is interesting to note that despite the obtained clinical improvements, changes of microbiological parameters were only found in some of the studies (Braun et al. 2008; Christodoulides et al. 2008; Sigusch et al. 2010; Ge et al. 2011; Alwaeli et al. 2015).

A very recent systematic review has investigated the adjunctive effects of PDT application to nonsurgical mechanical instrumentation. Only studies including at least 20 patients with untreated periodontitis and with a follow-up period of six months were included, while PDT has only been used once after mechanical debridement. The results failed to reveal statistically significant additional clinical improvements following a single application of PDT to nonsurgical mechanical instrumentation compared to mechanical debridement alone (Salvi et al. 2019).

However, in periodontal patients enrolled in a maintenance program (i.e. patients with treated periodontitis), the additional application of PDT to mechanical debridement has been shown to stabilize tissue inflammation, evidenced by higher values of BOP reduction (Chondros et al. 2009; Lulic et al. 2009; Cappuyns et al. 2012; Campos et al. 2013; Kolbe et al. 2014; Petelin et al. 2014; Muller Campanile et al. 2015).

Increasing evidence also suggests that in periodontal patients enrolled in maintenance, the repeated application (i.e. two, three, or even five times) of PDT to mechanical debridement may yield better outcomes in terms of pocket depths and inflammation (i.e. BOP), compared to single applications (Lulic et al. 2009; Muller Campanile et al. 2015; Grzech-Leśniak et al. 2019).

A very recent study has evaluated clinically and microbiologically the outcomes following one single session of subgingival mechanical debridement (scaling and root planing; e.g. SRP) followed by 1× immediate use of PDT and 2 × subsequent use of PDT without SRP. Forty patients diagnosed with generalized chronic periodontitis who were enrolled in a periodontal maintenance (recall) program were randomly assigned to one of the two treatments: (i) SRP by means of ultrasonic and hand instruments followed by one single session of SRP followed by 1× immediate use of PDT and 2 × subsequent use of PDT without SRP (test) or (i) SRP alone (control) (Grzech-Leśniak et al. 2019).

The results revealed that both treatments improved statistically significantly in most of the evaluated parameters. In the test group, BOP decreased statistically significantly ($p < 0.05$) after three and six months, while in the control group the respective values decreased statistically significantly only at three months. The results have provided additional evidence of the potential clinical benefit of repeated PDT applications indicating that the repetition of this treatment may additionally improve clinical outcomes, in particular the gingival inflammation evidenced by a decrease in BOP (Figures 7.1 and 7.2).

7.2 Use of PDT as an Alternative to Systemic or Local Antibiotics

An extremely important aspect which needs to be kept in mind when considering the use of PDT is the lack of bacterial resistance, which gains even more importance in light of the worldwide increase in bacterial resistance against antibiotics (Rams et al. 2014; Olsen 2015).

Thus, its repeated application in conjunction with mechanical debridement may represent a potential alternative which is worthwhile to consider for treating periodontal and peri-implant infections (Sculean et al. 2015).

A randomized controlled trial has evaluated the treatment of patients diagnosed with aggressive periodontitis (AgP) by means of nonsurgical periodontal therapy in conjunction with either systemic administration of amoxicillin and metronidazole or two-times topical application of PDT (Arweiler et al. 2014).

The results have shown that both treatment protocols resulted in statistically significant improvements in PD reduction, gain of CAL, and improvement in BOP compared to baseline. The systemic use of amoxicillin and metronidazole yielded however, at both three and six months, statistically significant higher reductions in mean PD compared with the treatment using PDT. The most important clinical finding was the change in the total number of pockets ≥7 mm following both treatment protocols. In the PDT group, the total number of pockets ≥7 mm was reduced from 137 to 45 with the corresponding values of 141 and 3 in the amoxicillin and metronidazole group. Moreover, compared to the results at three months and at six months, an additional decrease in the number of pockets ≥7 mm was measured. On the other hand, the use of PDT has also led to statistically and clinically significant improvements compared to baseline, although the number of residual pockets needing further therapy was substantially higher compared with the use of systemic antibiotics (e.g. 45 vs. 3) (Arweiler et al. 2014).

The changes in clinical parameters were also accompanied by changes in the concentration of matrix metalloproteinases 8 and 9 (MMP-8 and -9) in the gingival crevicular fluid (GCF). However, while in the antibiotic group, a statistically significant decrease of MMP-8 GCF level at both three and six months posttreatment was

observed, these changes were not significant in the PDT group (Skurska et al. 2015).

Taken together, the available data suggest a rather limited clinical benefit of using PDT in the treatment of patients with AgP (de Oliveira et al. 2007; Novaes Jr. et al. 2012; Arweiler et al. 2014; Moreira et al. 2015). Therefore, at present, PDT cannot be recommended as a replacement for systemic antibiotics in patients with AgP.

The use of PDT as a potential alternative to local antibiotics has been evaluated in an RCT study comparing nonsurgical treatment of incipient peri-implantitis (sites with PD 4–6 mm, BOP positive, and radiographic bone loss ≥2 mm) by means of mechanical debridement followed by either use of local antibiotics (e.g. minocycline) or application of PDT. The results at six months and at one year have failed to reveal statistically or clinically significant differences between the two treatment protocols, thus suggesting that PDT may represent a valuable alternative to local antibiotics during nonsurgical treatment of incipient peri-implantitis (Schär et al. 2013; Bassetti et al. 2014).

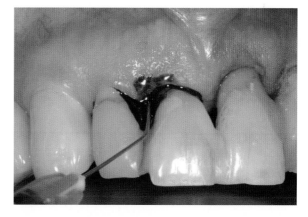

Figure 7.1 Application of the phenothiazine chloride dye following subgingival SRP. *Source:* Dr. Anton Sculean.

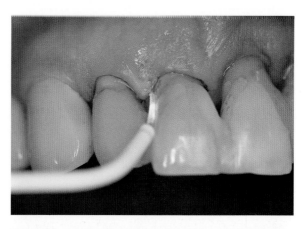

Figure 7.2 Application of the low level-laser light into the pocket. *Source:* Dr. Anton Sculean.

7.3 Conclusions

Based on the available evidence from the literature the following conclusions can be drawn:

- The primary indication for PDT is the treatment of periodontal patients enrolled in maintenance (i.e. recall).

- The repeated application of PDT to mechanical debridement appears to additionally improve the clinical outcomes compared to single applications.
- Increasing evidence appears to indicate that PDT may represent a possible alternative to local antibiotics.

References

Adriaens, P.A. and Adriaens, L.M. (2004). Effects of nonsurgical periodontal therapy on hard and soft tissues. *Periodontology 2000 36*: 121–145.

Alwaeli, H.A., Al-Khateeb, S.N., and Al-Sadi, A. (2015). Long-term clinical effect of adjunctive antimicrobial photodynamic therapy in periodontal treatment: a randomized clinical trial. *Lasers Med. Sci. 30* (2): 801–807.

Al-Zahrani, M.S. and Austah, O.N. (2011). Photodynamic therapy as an adjunctive to scaling and root planing in treatment of chronic periodontitis in smokers. *Saudi Med. J. 32* (11): 1183–1188.

Andersen, R., Loebel, N., Hammond, D. et al. (2007). Treatment of periodontal disease by photodisinfection compared to scaling and root planing. *J. Clin. Dent. 18* (2): 34–38.

Arweiler, N.B., Pietruska, M., Pietruski, J. et al. (2014). Six-month results following treatment of aggressive periodontitis with antimicrobial photodynamic therapy or amoxicillin and metronidazole. *Clin. Oral Investig. 18*: 2129–2135.

Badersten, A., Nilveus, R., and Egelberg, J. (1981). Effect of nonsurgical periodontal therapy. I. Moderately advanced periodontitis. *J. Clin. Periodontol. 8* (1): 57–72.

Badersten, A., Nilveus, R., and Egelberg, J. (1984). Effect of nonsurgical periodontal therapy. II. Severely advanced periodontitis. *J. Clin. Periodontol. 11* (1): 63–76.

Balata, M.L., Andrade, L.P., Santos, D.B. et al. (2013). Photodynamic therapy associated with full-mouth ultrasonic debridement in the treatment of severe chronic periodontitis: a randomized-controlled clinical trial. *J. Appl. Oral Sci.*: revista FOB *21* (2): 208–214.

Bassetti, M., Schär, D., Wicki, B. et al. (2014). Anti-infective therapy of peri-implantitis with adjunctive local drug delivery or photodynamic therapy: 12-month outcomes of a randomized controlled clinical trial. *Clin. Oral Implants Res. 25* (3): 279–287.

Bassir, S.H., Moslemi, N., Jamali, R. et al. (2013). Photoactivated disinfection using light-emitting diode as an adjunct in the management of chronic periodontitis: a pilot double-blind split-mouth randomized clinical trial. *J. Clin. Periodontol. 40* (1): 65–72.

Betsy, J., Prasanth, C.S., Baiju, K.V. et al. (2014). Efficacy of antimicrobial photodynamic therapy in the management of chronic periodontitis: a randomized controlled clinical trial. *J. Clin. Periodontol. 41* (6): 573–581.

Bonito, A.J., Lux, L., and Lohr, K.N. (2006). Impact of local adjuncts to scaling and root planing in periodontal disease therapy: a systematic review. *J. Periodontol.* 2005;76(8):1227-36. Review. Erratum in: J Periodontol 2006;77(2):326. Erratum in: J Periodontol 77: 326–327.

Bostanci, N. and Belibasakis, G.N. (2012). Porphyromonas gingivalis: an invasive and evasive opportunistic oral pathogen. *FEMS Microbiol. Lett. 333* (1): 1–9.

Braun, A., Dehn, C., Krause, F. et al. (2008). Short-term clinical effects of adjunctive antimicrobial photodynamic therapy in periodontal treatment: a randomized clinical trial. *J. Clin. Periodontol. 35* (10): 877–884.

Campos, G.N., Pimentel, S.P., Ribeiro, F.V. et al. (2013). The adjunctive effect of photodynamic therapy for residual pockets in single-rooted teeth: a randomized controlled clinical trial. *Lasers Med. Sci. 28* (1): 317–324.

Cappuyns, I., Cionca, N., Wick, P. et al. (2012). Treatment of residual pockets with photodynamic therapy, diode laser, or deep scaling. A randomized, split-mouth controlled clinical trial. *Lasers Med. Sci. 27* (5): 979–986.

Chan, Y. and Lai, C.H. (2003). Bactericidal effects of different laser wavelengths on periodontopathic germs in photodynamic therapy. *Lasers Med. Sci. 18* (1): 51–55.

Chondros, P., Nikolidakis, D., Christodoulides, N. et al. (2009). Photodynamic therapy as adjunct to non-surgical periodontal treatment in patients on periodontal maintenance: a randomized controlled clinical trial. *Lasers Med. Sci. 24* (5): 681–688.

Christodoulides, N., Nikolidakis, D., Chondros, P. et al. (2008). Photodynamic therapy as an adjunct to non-surgical periodontal treatment: a randomized, controlled clinical trial. *J. Periodontol. 79* (9): 1638–1644.

Cobb, C.M. (1996). Non-surgical pocket therapy: mechanical. *Ann. Periodontol. 1* (1): 443–490.

de Oliveira, R.R., Schwartz-Filho, H.O., Novaes, A.B. Jr. et al. (2007). Antimicrobial photodynamic therapy in the non-surgical treatment of aggressive periodontitis: a preliminary randomized controlled clinical study. *J. Periodontol. 78* (6): 965–973.

Dilsiz, A., Canakci, V., and Aydin, T. (2013). Clinical effects of potassium-titanyl-phosphate laser and photodynamic therapy on outcomes of treatment of chronic periodontitis: a randomized controlled clinical trial. *J. Periodontol. 84* (3): 278–286.

Dougherty, T.J., Gomer, C.J., Henderson, B.W. et al. (1998). Photodynamic therapy. *J. Natl. Cancer Inst. 90* (12): 889–905.

Drisko, C.H. (1998). Root instrumentation. Power-driven versus manual scalers, which one? *Dent. Clin. N. Am. 42* (2): 229–244.

Ge, L., Shu, R., Li, Y. et al. (2011). Adjunctive effect of photodynamic therapy to scaling and root planing in the treatment of chronic periodontitis. *Photomed. Laser Surg. 29* (1): 33–37.

Gillies, M., Ranakusuma, A., Hoffmann, T. et al. (2015). Common harms from amoxicillin: a systematic review and meta-analysis of randomized placebo-controlled trials for any indication. *CMAJ 187* (1): E21–E31.

Grzech-Lesniak, K. (2017). Making use of lasers in periodontal treatment: a new gold standard? *Photomed. Laser Surg. 35* (10): 513–514.

Grzech-Leśniak, K., Gaspirc, B., and Sculean, A. (2019). Clinical and microbiological effects of multiple applications of antibacterial photodynamic therapy in periodontal maintenance patients. A randomised controlled clinical study. *Photodiagn. Photodyn. Ther. 27*: 44–50.

Javed, F. and Romanos, G.E. (2013). Does photodynamic therapy enhance standard antibacterial therapy in dentistry? *Photomed. Laser Surg. 31* (11): 512–518.

Keestra, J.A., Grosjean, I., Coucke, W. et al. (2015a). Non-surgical periodontal therapy with systemic antibiotics in patients with untreated aggressive periodontitis: a systematic review and meta-analysis. *J. Periodontal Res. 50* (6): 689–706.

Keestra, J.A., Grosjean, I., Coucke, W. et al. (2015b). Non-surgical periodontal therapy with systemic antibiotics in patients with untreated chronic periodontitis: a systematic review and meta-analysis. *J. Periodontal Res. 50* (3): 294–314.

Kikuchi, T., Mogi, M., Okabe, I. et al. (2015). Adjunctive application of antimicrobial photodynamic therapy in nonsurgical periodontal treatment: a review of literature. *Int. J. Mol. Sci. 16* (10): 24111–24126.

Kolbe, M.F., Ribeiro, F.V., Luchesi, V.H. et al. (2014). Photodynamic therapy during supportive periodontal care: clinical, microbiologic, immunoinflammatory, and patient-centered performance in a split-mouth randomized clinical trial. *J. Periodontol. 85* (8): e277–e286.

Lindhe, J., Westfelt, E., Nyman, S. et al. (1984). Long-term effect of surgical/non-surgical treatment of periodontal disease. *J. Clin. Periodontol. 11* (7): 448–458.

Luchesi, V.H., Pimentel, S.P., Kolbe, M.F. et al. (2013). Photodynamic therapy in the treatment of class II furcation: a randomized controlled clinical trial. *J. Clin. Periodontol. 40* (8): 781–788.

Lui, J., Corbet, E.F., and Jin, L. (2011). Combined photodynamic and low-level laser therapies as an adjunct to nonsurgical treatment of chronic periodontitis. *J. Periodontal Res. 46* (1): 89–96.

Lulic, M., Leiggener Gorog, I., Salvi, G.E. et al. (2009). One-year outcomes of repeated adjunctive photodynamic therapy during periodontal maintenance: a proof-of-principle randomized-controlled clinical trial. *J. Clin. Periodontol. 36* (8): 661–666.

Moan, J. and Berg, K. (1991). The photodegradation of porphyrins in cells can be used to estimate the lifetime of singlet oxygen. *Photochem. Photobiol. 53* (4): 549–553.

Moreira, A.L., Novaes, A.B. Jr., Grisi, M.F. et al. (2015). Antimicrobial photodynamic therapy as an adjunct to non-surgical treatment of aggressive periodontitis: a split-mouth randomized controlled trial. *J. Periodontol. 86* (3): 376–386.

Muller Campanile, V.S., Giannopoulou, C., Campanile, G. et al. (2015). Single or repeated antimicrobial photodynamic therapy as adjunct to ultrasonic debridement in residual periodontal pockets: clinical, microbiological, and local biological effects. *Lasers Med. Sci. 30* (1): 27–34.

Nagahara, A., Mitani, A., Fukuda, M. et al. (2013). Antimicrobial photodynamic therapy using a diode laser with a potential new photosensitizer, indocyanine green-loaded nanospheres, may be effective for the clearance of Porphyromonas gingivalis. *J. Periodontal Res. 48* (5): 591–599.

Noro Filho, G.A., Casarin, R.C., Casati, M.Z., and Giovani, E.M. (2012). PDT in non-surgical treatment of periodontitis in HIV patients: a split-mouth, randomized clinical trial. *Lasers Surg. Med. 44* (4): 296–302.

Novaes, A.B. Jr., Schwartz-Filho, H.O., de Oliveira, R.R. et al. (2012). Antimicrobial photodynamic therapy in the non-surgical treatment of aggressive periodontitis: microbiological profile. *Lasers Med. Sci. 27* (2): 389–395.

Ochsner, M. (1997). Photophysical and photobiological processes in the photodynamic therapy of tumours. *J. Photochem. Photobiol. B 39* (1): 1–18.

Olsen, I. (2015). Biofilm-specific antibiotic tolerance and resistance. *Eur. J. Clin. Microbiol. Infect. Dis.* *34* (5): 877–886.

Olsen, C.E., Weyergang, A., Edwards, V.T. et al. (2017). Development of resistance to photodynamic therapy (PDT) in human breast cancer cells is photosensitizer-dependent: possible mechanisms and approaches for overcoming PDT-resistance. *Biochem. Pharmacol.* *144*: 63–77.

Page, R.C. and Kornman, K.S. (1997). The pathogenesis of human periodontitis: an introduction. *Periodontology 2000* *14*: 9–11.

Petelin, M., Perkic, K., Seme, K. et al. (2014). Effect of repeated adjunctive antimicrobial photodynamic therapy on subgingival periodontal pathogens in the treatment of chronic periodontitis. *Lasers Med. Sci.*

Pfitzner, A., Sigusch, B.W., Albrecht, V. et al. (2004). Killing of periodontopathogenic bacteria by photodynamic therapy. *J. Periodontol.* *75* (10): 1343–1349.

Polansky, R., Haas, M., Heschl, A. et al. (2009). Clinical effectiveness of photodynamic therapy in the treatment of periodontitis. *J. Clin. Periodontol.* *36* (7): 575–580.

Queiroz, A.C., Suaid, F.A., de Andrade, P.F. et al. (2015). Adjunctive effect of antimicrobial photodynamic therapy to nonsurgical periodontal treatment in smokers: a randomized clinical trial. *Lasers Med. Sci.* *30* (2): 617–625.

Rams, T.E., Degener, J.E., and van Winkelhoff, A.J. (2014). Antibiotic resistance in human chronic periodontitis microbiota. *J. Periodontol.* *85* (1): 160–169.

Romanos, G.E. and Brink, B. (2010). Photodynamic therapy in periodontal therapy: microbiological observations from a private practice. *Gen. Dent.* *58* (2): e68–e73.

Rudney, J.D., Chen, R., and Sedgewick, G.J. (2001). Intracellular Actinobacillus actinomycetemcomitans and Porphyromonas gingivalis in buccal epithelial cells collected from human subjects. *Infect. Immun.* *69* (4): 2700–2707.

Salvi, G.E., Stähli, A., Schmidt, J.C. et al. (2019 Dec 20). Adjunctive laser of antimicrobial photodynamic therapy to non-surgical instrumentation in patients with untreated periodontitis. A systematic review and meta-analysis. *J. Clin. Periodontol.* https://doi.org/10.1111/jcpe.13236. [Epub ahead of print.]

Schär, D., Ramscier, C.A., Eick, S. et al. (2013). Anti-infective therapy of peri-implantitis with adjunctive local drug delivery or photodynamic therapy: six-month outcomes of a prospective randomized clinical trial. *Clin. Oral Implants Res.* *24*: 104–110.

Sculean, A., Aoki, A., Romanos, G. et al. (2015). Is photodynamic therapy an effective treatment for periodontal and Peri-implant infections? *Dent. Clin. N. Am.* *59* (4): 831–858.

Sharman, W.M., Allen, C.M., and van Lier, J.E. (1999). Photodynamic therapeutics: basic principles and clinical applications. *Drug Discov. Today* *4* (11): 507–517.

Sigusch, B.W., Engelbrecht, M., Volpel, A. et al. (2010). Full-mouth antimicrobial photodynamic therapy in Fusobacterium nucleatum-infected periodontitis patients. *J. Periodontol.* *81* (7): 975–981.

Skurska, A., Dolinska, E., Pietruska, M. et al. (2015;26). Effect of nonsurgical periodontal treatment in conjunction with either systemic administration of amoxicillin and metronidazole or additional photodynamic therapy on the concentration of matrix metalloproteinases 8 and 9 in gingival crevicular fluid in patients with aggressive periodontitis. *BMC Oral Health* *15*: 63.

Theodoro, L.H., Silva, S.P., Pires, J.R. et al. (2012). Clinical and microbiological effects of photodynamic therapy associated with nonsurgical periodontal treatment. A 6-month follow-up. *Lasers Med. Sci.* *27* (4): 687–693.

Umeda, M., Takeuchi, Y., Noguchi, K. et al. (2004). Effects of nonsurgical periodontal therapy on the microbiota. *Periodontology 2000* *36*: 98–120.

von Tappeiner, H.J.A. (1904). On the effect of photodynamic (fluorescent) substances on protozoa and enzymes. *Arch. Klin. Med.* *39*: 427–487. (German).

Wilson, M., Dobson, J., and Harvey, W. (1992). Sensitization of oral bacteria to killing by low-power laser radiation. *Curr. Microbiol.* *25* (2): 77–81.

8

Understanding Laser Safety in Dentistry

Vangie Dennis[1], Patti Owens[2] and Georgios E. Romanos[3]

[1] *Executive Director Perioperative Services, Atlanta Medical Center, Atlanta, GA, USA*
[2] *President of Aesthetic Med Consulting International, LLC*
[3] *Stony Brook University, School of Dental Medicine, Stony Brook, NY, USA*

8.1   Laser Safety

When lasers are introduced into a healthcare environment, whether in a hospital, surgery center, physician's office, or a dental office, healthcare professionals must be prepared to address issues of safety for both the staff and the patient. All lasers present hazards to patients and to the individuals utilizing them as well as anyone present in the area in which they are being activated. This equipment should be utilized in accordance with established regulations, standards and recommended practices, manufacturer's recommendations, and institutional policies. Laser safety is based on knowledge of the specific laser being utilized, its instrumentation, mode of operation, power densities, action in tissues, and risk assessment.

8.2   International Laser Standards

The International Electrotechnical Commission (IEC). IEC 60825-1 3.0:2014, 60601-2-22 Ed. 3.1:2011 and 60825-8:2006 are international standards that provide the safe manufacturing and use of medical-surgical, cosmetic, and therapeutic lasers. Since this is a global economy, dental lasers manufacturers will need to be aware of the numerous international specifications and performance standards.

8.3   Regulatory Agencies and Nongovernmental Organizations

8.3.1   Food and Drug Administration

All laser products manufactured or imported into the United States are subject to the Food and Drug Administration's (FDA) Radiological Health Regulations (21 CFR Parts 1000–1050). The FDA's authority to regulate laser products is granted by the Federal Food, Drug, and Cosmetic Act. Under these regulations, the manufacturer must build their product to comply with a performance standard (1040.10 & 1040.11), self-certify the product complies to the applicable parts of the performance standard (1010.2), affix identification information to the product (1010.3), and submit reports and maintain records (1002). These requirements must be met before the manufacturer can leave the product with another entity. Medical laser products are subject to additional requirements (21 CFR Parts 800–1299). Some requirements apply to medical devices before they are marketed (premarket requirements), and others apply to medical devices after they are marketed (postmarket requirements). It is important to be acquainted with the organizations, laws, and standards regulating or affecting the use of lasers in a medical setting. Healthcare professionals can then develop and implement an appropriate laser safety program.

8.3.2 FDA Center for Devices and Radiological Health

All medical lasers are regulated by the FDA under the Medical Device Amendments to the Food and Drug Act. Any medical device that is manufactured, repackaged, relabeled, or imported into the US must meet FDA regulations. These regulations are enforced by the National Center for Devices and Radiological Health (CDRH), which is a regulatory bureau of the FDA. The FDA regulates more than 250 types of lasers including those intended for medical and surgical use. Medical, surgical, aesthetic, and dental lasers are usually classified as class II medical devices, which indicate that they have a moderate to high risk to the patient. Manufacturers must conform to all of the federal safety requirements including performance standards involving compliance with engineering, electronics, and hardware specifications. Manufacturers are also required to conform with FDA labeling requirements along with supplying maintenance and procedure manuals. Medical laser devices must be cleared or approved by the CDRH prior to any marketing or testing of a laser for a particular clinical application or use.

In addition, the FDA has been empowered by the US Congress to provide regulations for electronic products that emit radiation. The regulations created by the FDA require the manufacture of laser products to produce a product that complies with the performance standard for laser products 21CFR 1040.10 and.11. This standard is referred to as the Federal Laser Product Performance Standard (FLPPS). The FLPPS specifies a hazard classification scheme based on a laser product's ability to cause damage to the eye and skin It also provides requirements for hazard labels, user information, and performance requirements for engineering features such as protective housings, safety interlocks, and viewing optics incorporated into the product. The control measures specified in the ANSI standard can be applied to the products classified under the FLPPS or the conditions of Laser Notice No. 56.

8.3.3 American National Standards Institute

The American National Standards Institute (ANSI) is a voluntary organization of experts, including manufacturers, consumers, scientific-technical and professional organizations, and government agencies who determine industry consensus standards in technical fields. ANSI's mission is to provide a practice standard for the safe use of lasers and laser systems for diagnostic and therapeutic use in healthcare facilities. The ANSI Z136.3-12018 "American National Standard for Safe Use of Lasers in Health Care" is the national benchmark standard. The first cohesive blueprint for building a safe and effective dental laser program is outlined in the ANSI Z136.3 Standard. ANSI states that an adequate program for control of laser hazards be established in every healthcare facility that utilizes medical lasers. The program must include provisions for a laser safety officer, education of users, protective measures, and management of accidents. ANSI Z136.3 covers many areas of lasers and their safe use including terminology, hazard evaluation, classification, control measures, and administrative controls. Federal legislation and state laser safety regulations, as well as professional and advisory standards, are based on the ANSI standard. This standard of practice is also the most cited source during medical litigations.

8.3.4 Occupational Safety and Health Administration

With the Occupational Safety and Health Act of 1970, Congress created the Occupational Safety and Health Administration (OSHA). OSHA's primary goal is for employers to keep their workplace free of serious recognized hazards. OSHA is concerned primarily with the safety of healthcare workers, and their enforcement can be administered on a national or state level. OSHA can enforce the ANSI standards even though they do not have specific legislated regulations governing laser safety in healthcare facilities. OSHA can cite violations under the General Duty clause if the level of compliance is not satisfactory, and they view employees are at risk.

OSHA can also issue citations utilizing CFR Part 1910, which provides the general industry standards for employee protection. Under the 1910.132 Personal Protective Equipment, this regulation addresses the need for the appropriate protectant safeguards, including laser safety eyewear, face shields, masks, and protective clothing. OSHA furthermore states under 1910.133(a) (1), that "the employer shall ensure that each affected employee use appropriate eye and face protection when exposed to eye or face hazards from flying particles, molten metal, liquid chemicals, acids or caustic liquids, chemical gases or vapors, or *potentially injurious light radiation.*" In addition, the employer needs to aware of the blood-borne pathogen regulation 1910.1030, pertaining to employee exposure to blood and other potentially infectious material (OPIM). Laser plume is

FDA Classification of Medical Devices
Medical devices were classified in 1976 by the FDA according to their safety factors
Class I   Subject to general controls
Class II   Devices for which general controls are not enough
Class III   Implant and life support devices

Laser Classification Systems

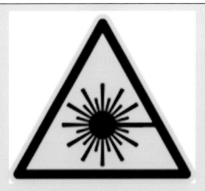

Warning label for class 2 and higher

Listed below is a summary of common characteristics for the laser classification systems as specified by the International Electrotechnical Commission (IEC) 60825-1 and ANSI Z136.3.1-2014 standards along with the U.S.FDA-CDRH (21CFR1040.10) requirements.

Class 1 – IEC, FDA, ANSI Z136

A **Class 1** laser is safe under all conditions of normal operation. This means it is safe when viewing a laser with the naked eye or with the aid of typical magnifying optics (e.g. telescope or microscope). No administrative controls required.

Class 1M – ANSI Z136, IEC

A **Class 1M** laser is safe for all conditions of use except when passed through magnifying optics such as microscopes and collecting optics. Administrative controls required when viewing with magnifying optical aids.

Class 1C – IEC, ANSI Z136.3

A **Class 1C** laser is safe under all conditions of normal use. These devices are designed for direct contact with the skin and are apt to be home laser devices. Higher classified lasers tend to be embedded in "eye-safe" devices that do not allow any emission of radiation which would exceed Class 1 level laser. No administrative controls required.

Class 2 – IEC, FDA, ANSI Z136

A **Class 2** laser is considered to be safe due to the blink reflex (glare aversion response to bright lights) that will limit the exposure to no more than 0.25 seconds. It only applies to visible-light lasers (400–700 nm). (400–780 nm). AEL (Accessible Emission Limit) is typically 1 mW or less for CW lasers. No administrative controls required.

Class 2a – FDA

A **Class 2a** is a low powered visible laser where the laser requires in excess of 1000 seconds of continuous viewing to produce a burn to the retina. No administrative controls required.

Class 2M - IEC, ANSI

A **Class 2M** laser is safe due to the blink reflex, if not viewed through magnifying optical instruments. Visible low power lasers; either collimated with large beam diameter or highly divergent beam. Administrative controls required if viewed with collecting optics.

Class IIIa - FDA

A **Class 3a** lasers are visible lasers in this class, and they can be momentarily hazardous when viewed directly for extended periods of time. Hazards increase if staring directly at the beam without eye protection. Lasers similar to the Class 2 with the exception that collecting optics cannot be used to directly view the beam. No administrative controls are usually required.

Class 3R – IEC, ANSI

A **Class 3R** laser is considered relatively safe if handled carefully, with restricted beam viewing. They have reduced (therefore 3R) requirements from those lasers that they have associated risks. Possibility of ocular hazards can occur under direct or specular viewing if the eye is dilated and focused. AEL is typically 5 mW or less for CW lasers. Class 3R does not create fire hazards or diffuse beam hazards. No administrative controls are usually required.

Class 3B – IEC, FDA, ANSI

A **Class 3B** laser is a medium-powered visible or invisible laser that can be hazardous with ocular injuries resulting from a direct viewing or specular reflections. However, a Class 3 laser exposure is not considered hazardous from a diffuse reflection. Class 3B lasers also do not create nonbeam hazards. AEL is typically 5 mW to 500 mW for CW lasers. Administrative controls are required.

Class 4 – IEC, FDA, ANSI

A **Class 4** laser is a high-power visible or invisible laser and the most dangerous classification. By definition, a Class 4 laser can burn the skin or can cause devastating and permanent eye damage as a result of direct, specular reflected, or diffuse beam viewing. These hazards may also apply to indirect or nonspecular reflections of the beam. These lasers may ignite combustible materials, and thus may represent a fire risk along with other nonbeam hazards. AEL is typically greater than 500 mW for CW lasers. Administrative controls are required. Chart adapted from the RLI, FDA, ANSI, and Wikipedia – https://en.wikipedia.org/wiki/Laser_safety, https://www.rli.com/resources/articles/classification.aspx

generated from vaporizing laser devices, such as the CO_2, Er:YAG, Ho:YAG, Er,Cr:YSGG lasers, which produce airborne contaminants, toxic gases, organic compounds, and splatter of blood-borne particles.

8.4 State Regulations

State regulations, including FDA, are the only guidelines for laser safety that are backed by legislative action. The concern over laser safety is reflected in the increasing number of states that are enacting medical laser safety legislation. Regulations governing the safe use of lasers present healthcare personnel with a complex set of guidelines. Only FDA and individual state enactments are supported by legislation. All other guidelines are recommended practices or standards and are based on the ANSI Z136.3 practices.

8.5 Nongovernmental Controls and Professional Organizations

8.5.1 American Society for Lasers in Medicine and Surgery

The American Society for Lasers in Medicine and Surgery (ASLMS), in 1980, issued reports that were adopted as recommendations by the society's members. In 1990, the board of directors released nine recommended perioperative practices relating to patients undergoing laser procedures. This included assessment, nursing diagnosis, planning, implementation, and evaluation of nursing care. Position statements are available to provide practice guidelines for physician education and credentialing along with nonphysician laser use. In 2017, ASLMS drafted and approved their "Position Statement on Lasers and Energy Device Plume" addressing the hazards of working with devices that caused vaporization and ejected tissue plume. The utilization of a plume evacuator, the appropriate personal protective equipment (PPE), and the possible use of a debris barrier is advocated to mitigate potential employee risks.

8.5.2 Association of periOperative Registered Nurses (AORN)

The Association of periOperative Registered Nurses' (AORN) "Recommended Practices for Laser Safety in the Practice Setting" was first published in 1989. These broad recommended practices provide guidelines to support perioperative nurses in developing policies and procedures for the safe use of lasers in their practice

setting. These guidelines represent evidence-based practices for laser use in surgical, ambulatory, and clinic facilities.

8.6 The Joint Commission (TJC)

The Joint Commission (TJC) mandates that facilities conduct a safety assessment to determine any potential risks from hazardous energy. In the "Environment of Care" chapter, Element of Performance (E.P.) 7 EC.02.02.01, the standard does state, "The critical access hospital minimizes risks associated with selecting and using hazardous energy sources." TJC can also refer to ANSI Z136.3-2018 in regard to the control of laser hazards concerning the management of laser plume of smoke. The Element of Performance 9 states that critical hospitals should also minimize risks associated with disposing of hazardous gases and vapors:

> "NOTE: hazardous gases and vapors include, but are not limited to: ethylene oxide and nitrous gases, vapors generated by glutaraldehyde; cauterizing equipment, such as *lasers*."

8.7 Standards and Practice

Control of potential health hazards associated with the use of dental laser systems requires the adoption of appropriate safety standards and policies that are relevant to the specific laser situation. It is imperative that, for the safety of patients, physicians, hygienists, and other medical personnel, everyone involved with medical lasers understands how to safely manage each type of laser in a medical setting. Before a laser is utilized clinically, a laser safety program should be established with written policies and procedures to establish authority, responsibility, and accountability.

8.7.1 Laser Safety Officer

The laser safety officer (LSO) is a person appointed by the administration that has attained the training and education to administer a laser safety program. The LSO has the authority to suspend, restrict, or terminate a laser procedure if they determine that the hazard controls are not adequate. This does not mean the LSO must be present during every laser procedure. The LSO is responsible for the appropriate classification of lasers within the facility, hazard evaluation, control measures, procedural approval, protective equipment, maintenance of equipment, and training for all personnel associated with lasers and medical surveillance (ANSI 2018). The job description and responsibilities can be daunting; however, the LSO can utilize qualified personnel, technical support, and other resources if necessary. ANSI does state that the LSO can be a laser user, operator, or any other trained individual who is qualified to administer a laser program. ANSI Z136.3-2018 Appendix A describes the specific duties and responsibilities:

a) **Safety Program.** The LSO is the designated individual who has the responsibility to administer the facility's laser safety program. Advanced training and education are required along with the skill set to knowledgeably assess the laser hazards and institute the necessary safety controls.

b) **Hazard Classification.** The LSO assesses all laser devices to determine appropriate labeling that is FDA/CDRH required. Also, the LSO should note correct classification of each laser system and instigate safety controls for all Class 3B and 4 lasers.

c) **Hazard Evaluation.** The LSO will conduct a hazard evaluation of all new and existing laser devices.

d) **Hazard Response.** The LSO, or designee, will immediately communicate to the user any danger or hazards that could occur in use of a laser device.

e) **Control Measures.** The LSO will verify that all safety controls determined by the manufacturer or established by the LSO be employed.

f) **Procedure Approvals.** The LSO will establish, approve and enforce the facility's policies and procedures.

g) **Protective Equipment.** The LSO will confirm that all PPE is available and functional for all members of the laser team.

h) **Signs and Labels.** The LSO will verify that all laser signs follow the ANSI Z136.1 and.3, Section 4.7.

i) **Facilities and Equipment.** The LSO will approve all laser installation In accordance with the manufacturer's safety information. Any modifications will be reviewed and documented by the LSO. Required servicing and preventative maintenance will be performed by qualified technicians per manufacturer's protocol.

j) **Training.** The LSO confirms that the required laser safety education and training is provided to all members of the laser team including the laser user, operators, student, technicians, hygienist, and other ancillary staff. Records will be maintained.

k) **Records.** The LSO will verify that all national, state, and local required records are maintained along with facility audits and policies and procedures.

8.8 Hazard Evaluation and Control Measures

Hazard evaluation is influenced by various factors of the laser system being utilized. The classification of the laser and the wavelength of the laser may also assist in defining the necessary control measures to be incorporated into the safety program. These factors affect which safety controls need to be incorporated into the laser safety program and implemented into practice. Control measures are those procedures or methods implemented to minimize hazards associated with a particular laser when it is in the operational mode. Control measures may be influenced by the ability of the laser energy to injure, the environment in which the laser will be activated, personnel that may use or be exposed within the nominal hazard zone (NHZ), the delivery systems, and the nonbeam hazards associated with the specific laser. Ancillary hazards create the potential for significant injuries to occur. Injuries, including death, may occur during testing of laser equipment, during electrical equipment checks and servicing, from fires, explosions, and even embolisms.

8.9 Administrative Controls

Administrative controls are those methods or procedures specifying explicit criteria that determine the implementation of engineering controls or work practices for personnel protection. Standard operating procedures (SOP's) are established from institutional policies and procedures. Safety controls, maintenance, and service, as well as the function of the laser, should be incorporated into the facilities SOPs. SOP's may also include documentation requirements for pre-procedure safety checklists, and intraprocedural laser operation and safety. The LSO is responsible for the execution of the SOP's.

8.10 Procedural and Equipment Controls

Engineering and procedural controls are determined by the LSO and must be implemented when appropriate to circumvent potential hazards. Procedural controls require adherence to written SOP's to ensure the safety of all personnel working in the region of lasers. SOP's should provide for operational guidelines, emergency shut-off mechanisms, stand-by functions, use of low reflective materials near the laser beam path, and storage.

Operational guidelines should require switches, whether foot pedal or finger trigger, which control the laser energy be guarded to prevent accidental activation. This may necessitate one foot pedal access for the individual controlling the delivery device to prevent inadvertent activation of the laser (Castelluccio 2012). Accessory attachments to lasers must also be compatible with the laser safety guidelines. This includes laser filters on operating microscopes that protect the operator at the binocular viewing tube and through the accessory viewing tubes.

Lasers should be placed in the stand-by mode when the laser is on but not being fired, or when the user is no longer in control of the delivery device, to prevent accidental discharge. When not in use, storage of the laser and/or disabling of the laser is necessary to prevent inadvertent activation of the laser by nonauthorized personnel. Lasers should be stored in secured areas.

Nonreflective instruments (dull, anodized, or matte-finished) should be used in or near the laser beam to defocus or disperse the laser beam (Fencl 2017). Appropriate backstops or guards should be used to prevent the laser beam from striking normal tissue, nontargeted teeth, or tissues.

8.11 Laser Treatment Controlled Area

The nominal hazard zone (NHZ) is the space in which the level of the direct, reflected, or scattered radiation used during the normal laser operation exceeds the applicable maximum permissible exposure (MPE) (Spratt et al. 2012). An NHZ should be identified by the LSO to prevent unintentional exposure to the laser beam. Determination of the NHZ should take into consideration information gathered from the manufacturer's labeling, by analysis, to radiation transmission of the beam and the potential for equipment failure. The NHZ is usually contained within the room but may extend through open doors or transparent windows, depending on the type of laser used. It is the LSO's responsibility to define the NHZ and ensure that the proper safety practices are adhered to in the NHZ.

The appropriate warning signs posted at every entryway into the laser treatment–controlled area should define the NHZ (Figures 8.1–8.3). The symbols and wording on the warning signs should be specific for the type of laser used and designed according to the information described in the ANSI standard for the Safe Use of Lasers in Health Care Facilities. New signs should be compliant with the ANSI Z535.2 even though older signs will be grandfathered in.

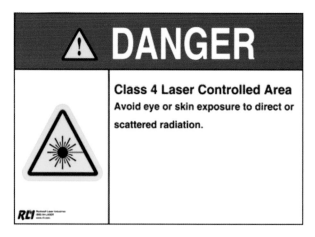

Figure 8.1 ANSI Z535.2 new laser signs. *Source:* Rockwell Laser Industries (RLI).

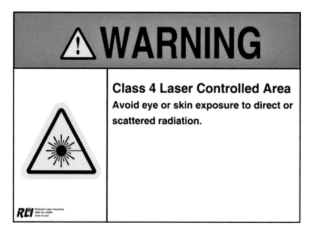

Figure 8.2 ANSI Z535.2 new sign example. *Source:* Rockwell Laser Industries (RLI).

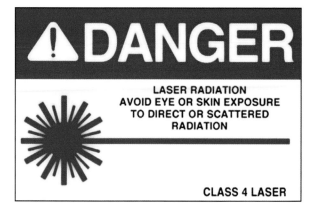

Figure 8.3 ANSI Z136.12014 grandfathered sign. *Source:* Vangie Dennis.

Windows and viewing areas should be limited because the NHZ may reach beyond the room in which the laser is in use. Additional safety controls, such as closing doors and covering windows with applicable filters or barriers or restricting traffic, may need to be implemented dependent on the laser used. Screens, curtains, or a blocking barrier may be placed near entryways to avert laser radiation (Figures 8.4 and 8.5).

Only authorized persons (including patients), approved by the laser safety officer, should be in the vicinity of the NHZ. Only authorized laser operators who have been delegated specific responsibilities by the laser safety officer may operate a laser. An authorized laser operator is a person trained in laser safety and approved by the facility to operate the laser. This person is responsible for the safety of the equipment and the treatment environment in the NHZ. They must remain at the laser control while the laser is in use. Their responsibilities include:

- Assessment of the procedure needs including anesthesia needs, type of laser, and accessory equipment,
- Equipment checks prior to use including accessories, operation, and safety equipment to ensure safe working conditions,
- Safety controls for all personnel (including the patient) in the treatment area, such as wearing appropriate eyewear,
- Appropriate signage displayed with the appropriate laser protective eyewear (LPE),
- Setting the laser wattage and exposure appropriately and monitoring activation of the laser and observation of team members for breaks in safety,
- Completing a safety checklist and laser log.

All healthcare personnel in the vicinity of the NHZ should be trained in the implementation of all laser safety precautions to avoid inadvertent exposure to laser hazards. All personnel, including the patient, within the NHZ should use appropriate PPE.

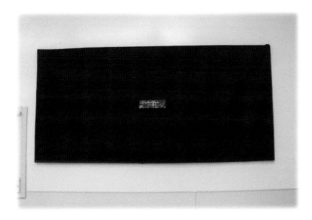

Figure 8.4 Example of occlusive tested laser window covers. *Source:* Vangie Dennis.

8.12 Maintenance and Service

Preventative maintenance should be done every six months. Only properly educated, trained, and approved technicians should be allowed to work on the laser or handle the electrical components (Takac and Stojanović 1999). Thorough documentation of all fault codes, equipment malfunctions, technical support, and servicing needs to be conducted and maintained for audits and future reference.

8.13 Beam Hazards

8.13.1 Eye Protection

Patient eyes should be protected when in the NHZ. Everyone in the NHZ should wear appropriate eyewear approved by the laser safety officer (Figure 8.6). The eye is the organ that is most susceptible to laser injury. The optics of the eye can concentrate and focus laser light at wavelengths ranging from 400 to 1400 nm on the retina, which increases the potential ocular hazard. Ultraviolet and far-infrared wavelength regions (outside 400–

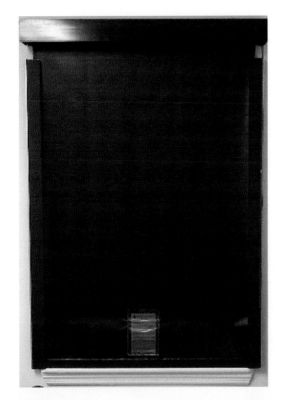

Figure 8.5 Example of occlusive tested laser covers. *Source:* Patti Owens.

1400 nm) principally produce corneal effects. Also, laser radiation at certain wavelengths may cause damage to the lens of the eye (AORN Recommended Practices 2017). Appropriate laser safety eyewear filters out the hazardous wavelength of laser radiation (Figures 8.7 and 8.8). In addition to direct exposure from misdirected and damaged fibers, scattered, diffused, and reflected laser beams can cause eye injuries. LPE for the laser staff may include laser goggles, laser glasses with side shields, and prescription glasses with special filters or coatings.

The patient's eyes and eyelids should be protected from the laser beam by appropriate methods when the eyes are in the NHZ. Protective methods may include wet eye pads, laser protective eyewear, or laser metal occlusive eye shields (Figures 8.9–8.11). Metal FDA-approved and tested corneoscleral eye shields may be necessary when the laser treatment is performed around the ocular ridge, corneal adnexa, and on the eyelids. Best practices indicate the use of water-based anesthetic drops and lubricant. Corneoscleral shields should be selected based on the patient's ocular size, should be inserted and removed by a trained professional to prevent corneal abrasions, and should be sterilized in between use per manufacturer's instructions for use (IFU).

All personnel in the NHZ should wear protective eyewear that is labeled with the appropriate optical density and wavelength while the laser is in use. Ocular hazards

may transpire during operational pretesting of the laser to confirm beam alignment and calibration. One should never look directly into the beam. Most LPE is tested for an indirect or reflected exposure. Potential for ocular hazards is also present during fiberoptic procedures as a result of the fiber becoming disconnected or breaking. Both instances also require protective eyewear to be utilized to prevent exposure of the eye. Protective eyewear should be available outside the room near the posted warning signs

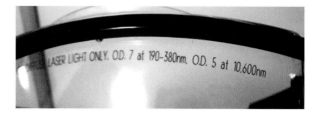

Figure 8.8 Example of laser wavelength and O.D. imprinted on eyewear. *Source:* Patti Owens.

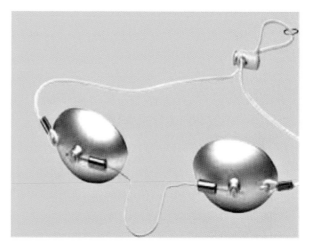

Figure 8.9 Example of occlusive metal laser eyewear. *Source:* Vangie Dennis.

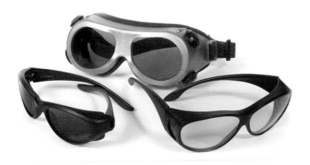

Figure 8.6 Appropriate eye protection (goggles) specific for different wavelengths. *Source:* Vangie Dennis.

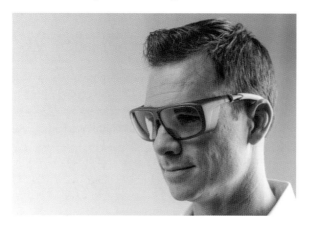

Figure 8.7 Laser protective eyewear (LPE). *Source:* Innovative Optics.

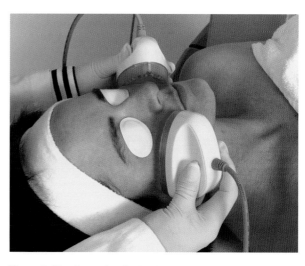

Figure 8.10 Example of adhesive laser protective eyewear. *Source:* Rockwell Laser Industries (RLI).

Figure 8.11 Example of corneoscleral patient eye shields. *Source:* Vangie Dennis.

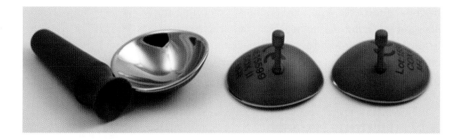

designating the specific type of laser in use. For optimal protection, inspect eyewear for pitting, cracking, discoloration, coating damage, frame condition, and light leaks. If any of these are present, the eyewear is considered inadequate for eye protection and should be discarded.

8.13.2 Skin Protection

Whenever there is a potential hazard of thermal burns from high-powered lasers, all persons in the laser treatment area should be protected from the laser beam exposures to their skin and other nontargeted tissues. Overexposure to ultraviolet radiation can lead to skin sensitivities or even burns from direct or reflected laser energy. Surgical gloves, tightly woven fabrics, and flame-retardant material, dependent of the laser being utilized, may provide skin protection. Protection of exposed tissues around the operative site may be accomplished by covering the areas with saline-saturated or water-saturated, fire/flame-retardant materials (e.g. towels, sponges, drapes, fabrics). These materials must remain moist to absorb or disperse the energy of the laser beam. Polypropylene or plastic drapes can melt if a laser beam strikes them and woven or nonwoven fabrics can be ignited. Laser handpieces or fiber tips should be placed on a moistened surface to prevent a fire from the hot tip or shatter of the tip if placed on a cold surface.

8.14 Laser Safety and Training Programs

A laser safety program establishes and maintains policies and procedures to ensure control of laser hazards. Laser safety programs policies and procedures should include, but are not limited to, the following:

- LSO guidelines defining the authority and responsibility for evaluation and control of laser hazards. A laser committee may need to be developed when increased laser usage necessitates maintaining enforcement of SOP's.
- Criteria and education for procedures for all personnel working in a NHZ. All personnel working with lasers should attend laser safety education courses periodically.
- Credentialing and clinical practice privileges of the medical staff are the facility's responsibilities. Credentialing should be for specific laser procedures with specific laser types.
- Implementation of laser hazard control measures.
- A continuous quality improvement program to include appropriate use and maintenance of equipment, management, and reporting of accidents and well as prevention.

A laser education program for personnel working on or around lasers, for a facilities specific laser(s) and for specific to the procedures being performed in the facility, must be implemented. The program must comply with applicable standards and regulations covering all procedures necessary to provide a safe environment. Personnel should demonstrate and complete competency skills periodically.

8.15 Medical Surveillance

Medical surveillance for all class 3b and class 4 laser users exposed to laser radiation in the NHZ should be performed when abnormal exposures have occurred. Surveillance is specific to the personnel category and the known risks associated with the particular laser operated. Personnel categories are broken into laser personnel who routinely work in the NHZ and incidental personnel who are unlikely to be exposed to laser energy (e.g. custodial, supervisory, clerical). Surveillance may be required to assess a baseline level of visual performance, pre-employment, to assist in the evaluation of laser damage in the case of inadvertent exposure to the eye. Surveillance can also identify those individuals who may be at risk from ultraviolet hazards, specifically to the skin. Laser accidents must be documented to define the need for further evaluation of the injured person. Suspected exposures and potential injuries from retinal hazardous laser wavelengths (400–1400 nm) should be followed up by an ophthalmologist examination within 48 hours postaccident.

8.16 Nonbeam Hazards

Hazards other than directly related to exposure to the laser (e.g. eye, skin, and other tissues) are known as nonbeam hazards. Potential hazards related to nonbeam hazards are diverse, and the LSO must determine the appropriate control methods to be implemented. Evaluations of the hazards may necessitate the need to enlist the assistance of safety and/or industrial hygiene personnel from OSHA.

8.17 Electrical Hazards

Lasers contain high-voltage electrical circuits that may lead to shock, electrocution, or fire. Injuries from these types of hazards are some of the leading causes of laser-related accidents and deaths. Potential electrical hazards from damaged electrical cords, faulty grounding, lack of compliance with training programs, and inadequate or inappropriate use of lockout/tagout procedures can be prevented by adherence to SOP's of the facility. Visual inspection of the laser including electrical, plumbing, accessory equipment, delivery systems, gas supply, and sterile draping prior to use may prevent injuries from occurring. Observance of general electrical safety (e.g. no fluids placed on or near lasers, extension cords not used to power lasers) will also support the maintenance of safety.

Most medical lasers also require sophisticated cooling systems involving a coolant and fans. Do follow manufacturer's IFU for replacing coolant, if necessary, and keep the lasers at distance from any walls or obstruction that would prevent cooling ventilation to occur.

8.18 Smoke Plume

Vaporization of tissues may release toxic gases (e.g. acetone, isopropanol, toluene, formaldehyde, metal fumes, and cyanide), noxious organic compounds, and cellular nanoparticles, including carcinogens and viruses. This laser plume contains water, carbonized particles, mutated deoxyribonucleic acid (DNA), and intact cells. At certain concentrations, ocular, upper respiratory tract irritation, and unpleasant odors may transpire. These substances should not be inhaled, thereby, initiating the need for some type of smoke evacuation system to be utilized to prevent personnel and the patient from inhaling plume. Removal of plume will also enhance the visualization of the dental treatment site and may prevent the laser beam from potentially being reflected.

Smoke plume inhalation should be reduced to a minimum by utilizing multiple controls. These controls may include the use of high-filtration masks, wall suction units with in-line filters, and smoke evacuators (Figure 8.12). High-filtration or N-95 masks should be used in conjunc-

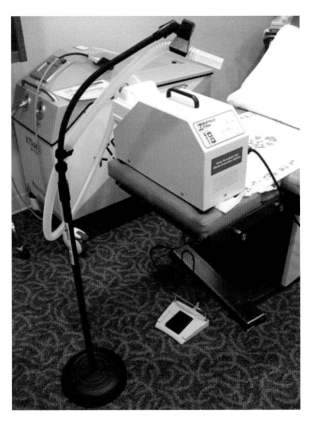

Figure 8.12 Example of portable plume evacuator with support clamp. *Source:* Patti Owens.

tion with other controls and not as a sole means for protection. These masks should be tight fitting and filter particles as small as 0.1 μm. Wall suction systems may be used when the generation of a minimal amount of plume is expected, such as laparoscopic cases. Wall suctions generate low suction rates and are designed for fluids, thus an in-line filter should be used to collect particulate matter. A mechanical smoke evacuator or suction with a high-efficiency ultra-low penetrating air filter (ULPA), having filtration of particles at 0.12 μm at 99.999% efficacy, should be used when a large amounts of laser plume is expected. These systems should be turned on simultaneously with the activation of the laser energy and placed as close as possible to the laser site. Standard precautions (gloves and mask) should be taken when using lasers, as well as when handling contaminated filters due to the amount of potential generated contaminants.

8.19 Fire and Explosion Hazards

All persons in the laser treatment area should be protected from flammability hazards associated with laser usage. Fire is a potential hazard that can have devastating consequences. Laser energy can ignite flammable liquids, solids, and gases. A fire occurring with these types of materials most often materializes outside the patient, but fires can ignite with materials in the patient. Becoming aware of the safeguards and adherence to them can protect the patient as well as healthcare personnel.

Personnel should be aware of the items that have a potential for causing fire, burns, or explosions. These may include clothing, teeth protectors, drapes, hair, endotracheal tubes, paper or gauze materials, gases (e.g. oxygen, methane, anesthetic gases), and flammable liquids or ointments (e.g. skin prep solutions, oil-based lubricants). Water or saline and fire extinguishers should be readily available where lasers are used. Any compound or solution containing alcohol (e.g. Hibiclens, Hibitane, tape removers, degreasers, benzoin, tinctures, etc.) can ignite from contact with laser energy. Alcohol vapors should not be allowed to accumulate under drapes or clothing. Overheating of iodoforms, that is to pool on or around the skin, or aerosolized Betadine can lead to flash fires when laser energy is utilized.

Oxygen concentration in the room should be kept to a minimum. The anesthesia provider should be aware of the hazards of oxygen leaking from around a patient's face mask or nasal cannula. They should be prepared to turn off the free flow of oxygen during laser activation. Various 50% nitrous and 50% oxygen devices are now being used for pain control during dental procedures. Extreme care needs to be taken that the laser is not activated while the patient is inhaling on the mouthpiece. Remember, nitrous with oxygen can potentiate an ignition! The mouthpiece needs to be removed from the laser site during laser activation.

8.20 Shared Airway Procedures

Guidelines to minimize the risks associated with lasers and other energy modalities should be incorporated into the dental team's practices. There are various types of laser-dedicated endotracheal tubes. The type of laser wavelength utilized dictates the brand of endotracheal tube used. Some tubes have FDA clearances for specific wavelengths of lasers. The red rusch reusable tube wrapped in the 3 m foil tape is not an acceptable laser tube and is not an FDA approved tube. This tube is an evolved practice for which there are initial articles published in the medical literature stating this is an acceptable tube in the beginning of laser ENT airway applications. However, with the advent of new FDA-approved laser tubes for specific wavelengths, this wrapped tube should NEVER be used. The PVC endotracheal tube is contraindicated with laser airway procedures when the tube is in direct contact with the laser beam. PVC material is very flammable, and the by-products are hydrochloric gas and, in the presence of fluid, hydrochloric acid. There are no laser resistant tubes presently on the market. All tubes under pressure are explosive.

Considerations should be taken when choosing the appropriate anesthetic agent. No one anesthetic technique is used to the exclusion of others. Helium and compressed air are acceptable gases to use in laser procedures. Helium is a less dense gas and has the ability to flow through compromised airways easier than compressed air. Helium will also retard burning, but the risks of delivering hypoxic levels can be a problem. Pulse oximetry should always be utilized with helium delivery. Nitrous oxide is contraindicated in upper airway laser surgery. Nitrous oxide, in the presence of oxygen, will present as if 100% oxygen is being delivered. The FIO_2 of the oxygen range should be no higher than 30%. Above the 30% range supports combustion.

The cuff of the endotracheal tube should be instilled with normal saline or water and methylene blue dye. The saline or water will serve as an extinguisher and the methylene blue dye as an indicator the cuff has been breached. The endotracheal tube cuff is hit 2% of the time even when lasers are utilized by the best technicians.

Areas of the patient's face accessible to the laser should be protected from stray beams. The patient's eyes should be covered with wet sponges or laser conformers as indicated by the surgical procedure. Water-soluble lubricant is indicated if a laser is used. Petroleum-based lubricant is flammable and, therefore, contraindicated.

Before any laser airway procedure, staff should familiarize themselves with the procedural steps to managing an airway fire. The steps are as follows:

1) Stop the gas flow to the tube: Disconnection of the breathing circuit is the quickest method of stopping the gas flow.
2) Extinguish the fire with water/saline. The operating room staff and anesthesia should have water/saline readily available on the operating room back table and anesthesia cart. Removing the tube without extinguishing the fire will allow the tube to continue to burn on extubation.
3) Access of the bronchoscopes and trach trays should be readily available. The location of the instruments should be established before any airway procedure. Failure to remove any pieces of the tube will allow the tube to continue to burn in the patient.

During head and neck surgeries, the patient is mechanically ventilated in the majority of the procedures. If precautionary protocols are not followed and instantaneous action not taken if an airway fire occurs, hot gases can be forced deep into the lungs, causing extensive injuries. Seconds of indecision or confusion can cause irreparable damage or death to the patient. The avoidance, recognition, and management of airway procedures, as well as the collaborative communication between the operating team, is essential in increasing patient safety and improved care.

8.21 Conclusion

Lasers are a remarkable tool and are becoming an accepted mode of operation. The laser's limits are endless and have been an asset in industry, armed forces, and medicine. Seldom in our century has a new technology brought so many benefits and enhanced our lives. It's important to keep in mind that technology such as the laser has an enormous value and has made a difference in our healthcare arena. That it was even discovered says so much about the depth of human scientific and creative potential. How we ultimately use it says much about our human character. L. Beecher said that no great advance has ever been made in science, politics, and religion without controversy, but technology leads to the further growth of technology.

It is important to understand that regardless of the clinical setting, the presence of laser equipment creates a need for unique control measures and work practice controls to be developed and implemented. Whether your setting is a small dental clinic, a doctor's office, or large hospital, laser safety is not the responsibility of one individual, but the obligation and duty of everyone involved in the laser surgery process.

All personnel involved in the care of a patient may be in the vicinity of the NHZ and thus should be educated appropriately to maintain a safe environment for patient care. A well-developed laser safety program that is compliant with the ANSI Z136 series can assure safety when implemented properly. When everyone knows the fundamentals of maintaining a laser-safe environment, risk of accidents, resulting from ignorance or noncompliance with policy, is greatly reduced (Table 8.1).

Table 8.1 Related links.

http://www.oshs-slc.gov/sltc/laserhazards
http://www.fda.gov/cdrh/radhlth/laser.html

References

ANSI, Z. (2018). 136.3 for the Safe Use of Lasers in Health Care Facilities. New York: American National Standards Institute.

AORN Recommended Practices. (2017). *Perioperative Standards and Recommended Practices*. doi:10.6015/psrp.13.01.0043

Castelluccio, D. (2012). Implementing AORN recommended practices for laser safety. *AORN J. 95* (5): 612–627.

Fencl, J.L. (2017). Guideline implementation: surgical smoke safety. *AORN J. 105* (5): 488–497.

Spratt, D., Cowles, C.E., Berguer, R. et al. (2012). Workplace safety equals patient safety. *AORN J. 96* (3): 235–244.

Takac, S. and Stojanović, S. (1999). Characteristics of laser light. *Med. Pregl. 52* (1–2): 29–34.

Appendix A

Suggested Reading

Al Bayaty F. Applications of Dental Lasers in Periodontal Therapy. An Overview. 2012.

American National Standard for Safe Use of Lasers in Health Care. (2011) ANSI Z136.3-2011. Laser Institute of America.

Barat, K. (2014). Laser Safety. Tools and Training. 2nd. edition. CRC Press.

Berns, M.W. and Greulich, K.O. (eds.) (2007). Laser manipulation of cells and tissues. In: Methods of Cell Biology, vol. 82. Elsevier.

Bogdan Allemann, I. and Kaufman, J. (2011). Laser principles. In: Basics in Dermatological Laser Applications. Curr Probl Dermatol, vol. 42 (eds. I. Bogdan Allemann and D.J. Goldberg), 7–23. Basel: Karger.

Bretenaker, F. and Treps, N. (2015). Laser. 50 Years of Discoveries. World Scientific Publ.

Brugnera, A. Jr. and Nammour, S. (eds.) (2018). World Federation for Laser Dentistry (WFLD). Laser Dentistry: Current Clinical Applications.

Catone, G.A. and Alling, C.C. (1997). Laser Applications in Oral and Maxillofacial Surgery. Saunders Publ.

Coluzzi, D.J. and Parker S.P.A. (2017). Lasers in Dentistry—Current Concepts (Textbooks in Contemporary Dentistry). Springer Publ.

Convissar, R.A. (ed.) (2000). Lasers and Light Amplification in Dentistry. Dental Clinics of North America. Saunders Co.

Convissar, R.A. (2015). Principles and Practice of Laser Dentistry, 2e. Mosby Elsevier.

Dinstl, K. and Fischer, P.L. (1981). Der Laser. Grundlagen und klinische Anwendung. Springer Publ (German).

Fowles, G.R. (1975). Introduction to Modern Optics, 2e. Dover Publ.

Franzen, R. (2011) Principles of Medical and Dental Lasers. An Introduction to Laser Medicine and Laser Dentistry.

Freitas, P.M. and Simoes, A. (eds.) (2015). Lasers in Dentistry. Guide for Clinical Practice. Wiley Publ.

Gutknecht, N. (ed.) (2007). Proceedings of the 1st International Workshop of Evidence-Based Dentistry on Lasers in Dentistry. Quintessence Publ.

Hamblin, M.R. and Huang, Y.-Y. (eds.) (2020). Handbook of Photomedicine. CRC Press.

Hecht, J. (1986). The Laser Guidebook. New York: McGraw-Hill Co.

Ishikawa, I, Frame, J.W., Aoki, A., (2003). Lasers in Dentistry. Revolution of Dental Treatment in the New Millennium. Proceedings of the 8th International Congress on Lasers in Dentistry. Excerpta Medica, Int. Congress Series 1248, Elsevier.

Milonni, P.W. and Eberly, J.H. (2010). Laser Physics. Wiley Publ.

Moritz, A. (2006). Oral Laser Applications. Chicago: Quintessence Publ.

Niemz, M. (2019). Laser-Tissue Interactions. Fundamental and Applications, 4e. Springer Publ.

Rockwell, B. (2015). Laser Safety Guide, 12e. Laser Institute of America.

Simunovic Z. (2009) Lasers in Medicine Science and Practice in Medicine, Surgery, Dentistry and Veterinary. Trilogy Updates. European Medical Laser Association.

Sliney, D.H. and Trokel, S.L. (1993). Medical Lasers and their Safe Use. Springer Publ.

Smith, K.C. (1989). The Science of Photobiology, 2e. Plenum Press.

Thakare, K.M., Charde, P., and Bhongade, M.L. (2017). Applications of Lasers in Periodontal and Implant Therapy. Scholar's Press.

Tuner, J. and Hode, L. (2002). Laser Therapy. Clinical Practice and Scientific Background. Prima Books.

Vitale MC, Caprioglio C. (2010) *Lasers in Dentistry. Practical Textbook*. Editioni Martina.

Welch, A.J. and Van Gemert, M.J.C. (2011). Optical-Thermal Responses of Laser-Irradiated Tissue, 2e. Springer Publ.

Appendix B

Physical Units

Mega 1 000 000	10^6
Kilo 1000	10^3
Centi 0,01	10^{-2}
Milli 0,001	10^{-3}
Micro 0,000 001	10^{-6}
Nano 0,000 000 001	10^{-9}
Pico 0,000 000 000 001	10^{-12}
Femto 0,000 000 000 000 001	10^{-15}
Atto 0,000 000 000 000 000 001	10^{-18}

Laser Parameters

Energy	joules $=$ watts $\times$ seconds
Fluence	energy density $=$ joules/cm^2 $=$ watts $\times$ seconds/cm^2
Power	watts $=$ joules/second
Irradiance	Power density $=$ watts/cm^2
Pulse duration	seconds, milliseconds, nanoseconds
Frequency	Hertz $=$ pulses per second
Wavelength	Nanometers (nm)
Spot size	Millimeters (mm)

Physical Parameters

Parameter	Symbol	Unit
Energy	E	J
Power	P	W
Power Density (Irradiance)	I	W/cm^2

Wavelength	lamda	nm (μm)
Laser Frequency	f	Hz
Time	t	second

Important Formulas

$$P = E/t \left(\text{Frequency} = 1/t, \text{in Hz} \right)$$

$$\text{meanP} = \text{Pmax} \times \text{tpulse} \times \text{frequency}$$

Pmax, is the maximum power (Watt)
tpulse, is pulse duration (second)

$$PD = \text{meanP}/S$$

PD is Power Density (Watt/cm^2); mean power (Watt);
S is the irradiated surface (cm^2)
r is the radius of the glass fiber;

$$\left(S = \pi r^2 \right), \pi = 3.14$$

Peak Power is the energy flow in every pulse

$$\text{Ppeak} : E/\Delta t$$

Average Power is the energy flow over one full time period.

$$\text{Pavg} = E/T$$

Therefore:

$$\text{Ppeak}\,\Delta t = \text{Pavg}\,T$$

Also, *Duty Cycle* is the fractional amount of time the laser is "on" during a specific given period.

$$\text{Duty Cycle} = \Delta t/t = \text{Pavg}/\text{Ppeak}$$

Advanced Laser Surgery in Dentistry, First Edition. Georgios E. Romanos.
© 2021 John Wiley & Sons, Inc. Published 2021 by John Wiley & Sons, Inc.

Index

Note: Page numbers in *italic* refer to figures.
Page numbers in **bold** refer to tables.

a

ablation 29–30, 33–34
  dentin 144
absorption
  energy 3
  light 24, 41–42
absorption spectrum *25*
  blood *21*
  water *21, 25*
accessories, safety 221
active medium 4
  laser types 11–24
adenomas 62
  palate 67, *68*
  sublingual salivary gland 79–80
administrative controls 219
Aggregatibacter
      actinomycetemcomitans 209
aggressive periodontitis, antibiotics
     vs photodynamic
     therapy 211
aging 41
air cooling, osteotomies 131
airways, shared 225–226
alcohol fire hazard 225
alexandrite lasers 17
  frequency-doubled, calculus
     removal 142–143
alveolar ridge, *see also* decortication
  fibroma 67
  leukoplakia 101, *102*
amalgam tattoos 108, 119, *120*
American National Standards
     Institute 216

American Society for Lasers in
     Medicine and Surgery 218
amlodipine, gingival hyperplasia
     80–81
amoxicillin 211
ancillary hazards 219
anesthesia 225
ANSI Z136.3 Standard 216
antibiotics 209, 211, *see also*
     bacteria
antioxidant activity 42
applicators 9–11
  burn from breakage *61*
argon lasers 13
  vascular lesions 107–108
articulated arms 7–8
Association of Perioperative
     Registered Nurses 218
authorized laser operators 221
average power 7, 229

b

bacteria
  enamel adhesion 29
  implants, CO_2 lasers 189, 190
  peri-implantitis 188–189
  periodontal tissues 139,
     140–142, 146
  photodynamic therapy on 28–29
  photo-elimination 31
     laser parameters **179**
bar restorations, lesions
     under 72–74
beam guide systems 7

beam profiles 7
biofilm 139
  removal from pockets 209–214
biopsy *see* excision biopsy
biostimulation 27–28, *see also*
     photobiomodulation therapy
bleeding on probing, photodynamic
     therapy on 210
blink reflex 217
blistering 50, *51*
block section *135*
blood, absorption spectrum *21*
blue lasers, wound healing 42
blue light diode lasers 18–19, *20*
blue-paper-initiated tips, peri-
     implant temperatures 202
bone
  augmentation 194, *196*, 197–199
  critical temperature 141
  defect, peri-implant 197–199
  healing 51–52, 129–130
     Nd:YAG lasers 50
  recontouring
     crown lengthening
       with 159–163
     laser parameters **179**
  regeneration, *see also* guided bone
     regeneration
     fractional thermolysis
       168–169, 171
     after peri-implantitis 189
  surgery 129–137, *see also*
     osteotomies
  thermal safety threshold 200

Advanced Laser Surgery in Dentistry, First Edition. Georgios E. Romanos.
© 2021 John Wiley & Sons, Inc. Published 2021 by John Wiley & Sons, Inc.

bone-to-implant contact
      percentage 204
brackets, orthodontic 122, *123*
breaking strengths, wound healing,
      Nd:YAG lasers 47–50
bubbles, Ho:YAG lasers on
      bone 130–131
buccal mucosa
    fibroma 66, 70–72
    hemangioma 109
    lipoma 76, *78*
burns, fiber applicator breakage *61*

c
calcium antagonists, gingival
      hyperplasia 80–81
calculus removal 142–144, *175*,
      209–214
    laser parameters **179**
CO_2 lasers 12–13
    bacteria reduction, tooth
      damage 142
    crown lengthening 158–159
    dermatology 33
    excision biopsy 60, 61
    flexible hollow guides 8
    frenectomy 88–90
    gingivectomy 81
    hemostasis 106
    implants
      bacteria 189, 190
      exposure 185–187
    leukoplakia 100
    malignant soft tissue tumors 106
    oral surgery 57
    osteotomies 129–130, **131**
    penetration depth 12, *58*
    peri-implant
      hyperplasias 192–193
    periodontics 144
      parameters **179**
    on roots 149–150
    vestibuloplasties 93–94
    wound healing 44–47
      osteotomies 52
carbonization 29, 58, 61
    CO_2 lasers, osteotomies 129
carbonized fibers, lasers 31
carcinoma in situ 100
caries
    CO_2 lasers 12
    pulse duration for 34

cementum
    calculus removal and 144
    resorption 141
char-free (ultrapulse) mode 5, 6, 23
chopped pulses 5
Cr^{+2}: Zn Ce laser 21
chromophores
    for hair removal 26
    selective thermolysis 24
    thermal relaxation time 5–6
class II medical devices 216
cleaving, glass fibers 150, 151
coagulation 106–107, 140
    after excisions 59, 60–61, *62, 83*
    implant exposure 187
coagulopathies 106–107, 154–156
coherence, light 3
cold sores, biostimulation 27
collagen 29, 33, 41
collagen membrane *194, 195,* 196,
    197, 198
collimation 4
color
    laser light, wound healing 44
    of tissues 88
conductivity, thermal 29
contact mode, tissue effects *32*
continuous-wave lasers 5, *6*
    CO_2 lasers
      excision biopsy 47
      osteotomies 129, **131**
    peri-implant temperatures 200
    thermal effects *30*
control measures, laser safety 219
controlled areas 220–221
cooling
    laser equipment 224
    osteotomies 131
cork tips, peri-implant
      temperatures 202
cornea, laser light interactions 26
corneoscleral shields 222, *223*
credentialing 223
critical temperature, bone 141
crown lengthening *134,* 135,
    157–164
crystal lasers 14–17
cuffs, endotracheal tubes 225
curettage 139, 140, 144–149, *178*
    laser parameters **179**
cyclosporine-A, gingival
      hyperplasia 80–81

cysts, salivary glands 83–87
cytotoxic products,
      photosensitizers 210

d
danger signs 220
debridement
    diode lasers with *166, 173*
    Nd:YAG lasers with 140, 149
    photodynamic therapy with 210
    power 200
decontamination *see* bacteria
decortication for implants
    Er,Cr:YSGG lasers *134,* 135–136
    Er:YAG lasers 131, 135
dehiscence, prevention,
      vestibuloplasties 94
delivery systems 7–9
denaturation 29, 41
dentin, ablation 144
dentures, vestibuloplasties for 93,
    94–95
diabetic ulcers,
      biostimulation 27–28
diastema *see* median diastema
diffusivity, thermal 29
diltiazem, gingival
      hyperplasia 80–81
diode lasers 17–19, *see also* gallium
      arsenide diode lasers
    810nm
      frenectomy 90–93
      leukoplakia 100
    980nm
      on bacteria 142
      fractional thermolysis *170–171*
      peri-implant
        hyperplasias 191–192
      peri-implantitis 195–196
      pocket epithelium removal 146
      vestibuloplasties 95, *96*
      wound healing 50
    blue light diode lasers 18–19, *20*
    excision biopsy 58, 60–61
    hemangiomas 114–116
    implants, damage 186, *187*
    Nd:YAG lasers *vs,* wound
      healing 50
    peri-implant temperatures 202
    peri-implantitis 188
    on periodontal tissues,
      parameters **179**

superpulse diode lasers 22–23
vestibuloplasties 94
diphenylhydantoin, gingival
hyperplasia 80–81
direct coupling 7
dissociation, molecules 27
downgrowth of epithelium,
retardation 149–151
drug-induced hyperplasias,
gingiva 80–81, 152–153
duty cycle 7, 229
dye lasers 17
pulsed mode, vascular
lesions 108

e
education of practitioners, lasers in
periodontics 178–181
Einstein, Albert 3
electrical hazards 224
electrons
energy levels 3
free, photoablation 34
Elements of Performance (TJC) 218
enamel, heat on 29
endotracheal tubes 225–226
energy, *see also* photon energy
units **229**
energy density 4
energy levels, electrons 3
epidermoid cyst 85–87
epithelium, *see also* long junctional
epithelium
removal from pockets 144–151
980nm diode lasers 146
laser parameters **179**
retardation of
downgrowth 149–151
epulides 81–83, 157
erbium fiber laser 20
Er,Cr:YSGG lasers 16
bone repair 52
dermatology 33
implants
decortication for *134*,
135–136
exposure 185
placement 204
osteotomies 131, *132*, *133*,
135–136
penetration depth 14
peri-implant temperatures 202

periodontics 144
parameters **179**
Er:YAG lasers 14–16, *15*
bone repair 52
calculus removal 143, 144
dermatology 33
gingivectomy 159–160
implants
decontamination 190
decortication for 131, 135
exposure 187
placement 204
on long bones 135
osteotomies 16, 130, 131, *132*
periodontics 141–142, 148
parameters **179**
vestibuloplasties 96, *97*
wound healing 47, 50
esthetics, crown lengthening
for 159–164
etching, polymer films 34
excimer lasers
193 nm 34
calculus removal 142
308 nm, on bone 130, **131**
wound healing 50
excision biopsy 58–59, 60–61
leukoplakia 59–60
excision new attachment procedure
(ENAP) 140
excited states 3
exostoses, tongue *133*, *134*
explosion hazards 225
extracellular matrix formation 44
extravasation cysts, salivary
glands 83, 85
eye
excimer laser (193 nm) 34
laser light interactions 26, *27*
optical coherence tomography 2
photodisruption 35
protection 221–223
safety measures for 26–27
eye shields 222, *223*

f
Fabry-Perot cavity 5
FDA classification 216–217
FDA Radiological Health
Regulations 215
Federal Laser Product Performance
Standard 216

femtosecond lasers, wound
healing 51
fiber applicators 10–11
burn from breakage *61*
fiber lasers 19–21
ytterbium high-power 21, *22*
fiber waveguides 8–9
fibroblasts 142, 149–150
fibroepithelial hyperplasia of the
palate 62–63, 67–69
fibromas 59, 62, 63–66
alveolar ridge 67
buccal mucosa 66, 70–72
lingual, removal *65*, 66
palate 69–70
filters, suction systems 224
fire hazards 224–225
fire retardants 223
fires, in airways 225–226
flexible hollow guides 8–9
floor of mouth, leukoplakia *102*
flossing 148
focal spot 7
Food and Drug
Administration 215–216
foot pedals, operational
guidelines 220
foreign body reaction 44
400nm laser, calculus removal 143
fractional thermolysis 31–33,
165–178
free electrons, photoablation 34
free-electron laser 24
bone repair 51
free-running lasers 5
frenectomy 87–93, 156–157
implants and 188
vestibuloplasty after 95–96, *97*
frequency-doubled alexandrite
lasers, calculus
removal 142–143
fusion power, lasers for 1

g
gallium arsenide diode lasers 17–18
on tooth extraction sockets 42
gallium nitride diode lasers 19
gas lasers 11–14
nuclear-pumped 24
gas plasma technology 35
giant cell granuloma,
gingival 77–79

gingiva
  epulides   81–83
  giant cell granuloma   77–79
  hyperplasias   72, *73*, 80–81,
      152–153, *see also* peri-implant
      hyperplasias
    drug-induced   80–81, 152–153
  leukoplakia   101, 103–104, *105*
  troughing   165
  tumors, pregnancy   157
gingivectomy   81, 152–153
  crown lengthening after   159–163
  laser parameters   **179**
gingivoplasty   152–153
  implants and   187
  laser parameters   **179**
glass fibers   31
  cleaning   150
  cleaving   150, 151
  radius   229
glass plate, treatment of
    hemangioma   112
glass tubes, CO_2 lasers   12
goggles   26–27, 222
grafts
  bone augmentation   194, 196,
      197, 198–199
  vestibuloplasties   94
granulation tissue   57
granulomas   62, *see also* giant cell
    granuloma
  pyogenic   70, *71*
green lasers, wound healing   42
ground states   3
guide systems   7
guided bone regeneration   194
guided tissue regeneration   140,
    150–151
guidelines for safety   218, 220
gyroscopes, lasers for   2

h

hair removal, chromophore for   26
handpieces   9–10
  CO_2 lasers   8
hard lasers *see* high-power lasers
hazard classifications   219
hazard evaluation   219
hazardous gases and vapors   218
heat transfer   29
  bacteria reduction   141
  to implants   199–203

inflammation   57
  wound healing delay   44, 50
helium   225
He:Ne lasers   14
  wound healing   42
hemangiomas   62
  ice cube method   109–114
  lip   109–112, 114–116, *117–118*,
      119
  tongue   112–114, *119*
hematoporphyrin   28
hemoglobin
  absorption of light   24
  absorption spectrum   *25*
hemostasis   69, 106–107
  Nd:YAG lasers   14
  periodontics   154–156
high-power lasers
  incisions   44, *46*, 47
  malignant soft tissue tumors   106
  scars from   *62*, 70, *71*
  wound healing   44
  ytterbium fiber   21, *22*
Ho:YAG lasers   16–17
  osteotomies   130–131
  wound healing   50
hydroxyapatite-coated implants,
    damage from lasers   190
hyperkeratosis   *60*
hyperplasias
  gingiva *see* hyperplasias *under*
    gingiva
  peri-implant   72–74, 187,
    190–193
  removal   62–63

i

ice cube method   108–120
impacted teeth, exposure   121–123
implants   185–207, *see also*
    decortication; peri-implant
    hyperplasias; peri-implantitis
  exposure   190, *191*
  during function   187–188
  placement   204
  preparation for   185–187
  recent research   199–203
  removal   *134, 135*, 136, 204
  research on surface
      damage   185–186
impression material, salivary gland
    cyst   84, *85*

incisions   58
  frenectomies   88
  gingival hyperplasia   81
  high-power lasers   44, *46*, 47
  implant exposure   187
  implant placement   204
  salivary gland cysts   83
  vestibuloplasties   93, 94
indocyanine green   210
infection, *see also* bacteria
  peri-implantitis   188–189
inflammation, *see also*
      peri-implantitis
  heat transfer   57
  photodynamic therapy on   210
  pockets   144–145
  wound healing, Nd:YAG
      lasers   50
initiated tips   147, 200, 202
injection laser diodes   18
international laser standards   215
intraluminal method,
      hemangiomas   112
iodoform, fire hazards   225
ionization   27
ionizing radiation   1
irritation fibroma   63–66
isomerization   27

j

Joint Commission, The   218

k

keratinized tissue width,
      vestibuloplasties   95–96,
      156–157
KTP lasers   14
  wound healing   47

l

laser patterned microcoagulation
      (LPM)   33, *34*
laser periodontal therapy   148–149
laser plume   216, 224
laser protective eyewear   222–223
laser safety officers   218–219
laser safety programs   219, 223
laser-assisted new attachment
      procedure (LANAP)   149
lasers   1–40
  application modes   5–7
  applicators   9–11

biological tissue
　　interactions   24–40
　delivery systems   7–9
　photochemical effects   27–29
　power   1
　size   1
　storage   220
　types   11–24
　uses   1–2
leukoplakia   99–105
　excision biopsy   59–60
　multiple lesions   101
light, properties   1, 3–4, 24–27,
　　41–42
light-activated disinfection
　　(photodynamic
　　therapy)   28–29, 156–164,
　　209–214
lingual fibroma, removal
　　65, 66
lip
　burn   *61*
　frenectomy   90–92
　hemangiomas   109–112, 114–116,
　　117–118, *119*
　mucoceles   84–85
　nevi   119, *120*
　papillomas   75–76, *77*
lipomas   62, 76–77, *78*
liquid lasers *see* dye lasers
lithotripsy   17, 123–124
long bones, Er:YAG lasers on   135
long junctional epithelium   139
　removal   145
longitudinal modes   7
low power lasers, wound
　　healing   42–44
low-level-therapy lasers   **27**
　wound healing   42–44
lubricants   225

m

macula, laser light interactions   26
maintenance of equipment   221
malignant soft tissue tumors   106
mandible, frenectomy   88,
　　89, 90
masers   3
masks, smoke inhalation
　　prevention   224
matrix metalloproteinases,
　　antibiotics *vs* PDT   211

maxilla
　frenectomy   88, *89*, 90–93
　vestibuloplasties   94–95
measurement, lasers for   2
median diastema
　closure   158–159
　frenectomies and   88
Medical Device Amendments, Food
　　and Drug Act   216
medical surveillance   223
melanin, absorption spectrum   *25*
metal tubes, CO_2 lasers   12
methylene blue
　endotracheal tubes   225
　as photosensitizer   210
metric system   **229**
metronidazole   211
microthermal zones   32
molecular binding energy   34
molecular lasers   12
monochromatism   4
mucocele, lip   84–85
multimode beams   7
muscles, after vestibuloplasties   93
mutagenesis   34

n

nano-plasmonics   1
National Center for Devices and
　　Radiological Health   216
Nd:YAG lasers   14
　amalgam tattoos   119, *120*
　on bacteria   142, 146
　　peri-implantitis   189
　with debridement   140, 149
　excision biopsy   60–61
　on granulation tissue   57
　implants, damage   106,
　　187, 190
　leukoplakia removal   103–104
　penetration depth   *58*, 108
　on periodontal tissues   141, 145,
　　148–149
　　parameters   **179**
　on pockets   151
　vascular lesions   108
　vestibuloplasties   94, 95–96, *97*
　wound healing   47–50
　　osteotomies   52
nevi, lip   119, *120*
new attachment, periodontal
　　tissues   139

retardation of epithelial
　　downgrowth for   149–151
new bone formation, Nd:YAG
　　lasers   50
nifedipine, gingival
　　hyperplasia   80–81
nitrogen, CO_2 lasers   12
nitrous oxide, fire hazards   225
nominal hazard zones   220–221
nonbeam hazards   223–224
nongovernmental
　　organizations   215–217
nuclear-pumped gas lasers   24

o

Occupational Safety and Health
　　Administration   216
operating microscopes, laser
　　filters   220
operational guidelines   220
operculectomy   121–123
ophthalmology *see* eye
optical coherence tomography   2
optical discs, lasers for   2
optical scalpels *see* high-power lasers
oral hygiene, bar restorations   *73*, 74
oral surgery, basic principles   57
orthodontics, unerupted
　　teeth   122–123
Osler's disease, telangiectasias   111
ossifying fibromas   74–75
osteotomies   51–52, 129–137
　Er:YAG lasers   16, 130, 131, *132*
overheating of implants   205
overheating of tissues
　CO_2 lasers   60
　peri-implant, prevention   200
　periodontics, avoidance   180
over-the-counter lasers *see* low-level-
　　therapy lasers
oxidation   42
oxygen, fire hazards   225

p

palate
　adenomas   67, *68*
　fibroepithelial hyperplasia   62–63,
　　67–69
　fibromas   69–70
papillomas, lip   75–76, *77*
papillomatosis   59
peak power   7, 229

pedunculated tumors, removal 64, *65*

penetration depth *31*
    argon lasers 13, 107
    CO_2 lasers 12, *58*
    Er,Cr:YSGG lasers 14
    Er:YAG lasers 14
    Ho:YAG lasers 14
    Nd:YAG lasers *58*, 108

pericoronitis *121*

peri-implant hyperplasias 72–74, 187, 190–193

peri-implantitis 188–199
    bone defect with 197–199
    experimental temperature change 200
    before loading 193–196
    photodynamic therapy 209–214

periodontal tissues, leukoplakia 103

periodontics, basic principles 139–140

periodontitis 139
    photodynamic therapy 209–214

PerioLase Nd:YAG laser, periodontal therapy 148–149

personal protective equipment 216, 222–223

phenothiazine chloride dye *211*

photobiomodulation therapy 41

photochemical effects 27–29

photodisruption 34–35

photodynamic therapy (PDT) 28–29, 156–164, 209–214

photon energy 34

photosensitizers 28, 209, 210

photothermal effects 29–33

pigmented lesions 107–120

Planck's constant 3

plaque removal 140, *175, 176*

plasma (physics) 34

plasma cleaning 35

plasma surface technology 35

platelet-derived growth factor, osteotomies 135

plume (smoke) 216, 224

pockets 139–140
    antibiotics *vs* photodynamic therapy 211
    under bar restorations 72

biofilm and calculus removal 209–214

epithelium removal 144–151
    980nm diode lasers 146
    laser parameters **179**
    Er,Cr:YSGG lasers 144
    gingival hyperplasia 80–81
    leukoplakia 103

polymer films, etching 34

porosity, implants 205

Porphyromonas gingivalis 209

position statements (ASLMS) 218

postoperative care, excision biopsy 61

potassium triphosphate *see* KTP lasers

power
    CO_2 lasers, leukoplakia removal 100
    debridement 200
    defined 6
    formulae 229
    laser classification 217
    units **229**

power density 7
    units **229**

pregnancy
    gingival tumor 157
    impacted tooth 121–122

pregnancy epulis 81–83

probing depth 139

procedural controls 219–220

professional organizations 218

prostate surgery, thulium lasers 22

prostheses, fibroepithelial hyperplasia from 62–63

pseudo-pockets 72

pulp temperature
    bacteria reduction 141–142
    calculus removal 143

pulse duration 5, *6*, 229

pulsed mode 5, *6, 30*
    CO_2 lasers, excision biopsy 47
    diode lasers, peri-implant hyperplasias 191–192
    dye lasers, vascular lesions 108

pumping 3, 5
    dye lasers 17
    of fiber lasers 19
    by fiber lasers 20

PVC (polyvinyl chloride), endotracheal tubes 225

pyogenic granulomas 70, *71*

q

Q-switched lasers 5
    Nd:YAG lasers
        calculus removal 142
        vascular lesions 108

quasi continuous wave diode lasers 22–23

r

radiation, non-ionizing 1

Radiological Health Regulations (FDA) 215

radius 229

ranula 85, *86*

reactive oxygen species 42

reattachment, periodontal tissues 139, 144

receptors for light 28

record-keeping, laser safety 219

red lasers, wound healing 42

reflection of light 24, *27*
    off implants 185
    safety measures 220

regulatory agencies 215–217

relapse, vestibuloplasties 93

resonators, optical 5

resorption of bone, after vestibuloplasties 93

resorption of cementum 141

retardation, epithelial downgrowth 149–151

retention cysts, salivary glands 83–85

retina, laser light interactions 26

root planing 139, 141, 146–148
    photodynamic therapy with 210

roots, effect of CO_2 lasers 149–150

rutile 190

s

safety measures 215–226
    for eyes 26–27, 221–223

safety programs 219, 223

salivary duct stone lithotripsy, alexandrite lasers 17

salivary glands
    cysts 83–87
    sialoliths 123–124

sublingual
  adenoma 79–80
  cyst 85, *86*
sandblasted surface, damage from
    lasers 186
sapphire tips, calculus removal 144
scaling 139, 141, 146–147
  photodynamic therapy with 210
scalpels, optical *see* high-power lasers
scars
  fractional thermolysis for 32, 33
  from high-power lasers *62*, 70, *71*
scattering, light 24
Schneiderian membrane,
    perforation 135
selective thermolysis 24
semiconductor lasers, *see also* diode
    lasers
  wound healing 50–51
shared airway procedures
    225–226
shrinkage 41
shuttered pulses 5
sialoliths 123–124
signage 221
sinus augmentation, window
    preparation *134*, 135
skin protection 223
skin resurfacing 32–33
skip areas, fractional
    thermolysis 31–32
smoke plume 216, 224
soft diet, leukoplakia removal 100
SOLEA laser 12–13
solid-state lasers 14–17
spacer 1
spectrum (electromagnetic) 1, *2, see
    also* absorption spectrum
  fiber lasers *21*
splinted implants, heat transfer to
    neighbors 202, *203*
splitting of bone *135*
spontaneous emission 3
spot sizes 10–11
stable resonators 5
standard operating procedures 219
stand-by mode 220
state regulations 218
stimulated emission 3
storage of lasers 220
stress relaxation 41
sublingual salivary gland

adenoma 79–80
cyst 85, *86*
submandibular gland,
    sialoliths 123–124
suction, smoke inhalation
    prevention 224
sulcular epithelium 147
superpulse diode lasers 22–23
superpulse mode 5, *6*, 23, *30*
  CO$_2$ lasers
    implant damage 185
    osteotomies 129
surgery
  bone 129–137, *see also*
      osteotomies
  lasers for 2
  oral, basic principles 57
surveillance, medical 223

t

technology 226
telangiectasias, Osler's disease 111
temperature
  bacteria reduction 141
  calculus removal 143
  implants 186, 187
    safety threshold 200
  peri-implant 202
temporomandibular joint arthroscopy
  Er:YAG lasers 16
  Ho:YAG lasers 17
The Joint Commission (TJC) 218
thermal conductivity coefficient 29
thermal relaxation time 5–6
3D printing, implants 205
thulium (Tm) lasers 20, 21–22
tip angle, calculus removal 143, 144
tips
  for excision biopsy 61
  initiated 147, 200, 202
  lasers 31
tissue color 88
titanium, damage from lasers
    185–186, 190
toluidine blue 210
tongue
  exostoses *133*, *134*
  fibroma, removal *65*, 66
  frenectomy 88, *89*
  hemangiomas 112–114, *119*
  leukoplakia *102*, 104, *105*
  lipoma 76–77, *78*

tooth extraction sockets, low power
    laser therapy 42, 44
tooth protection, during
    gingivectomy 81
toothbrushing 148
Townes, Charles H. 3
training, laser safety 219, 223
transmission arms (articulated) 7–8
transmission of light 24–26
transverse electromagnetic mode
    5, 7
transverse excited atmospheric
    (TEA) pressure CO$_2$
    lasers 130
triplet state, photosensitizers 210
troughing, gingiva 165
tumors
  benign soft tissue
    removal 59–80
    vestibuloplasties with 96–99
  gingiva, pregnancy 157
  malignant soft tissue 106
two-stage implants, exposure 190

u

ultrapulse mode 5, *6*, 23
ultrashort pulses 5, *6*
ultrasonics, Er:YAG lasers *vs*,
    calculus removal 144
unerupted teeth, exposure 121–123
units (physics) **229**

v

vaporization 29, 58–59
vascular lesions 107–120
verrucous leukoplakia, alveolar
    ridge 101
vestibuloplasty 73, 87, 93–99,
    156–157
  implants and 188
  removal of irritation fibroma
      with 64, *65*
vitamin A, for leukoplakia 100
von Willebrand's disease 106–107

w

wall suction systems 224
warning signs 220
water
  absorption spectrum *21*, 25
  tissue content 41
  vaporization 29

water cooling, osteotomies   131

waveguides   8–9

wavelengths   1, *2, 25*

    fiber lasers   20

    periodontics   180

    for photosensitizers   210

    tissue color and   88

    tissue penetration   *31*

    units   **229**

wet gauze   149

Widman flap procedure
    139, 140

window preparation, sinus
    augmentation   *134*, 135

windows (viewing)   221

wound healing   41–56

    biostimulation   27–28

    delay   44, 50

      osteotomies   51, 52, 129

    fractional thermolysis   31–32

    high-power lasers   44

    laser patterned microcoagulation   33

    vestibuloplasties   93

wrinkles, fractional thermolysis for   32

x

X-ray lasers   24

y

YAG lasers   14–16

ytterbium fiber
    laser   20

   high-power
    21, *22*

Yb:YAG laser, 3D printing
    of implants
    205